LAPAROSCOPIC
COLORECTAL SURGERY
THE LAPCO MANUAL

LAPAROSCOPIC COLORECTAL SURGERY
THE LAPCO MANUAL

EDITED BY

MARK COLEMAN MBChB FRCS MD honFRCPSG
Consultant Colorectal Surgeon, Plymouth UK

TOM CECIL BM FRCS DM
Consultant Colorectal Surgeon, Basingstoke UK

INTERNATIONAL GUEST EDITOR

Dr Brian Dunkin MD, FACS
Head, Section of Endoscopic Surgery
Houston Methodist Hospital
Houston, Texas, USA

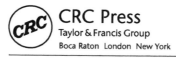

CRC Press
Taylor & Francis Group
Boca Raton London New York

CRC Press is an imprint of the
Taylor & Francis Group, an **informa** business

CRC Press
Taylor & Francis Group
6000 Broken Sound Parkway NW, Suite 300
Boca Raton, FL 33487-2742

© 2017 by Taylor & Francis Group, LLC
CRC Press is an imprint of Taylor & Francis Group, an Informa business

No claim to original U.S. Government works

Printed on acid-free paper

International Standard Book Number-13: 978-1-4987-1235-4 (Paperback)

Library of Congress Cataloging-in-Publication Data

Names: Coleman, Mark (Colorectal surgeon), editor. | Cecil, Tom (Colorectal surgeon), editor.
Title: Laparoscopic colorectal surgery / [edited by] Mark Coleman, Tom Cecil.
Other titles: Laparoscopic colorectal surgery (Coleman)
Description: Boca Raton : CRC Press, [2016] | Includes bibliographical references.
Identifiers: LCCN 2016024587| ISBN 9781498712354 (pack : alk. paper) | ISBN 9781498712378 (pdf)
Subjects: | MESH: Colorectal Surgery--methods | Laparoscopy--methods | Colorectal Surgery--education | Laparoscopy--education | Education, Medical, Continuing--methods | Great Britain
Classification: LCC RD543.C57 | NLM WI 650 | DDC 617.5/547--dc23
LC record available at https://lccn.loc.gov/2016024587

Visit the Taylor & Francis Web site at
http://www.taylorandfrancis.com

and the CRC Press Web site at
http://www.crcpress.com

This book is dedicated to Nick Taffinder who would have undoubtedly been part of the Lapco programme and contributed to this manual as if he were still with us today.

Contents

Foreword

Laparoscopy has been one of the major developments in colorectal surgery during the last 25 years. It transforms recovery after colorectal resection from a duration of months to weeks: with reduction in complications, hospitalisation, unsightly scars, and cost. This revolution started in the early 1990s but the complexity of the procedure limited uptake to relatively few enthusiasts.

By the early 2000s it became clear that a structured programme of training for consultants (senior specialists) was necessary to achieve wholesale change. It was also important to acknowledge and avoid the complications that accompany the introduction of a complex new technique when it is self-taught – 'the learning curve' This preceptorship commenced formally in 2004 with a dedicated band of 25 trainers who visited hospitals to provide training on a small number of cases. With involvement of the Department of Health's Cancer Action Team, under the leadership and vision of Professor Sir Mike Richards, this concept gained momentum and the process expanded: the National Training Programme was born.

The Programme was unique internationally for a number of reasons. It provided hands-on training for consultants in a complex surgical intervention, with established experts assisting during surgery. It ensured that a valid and reliable assessment of competence was developed by an internationally recognised academic training centre, Imperial College. Last, it required the consultants to pass the competency assessment prior to independent practice. We were greatly helped by Dr. Roland Valori who led Endoscopy Training in England, much of the surgical training mirroring that development.

This book describes how the programme was set up and run from 2007 onward. It includes the important issues of training efficacy and how we train trainers. It provides practical advice for trainees and established specialists on how operations should be undertaken. Last, it addresses other critical issues such as enhanced recovery care and the management of complications. The expert group of authors are to be congratulated on their contributions to laparoscopic colorectal surgery, so that patients worldwide may benefit from this transformational approach.

Professor Robin Kennedy, MBBS FRCS
Consultant Surgeon Adjunct Professor
Department of Surgery and Cancer
Imperial College London
London, United Kingdom

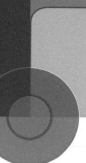

The USA Lapco Training Experience by Guest Editor Brian Dunkin

As the medical director of MITIE (Houston Methodist Institute for Technology, Innovation, and Education), a comprehensive education and research institute that trains over 6,000 health care professionals annually, I am dedicated to helping practicing surgeons stay abreast of their field. It is in this spirit that in 2012 I began a journey to create a pathway for surgeons in the US to up-skill in their ability to perform laparoscopic colon surgery. My plan was to pilot a novel program in my local area and, if successful, leverage that experience into a national training initiative with the help of professional surgical societies. When doing my due diligence on what had already been done in this area, I was introduced to the Lapco program and its leaders. Little did I know that attending my first Lapco train-the-trainers (TT) course in January of 2013 would begin a four year journey of amazing developments in surgical education.

Using the Lapco training program as an example of "best practice" we've worked in MITIE to import its model into the US and build on the experience. The "MITIE-Lapco" program includes a rigorous selection methodology for those who are chosen to attend the course as well as pre-course preparation with didactic material review, knowledge testing, and level setting of laparoscopic skills. Once surgeons come to MITIE for their hands-on training they are directed by Lapco TT trained faculty and evaluated using the rigorous Lapco assessment tools for formative and summative feedback. Finally, when we send these surgeons back to their home institutions, we support them with an expert mentor in the operating room just as Lapco did – but through the use of technology.

In the US it is almost impossible to have an in-person expert surgeon come to a trainee's operating room because of legal and regulatory barriers. As a result, we leveraged audio-visual communication to telementor surgeons in their own operating room while they are adopting MIS colon surgery. Through this process we learned that the Lapco TT methodology is ideally suited for telementoring. In fact, the MITIE-Lapco experience is not only serving as a platform for developing a national US training initiative to increase MIS colon surgery utilization, but has also led to the Society of American Gastrointestinal and Endoscopic Surgeons (SAGES) creating a telementoring task force that is leveraging the power of the society to advance the field of telementoring.

SAGES has also incorporated the Lapco TT methodology into its hands-on training courses. These special ADOPT programs have transformed the usual episodic post-graduate hands-on courses held at annual meetings into longitudinal training programs with multiple touch points throughout the year conducted by faculty with TT training. Successful procedural adoption from the SAGES ADOPT courses has been shown to far exceed that of standard post-graduate courses.

In addition, the Lapco TT program has been successfully imported into the US and its availability is expanding to surgeons across multiple specialties. As the first certified center outside of the UK approved to offer the Lapco TT course, MITIE has worked to develop multiple certified US trainers and to certify a second training site at the Center for Advanced Medical Learning and Simulation (CAMLS) in Tampa, Florida. It is planned for more centers and trainers to come on line in the coming months.

Finally, the Lapco TT methodology is being introduced into general surgical residency training programs in the US in an effort to improve intraoperative teaching and promote graduated independent practice. It is truly changing the culture of training to promote responsibility in the resident trainee and to allow them more independent work in the OR without sacrificing quality or outcomes.

In summary, the Lapco program is transforming how minimally invasive colon surgery is being taught in the US, expanding its availability to patients, fostering the advancement of telementoring, changing how a professional society trains colleagues to learn new procedures, and advancing graduate surgical training to promote safe, independent work by trainees in the operating room. This national impact is nothing short of astounding and the Lapco leaders as well as the National Health Service are to be commended for it.

Brain J. Dunkin, MD, FACS
Head, Section of Endoscopic Surgery
Houston Medical Hospital

Preface

The Lapco training programme for laparoscopic colorectal surgery (LCS) for specialists in England, United Kingdom helped to elevate the rate of laparoscopic colorectal resection from 5% to 50% between 2007 and 2014, respectively. Lapco employed a performance managed hands-on mentorship training network accompanied by rigorous assessment of educational and clinical outcomes. Over one-third of colorectal specialists in England were involved as trainers or trainees. This book is a comprehensive manual on how to train in and provide training in LCS. It also includes the evidence for and the complications from LCS. Colorectal surgeons have led the world in enhanced recovery, few more than the author of Chapter 11 in this book. LCS is also advancing rapidly and areas such as robotics and single-port surgery are also included here. The contributors to this book comprise the leading lights of LCS in the United Kingdom in the twenty-first century. The book has tried to follow the structure of the Lapco training methodology using a modular structure for the technical chapters based around the GAS forms (see Chapter 3) with learning points and a clear take home message for each chapter.

Acknowledgments

Tom and I would like to thank the following who participated in the Lapco programme and helped to complete this book. The programme would never have existed without the inspiration and leadership of Professor Sir Michael Richards at the National Cancer Action Team, Department of Health for England. There would be no educational or clinical outcomes to show the effectiveness and safety of the programme without Professor George Hanna at the Academic Department of Surgery, Imperial College, London. The Lapco Train the Trainers Course only came about with the help of Dr. Roland Valori and his colleagues from the National Endoscopy Training Programme, Dr. John Anderson and Dr. Siwan Thomas-Gibson. The programme was managed with characteristic vigour and sublime attention to detail by its National Manager, Mrs. Laura Langsford. Huge credit for the idea for the programme and the TT course must be given to Mr. Robin Kennedy, author of the book's Foreword. Since 2014, The Lapco organisation has attracted considerable international attention which has resulted in the development of similar programmes in Norway, USA and now, Australia. The key persons behind this international expansion have been Dr Ole Helmer Sjo from Oslo, Norway and our International Guest Editor for this book, Dr Brian Dunkin from Houston, USA. We would like to thank both for their enthusiasm and contribution to the success of Lapco worldwide. Finally, we would like to thank all the authors for their excellent and well-illustrated chapters, which we hope will be of help to those interested in training, or being trained, in LCS. It is a fitting way to underline the achievements of the Lapco programme. This manual is dedicated to the trainees, trainers, and patients who participated in one of the most successful surgical training programmes for established specialists in the world.

Mark Coleman, FRCS MD
Consultant Surgeon Plymouth Hospitals NHS Trust
Honorary Senior Lecturer (Associate Professor) PUPSMD

Contributors

Austin Acheson
Nottingham University Hospitals NHS Trust
Nottingham, United Kingdom

Steven J. Arnold
Basingstoke and North Hants Hospital
Basingstoke, United Kingdom

Tan Arulampalam
Colchester General Hospital
Colchester, United Kingdom

Tom Cecil
Basingstoke and North Hants Hospital
Basingstoke, United Kingdom

Mark Coleman
Derriford Hospital
Plymouth, United Kingdom

Chris Cunningham
Oxford University Hospitals
NHS Foundation Trust
Churchill Hospital
Oxford, United Kingdom

Tony Dixon
North Bristol NHS Trust
North Bristol, United Kingdom

Nuno Figueiredo
Colorectal Unit
Champalimaud Foundation
Lisbon, Portugal

Nader Francis
Yeovil District Hospital
Yeovil, United Kingdom

S Nadia Gilani
StR–General Surgery
East Sussex Healthcare Trust, KSS Deanery
Eastbourne, United Kingdom

Talvinder Singh Gill
University Hospital of North Tees
Stockton on Tees, United Kingdom

John Griffith
Bradford Royal Infirmary
Bradford, United Kingdom

Mark Gudgeon
Frimley Park Hospital
Frimley Park, United Kingdom

Sharmila Gupta
Colchester General Hospital
Colchester, United Kingdom

George Hanna
Imperial College London
London, United Kingdom

Paul Hendry
Freeman Hospital
Newcastle, United Kingdom

James Hollingshead
Chelsea and Westminster Hospitals NHS Trust
London, United Kingdom

Roel Hompes
John Radcliffe Infirmary
Oxford, United Kingdom

Alan Horgan
Newcastle Surgical Training Centre
Newcastle, United Kingdom

James Horwood
University Hospital of Wales
Cardiff, United Kingdom

David Jayne
Leeds Teaching Hospitals NHS Trust
Leeds, United Kingdom

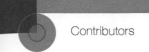

John T. Jenkins
St Marks Hospital
Northwick Park, United Kingdom

Joep Knol
Jessa Hospital
Hasselt, Belgium

Laura Langsford
Derriford Hospital
Plymouth, United Kingdom

Hugh Mackenzie
Imperial College
London, United Kingdom

Chris Mann
University Hospitals of Leicester NHS Trust
Leicester, United Kingdom

Charles Maxwell-Armstrong
Queens Medical Centre
Nottingham, United Kingdom

Andrew S. Miller
Leicester Royal Infirmary
Leicester, United Kingdom

Danilo Miskovic
St. James' University Hospital
Leeds Teaching Hospitals
Leeds, United Kingdom

Peter Alexander Newman
North Bristol NHS Trust
Bristol, United Kingdom

Gary Nicholson
Nuffield Department of Surgery
University of Oxford
Oxford, United Kingdom

Manfred Odermatt
Queen Alexandra Hospital
Portsmouth, United Kingdom

Amjad Parvaiz
Poole General Hospital
Poole, United Kingdom

Irshad Shaikh
St Marks Hospital
Northwick Park, United Kingdom

Shafaque Shaikh
University of Leeds
Leeds, United Kingdom

Kathryn Thomas
Nottingham University Hospitals NHS Trust
Nottingham, United Kingdom

Henry Tilney
Frimley Park Hospital
Frimley Park, United Kingdom

Jared Torkington
University Hospital of Wales
Cardiff, United Kingdom

Susannah M. Wyles
University of California, San Francisco
San Francisco, California

Abbreviations

ALaCaRT	Australasian laparoscopic cancer of the rectum trial
APER	Abdominoperineal resection
BMI	Body mass index
CAT	Competency assessment tool
CCIS	Cleveland clinic incontinence score
CEA	Carcinoembryonic antigen
CME	Complete mesocolic excision
CLASICC	Conventional vs laparoscopic assisted surgery in colorectal cancer
COLOR	Colon carcinoma laparoscopic or open resection
COREAN	Comparison of Open versus laparoscopic surgery for mid or low REctal cancer After Neoadjuvant chemoradiotherapy
COST	Clinical outcome of surgical therapy
CPEX	Cardiopulmonary exercise
CRC	Colorectal cancer
CTAF	Clinical teaching assessment form
CTEI	Clinical teaching effectiveness instrument
CTEQ	Clinical tutor evaluation questionnaire
CUSUM	Cumulative sum
ERAS	Enhanced recovery after surgery
ERP	External rectal prolapse
ERS	Emergency rotation scale
GAS	Generic assessment scale
GRS	Global rating scale
HD	High definition
IBD	Inflammatory bowel disease
ICA	Ileocolic artery
IMA	Inferior mesenteric artery
IRP	Internal rectal prolapse
JAG	Joint advisory group for gastrointestinal endoscopy
L-CAT	Laparoscopic competency assessment tool
LCS	Laparoscopic colorectal surgery
LVMR	Laparoscopic ventral mesh rectopexy
MAS	Minimal access surgery
MCA	Middle colic artery
MCV	Middle colic veins
MTEF	Mayo teaching evaluation form
NET	Neuroendocrine tumours
NHS	National health service
NOTES	Natural orifice trans-luminal endoscopic surgery
NTP	National training programme

NICE	National Institute for Clinical Excellence
OPG	Oxford prolapse grade
PCA	Patient controlled analgesia
PFD	Pelvic floor disorder
RCA	Right colic artery
RCT	Randomised controlled trial
RI	Rectal intussusception
ROLARR	RObotic versus LAparoscopic Resection for Rectal cancer
RUQ	Right upper quadrant
SFDQ	Stanford faculty development program
SILS	Single incision laparoscopic surgery
SMA	Superior mesenteric artery
SRUS	Solitary rectal ulcer syndrome
STEEM	Surgical theatre educational environment measure
STTAR	Structured training trainer assessment report
TAP	Transverse abdominus plane (blocks)
TATME	Transanal total mesorectal excision
TCT	Training the colonoscopy trainers
TEDS	Thromboembolic deterrent stockings
TME	Total mesorectal excision
UK	United Kingdom
VRAM	Vertical rectus abdominis muscle

PART 1

SET

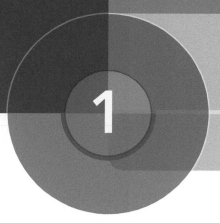

Evidence for laparoscopic surgery in the treatment of colorectal cancer

JAMES HORWOOD AND JARED TORKINGTON

1

LEARNING OBJECTIVES

- Understand the evolution of laparoscopic colorectal surgery.
- Review the major randomised trials upon which the National Institute for Health and Care Excellence (NICE) guidance regarding the introduction of laparoscopic colorectal surgery is based.
- Review the evidence behind short- and long-term outcomes and morbidity from the laparoscopic approach to colorectal resections.
- Provide an overview of ongoing clinical trials awaiting publication.
- Discuss future development of minimally invasive techniques.

INTRODUCTION

The first description of laparoscopic surgery in the treatment of colon cancer is usually credited to Jacobs and colleagues in 1991 (1). The authors from Florida described a variety of procedures in 20 patients for various indications, 12 of whom had adenocarcinomas or large adenomas. They concluded that 'although laparoscope-assisted colonic surgery may still be considered a procedure in evolution, we feel that in time it has the potential to be as popular as laparoscopic cholecystectomy'. Two decades later, laparoscopic colorectal surgery (LCS) has become the preferred surgical option for the treatment of colorectal cancer (CRC) when appropriate.

The subsequent uptake of LCS in the treatment of CRC was haphazard and generally slow. There were issues of standardising training and technique, rudimentary instrumentation, the difficulty of conceptualising anatomy in a different way, and significant concerns surrounding oncological safety. These fears of oncological compromise were fuelled by the emergence of cases of port site metastases (2), now clearly understood to be technique related but at the time multiple theories were proposed including the infamous 'chimney effect'.

The most significant moment in the United Kingdom in the transition of LCS from a technique employed by enthusiasts (sometimes even viewed as mavericks) to mainstream surgery was the publication in August 2006 of Technology Appraisal 105 (TA105) (3) from the National Institute for Health and Care Excellence (NICE) entitled 'Laparoscopic surgery for colorectal cancer'. These guidelines replaced those published in December 2000, TA17, which had called for laparoscopic surgery to only be carried out for colorectal cancer within the confines of a randomised controlled clinical trial. The new 2006 publication for NICE took advice from many surgeons and organisations and critically reviewed the results of those trials called for in the 2000 document to effectively open the door for LCS in the treatment of cancer. TA105 stated:

Laparoscopic surgery (including laparoscopically assisted surgery) is recommended as an alternative to open surgery for people with colorectal cancer if:

- Both laparoscopic and open surgery are suitable for the person and their condition.
- Their surgeon has been trained in laparoscopic surgery for colorectal cancer and performs the operation often enough to keep his or her skills up to date.

The decision about whether to use open or laparoscopic surgery should be made after informed discussion between the patient and the surgeon. In particular, they should talk about whether the patient's condition is suitable for laparoscopic surgery, the risks and benefits of the two procedures, and the surgeon's experience.

SHORT-TERM OUTCOMES

The critical trials in influencing this shift in policy were the Medical Research Council (MRC)-funded, UK-based Conventional versus Laparoscopic-Assisted Surgery in Colorectal Cancer (CLASICC) trial (4); the North American Clinical Outcomes of Surgical Therapy (COST) trial (5); the European Colon Carcinoma Laparoscopic or Open Resection (COLOR) trial (6); and the trial from Lacy which has become known as the Barcelona trial (7). All four trials, published in high-impact journals, demonstrated the anticipated short-term advantages from LCS for colon cancer such as reduced post-operative pain, less blood loss, early return of bowel function, and faster discharge from hospital. Crucially, the studies also showed no evidence for any detrimental effect in terms of oncological safety. Although these trials are never likely to be repeated in terms of design and critics have pointed to various flaws in each, they remain perhaps the most important and influential clinical studies in colorectal cancer of that time.

It is important to emphasise that only the CLASICC trial included rectal cancer patients (with a 34% conversion rate), and the main conclusions of the body of work of these trials collectively apply to colon cancer resection only. Each of these four trials was also carried out in a pre-enhanced recovery era, and evidence suggests that when laparoscopy is integrated into such a programme then discharge is even quicker (8).

The Cochrane Library published a review of the short-term benefits of laparoscopic colorectal resection in 2005 including 25 randomised controlled trials (9). The authors concluded that 'Under traditional perioperative treatment, laparoscopic colonic resections show clinically relevant advantages in selected patients. If the long-term oncological results of laparoscopic and conventional resection of colonic carcinoma show equivalent results, the laparoscopic approach should be preferred in patients suitable for this approach to colectomy'.

When looking for robust evidence for the use of LCS in rectal cancer specifically, we must turn to more recent studies. The first of these is the Comparison of Open versus Laparoscopic

Surgery for Mid and Low Rectal Cancer after Neoadjuvant Chemoradiotherapy (COREAN) trial (10), which randomised 340 patients with rectal cancer to open or laparoscopic surgery and replicated the earlier findings of reduced blood loss, reduced analgesic requirement, earlier return of bowel function, and a non-statistically significant shorter hospital stay but also showed a longer operating time for the LCS group. A second multicentre study from Europe, the Laparoscopic versus Open Rectal Cancer Removal (COLOR II) trial ($n = 739$ vs. $n = 364$) confirmed these findings (11). Both studies showed no difference in morbidity or mortality and crucially once again, no oncological differences between groups in terms of quality of specimen, lymph node harvest, or circumferential resection margin involvement.

The final group to consider separately where possible are patients undergoing abdominoperineal resection of low rectal cancer (abdominoperineal excision of rectum [APER]). In many ways, this is the one truly totally laparoscopic operation as the specimen is removed via the perineal incision negating the need for an abdominal extraction site. The CLASICC and COREAN trials (4,10) both demonstrated no statistical difference in circumferential positivity rates although the latter hinted at lower rates in the laparoscopic arms and in fact this was shown subsequently in the COLOR II trial (11). If one of the great advantages of laparoscopic surgery is the heightened visualisation deep in the pelvis, then this may be part of the explanation. It is also one of the arguments for the use of robotics where the 3D visualisation leads to further enhancement. Running parallel has been the re-focus on technique in the perineal part of the procedure and the tailoring of surgical options including the extra-levator excision (12).

LONG-TERM OUTCOMES AND COMPLICATIONS

A meta-analysis of 3-year outcomes for colon cancer in the CLASICC, COST, COLOR, and Barcelona trials by Bonjer et al. was published in 2007 (13). The analysis compared 796 patients in the laparoscopic arms of the trials and 740 patients undergoing open surgery. There was no difference in 3-year disease-free survival or overall survival.

The second meta-analysis published the same year considered colorectal cancer, included 10 studies, and revealed no significant differences in cancer mortality, recurrence, and lymph node harvest between the two groups of patients, concluding that laparoscopic surgery for colorectal cancer appears to be 'oncologically sound' (14).

Bonjer went on to lead a systematic review for the Cochrane Library published in 2008 (15). They considered 33 randomised controlled trials and concluded that 'Laparoscopic resection of carcinoma of the colon is associated with a long term outcome no different from that of open colectomy. Further studies are required to determine whether the incidence of incisional hernias and adhesions is affected by method of approach. Laparoscopic surgery for cancer of the upper rectum is feasible, but more randomised trials need to be conducted to assess long term outcome'.

Turning to rectal cancer, a Cochrane Library review in 2014 looking at laparoscopic versus open total mesorectal excision found 14 trials including 3528 patients. Their analysis of the data led to more cautious recommendations saying 'We have found moderate quality evidence that laparoscopic total mesorectal excision (TME) has similar effects to open TME on long term survival outcomes for the treatment of rectal cancer. The quality of the evidence was downgraded due to imprecision and further research could impact on our confidence in this result'. Since the publication of this review, the initial results of the Australian ALaCArt study and the similar US ACOSOG Z6051, both randomised non-inferiority studies comparing laparoscopic with open TME have been published (16,17). The authors of these studies should be commended on the attention to detail in ensuring the quality of both surgical resection and pathological assessment of the rectum. Combining both studies, over 900 patients with resectable rectal carcinoma were randomised, with a 30-day mortality <1%, circumferential resection margin (CRM) positivity <10% and clinical anastomotic leak rates of <3% with very high rates of sphincter preservation, representing the best results from rectal cancer surgery in the current literature.

However, in both studies, highly experienced surgeons were unable to produce as high a quality of rectal specimen when the TME was performed laparoscopically. Although under-powered for subgroup analysis, the studies suggest that in male and obese patients and those who have undergone neoadjuvant therapy, the laparoscopic approach to TME is associated with more breaches in the mesorectal fascia than occur at open surgery. Long-term results from these two influential studies are awaited to investigate whether this difference manifests as worse oncological outcomes.

The most recent published addition to this literature is the 3-year outcomes from the COLOR II trial (18). It was possible to analyse 699 patients in the laparoscopic arm and 345 in the open arm. The local recurrence rate in both groups was 5%. Disease-free survival (74.8% vs. 70.8%) and overall survival (86.7% vs. 83.6%) were similar. The same findings were reported for 3-year follow-up of the subjects included in the COREAN trial with disease-free survival at 79.2% versus 72.5%.

The laparoscopic approach to abdominoperineal resection (lap APR) is attractive, as previ-ously mentioned, employing specimen retrieval through the perineal wound, which negates the requirement for abdominal incision. The CLASICC study (4) included a subset, short-term outcome analysis of open versus lap APR (60 pts vs. 36 pts) for low rectal cancer. Although the CRM positivity rates were considerable in both groups (20% vs. 26%), there was no difference in 5-year disease-free and overall survival rates.

Ng et al. (19) undertook a randomised, prospective study of patients undergoing open ver-sus lap APR (48 pts vs. 51 pts). They reported an earlier return to bowel function (3.1 days vs. 4.6 days) and earlier return to independent ambulation (4.4 days vs. 5.9 days), however at the expense of longer operating time and higher overall costs. Importantly, the authors found no significant difference in 5-year survival rates (75% vs. 76%).

The laparoscopic approach to TME can facilitate dissection under vision to the pelvic floor even in the narrow pelvis and obese patients, however a concern surrounding lap APR is the risk of 'coning' the distal specimen as the dissection is completed to the pelvic floor. Many sur-geons believe that lap TME dissection should be stopped at the level of the seminal vesicles (in the male) and completed from the perineum, utilising an extralevator approach (possibly in the prone position) to reduce the incidence of positive CRM.

In addition, pathologies necessitating a more radical perineal dissection (squamous cell car-cinoma of the anus, recurrent rectal adenocarcinoma) that require an abdominal flap (vertical rectus abdominis myocutaneous [VRAM] flap) to enhance perineal healing will negate the potential benefits of the minimally invasive approach.

Attempts to improve perioperative staging, neoadjuvant therapy, and surgical quality to reduce the incidence of CRM positivity following abdominoperineal resection must also be applied to the laparoscopic technique. In addition, post-operative quality of life, sexual and uri-nary functions in this select group of patients need to be fully analysed in a prospective setting.

ADHESIONS AND SMALL BOWEL OBSTRUCTION

Adhesion-related complications have long blighted open abdominal surgery. Parker et al. (20) published a 10-year follow-up of over 12,500 patients undergoing open lower abdominal surgery, finding that 32% of patients were readmitted a mean of 2.2 times for adhesion-related complications in the 10-year follow-up period. These complications add to the morbidity, mortality, and expense of open colorectal surgery.

It has long been suspected that laparoscopic surgery would result in a significant reduction in adhesion formation and therefore adhesion-related complications. Dowson et al. (21) demonstrated a reduction in intra-abdominal adhesions in patients undergoing repeat laparoscopy following laparoscopic compared to open colorectal resections (0 vs. 7 lap vs. open $p = .001$). The clinical relevance of these findings has been confirmed by Rosin et al. (22), who reported an incidence of adhesion-related complications in only 1.3% of patients in their case series of over 300 consecutive laparoscopic resections. Subset analysis from the CLASICC study also demonstrated a non-significant trend towards a reduction in the incidence of adhesive intestinal obstruction and incisional hernia in the laparoscopic arms of the study (23).

FUNCTIONAL OUTCOMES

After the accepted short-term outcomes and the emerging oncological acceptability of LCS for rectal cancer, the next question is whether there may be functional improvement by a laparoscopic procedure. The Cochrane Review published in 2014 by Vennix et al. (24) cautiously confirmed the oncological equivalence and disease-free survival and improved short-term outcomes. They also concluded that there was no clear evidence of any differences in quality of life between open and LCS regarding functional recovery and bladder and sexual function.

EFFECT OF CONVERSION

There is no doubt that the oft-quoted studies from CLASICC, COLOR, COST, and Barcelona included surgeons who were, by and large, self-taught and at various stages of their learning curve using techniques that a decade on will have evolved and changed. This is most graphically illustrated by the 34% conversion rate in the rectal cancer patients included in the CLASICC trial.

In most studies of LCS, patients who require conversion fare worse in terms of blood loss, operating time, hospital stay, and oncological outcomes. Logically these are likely to be the most difficult operations and so poorer outcomes might be anticipated. Equally, conversion rates have come down significantly as training has improved and more patients fall into the NICE quoted category of being 'suitable for laparoscopic surgery'.

The 10-year follow-up of patients included in the CLASICC trial (25) shows no difference between overall survival or disease-free survival between laparoscopic or open procedures, but critically it demonstrates the poorer outcome in the conversion group. The median overall survival in these patients was 59.2 (38.8–73.5) months compared with 78.4 (66.1–106) months for open surgery and 94.8 (81.9–150.9) months for the laparoscopic group ($p = .001$). Although the conversion group in the original study has a higher percentage of Dukes C patients, the difference in survival remained when age, sex, and TNM stage were taken into account. Interestingly there was less effect in the rectal cancer converted group than the colon converted group but the same effect in surgeons with a lower conversion rate suggesting experience was unlikely to influence the outcome.

The literature is difficult to interpret as the criteria for conversion seem to vary, and there is no universally accepted definition of the terms *laparoscopic assisted* and *conversion*.

SUMMARY

Minimally invasive approaches to colorectal resection have enjoyed a rapid proliferation since first described in 1991 (1), particularly following the publication of NICE guidance (3) to become the gold standard approach for the majority of patients. Once the safety and efficacy of laparoscopic surgery for colonic carcinoma were established, improvements in technology, experience, and training have permitted minimally invasive options to be offered to the majority of patients.

Proctored training for established surgeons, followed by the establishment of fellowship positions, structured curricula, and training courses for trainee surgeons, have permitted the proliferation of laparoscopic colorectal surgery without the increase in surgical complications (26) that had been observed following the introduction of other minimally invasive procedures (27).

Colorectal surgery remains an exciting and dynamic specialty. We keenly await the long-term results of randomised trials demonstrating the safety and efficacy of laparoscopic approaches to rectal carcinoma, future developments in single incision laparoscopic surgery (SILS), robotic platforms (ROLARR study), and transanal total mesorectal excision (TATME), all of which have the potential to dramatically expand the boundaries of minimally invasive surgery, resulting in advances in both quality and safety, that will benefit future patients with both malignant and benign colorectal conditions.

KEY POINTS

- Considerable evidence from multicentre, randomised trials have demonstrated the short- and long-term benefits from laparoscopic colorectal surgery.
- Minimally invasive approaches to rectal resection require advanced laparoscopic skills. Evidence for oncological and functional equivalence between open and laparoscopic TME are awaited from multicentre studies.
- Robotic platforms and TATME have the potential to further improve outcomes from minimally invasive colorectal surgery.

TAKE-HOME MESSAGE

- Laparoscopic colorectal resection has evolved over two decades to become established as the evidence-based 'gold standard' approach for the majority of patients.

REFERENCES

1. Jacobs M, Verdeja JC, Goldstein HS. Minimally invasive colon resection (laparoscopic colectomy). *Surg Laparosc Endosc* 1991;1:144–50.
2. Wexner SD, Cohen SM. Port site metastases after laparoscopic colorectal surgery for cure of malignancy. *Br J Surg* 1995;82:295–8.
3. National Institute for Health and Clinical Excellence. *Colorectal Cancer: Laparoscopic Surgery (Review)*. Technology appraisal TA105. National Institute for Health and Clinical Excellence, London, 2006 (http://www.nice.org.uk/guidance/TA105).

4. Guillou PJ, Quirke P, Thorpe H, Walker J, Jayne DG, Smith AM et al. Short-term endpoints of conventional versus laparoscopic-assisted surgery in patients with colorectal cancer (MRC CLASICC trial): Multicentre, randomised controlled trial. *Lancet* 2005;365:1718–26.

5. COST Study Group. A comparison of laparoscopically assisted and open colectomy for colon cancer. *N Engl J Med* 2004;350:2050–9.

6. Veldkamp R, Kuhry E, Hop WC, Jeekel J, Kazemier G, Boner HJ et al. Laparoscopic surgery versus open surgery for colon cancer: Short-term outcomes of a randomised trial. *Lancet Oncol* 2005;6:477–84.

7. Lacy AM, Garcia-Valdecasas JC, Delgado S, Castells A, Taura P, Pique JM et al. Laparoscopy-assisted colectomy versus open colectomy for treatment of non-metastatic colon cancer: A randomised controlled trial. *Lancet* 2002;359:2224–9.

8. Wang Q, Suo J, Jiang J, Wang C, Zhao YQ, Cao X. Effectiveness of fast-track rehabilitation versus conventional care in laparoscopic colorectal resection for elderly patients: A randomised trial. *Colorectal Dis* 2012;14:1009–13.

9. Schwenk W, Haase O, Neudecker JJ, Müller JM. Short term benefits for laparoscopy colorectal resection. *Cochrane Database of Systematic Reviews* 2005, Issue 2. Art. No.: CD003145. DOI: 10.1002/14651858.CD003145.pub2.

10. Kang SB, Park JW, Jeong SY, Nam BH, Choi HS, Kim DW et al. Open versus laparoscopic surgery for mid or low rectal cancer after neoadjuvant chemoradiotherapy (COREAN trial): Short-term outcomes of an open-label randomised controlled trial. *Lancet Oncol* 2010;11:637–45.

11. Van der Pas MH, Haglind E, Cuesta MA, Furst A, Lacy AM, Hop WC et al. Laparoscopic versus open surgery for rectal cancer (COLOR II): Short term outcomes of a randomised phase 3 trial. *Lancet Oncol* 2013;14:210–8.

12. Martijinse IS, Dudink RL, West NP, Wasowicz D, Nieuwenhuijzen GA, van LI et al. Focus on extralevator perineal dissection in supine position for low rectal cancer has led to a better quality of surgery and oncologic outcome. *Ann Surg Oncol* 2012;19:786–93.

13. Bonjer HJ, Hop WC, Nelson H, Sargent DJ, Lacy AM, Catelis A et al. Laparoscopically assisted versus open colectomy for colon cancer: A meta-analysis. *Arch Surg* 2007;142:298–303.

14. Jackson TD, Kaplan GG, Arena G, Page JH, Rogers SO. Laparoscopic versus open resection for colorectal cancer: A meta-analysis of oncologic outcomes. *J Am Coll Surg* 2007;204:439–46.

15. Kuhry E, Schwenk W, Gaupset R, Romild U, Bonjer HJ. Long-term results of laparoscopic colorectal cancer resection. *Cochrane Database of Systematic Reviews* 2008, Issue 2. Art. No.: CD003432. DOI: 10.1002/14651858.CD003432.pub2.

16. Stevenson A, Solomon M, Lumley J, Hewett P, Clouston A, Gebski V, Davies L, Wilson K, Hague W, Simes J. Effect of laparoscopic assisted resection versus open resection on pathological outcomes in rectal cancer. *JAMA* 2015;34(13):1356–63.

17. Fleshman J, Branda M, Sargent D, Boller A, George V, Abbas M et al. Effect of laparoscopic assisted resection versus open resection of stage II or III rectal cancer on pathological outcomes. *JAMA* 2015;314(13):1346–55.

18. Bonjer HJ, Deijen CL, Abis GA, Cuesta MA, van der Pas MH, de Lange-de Klerk ES et al. A randomized trial of laparoscopic versus open surgery for rectal cancer. *N Engl J Med* 2015;372:1324–32.

19. Ng S, Leung K, Lee J, Yiu R, Li J, Teoh A, Leung W. Laparoscopic-assisted versus open abdominoperineal resection for low rectal cancer: A prospective randomized trial. *Ann Surg Oncol* 2008;15(9):2418–25.

20. Parker M, Ellis H, Moran B, Thompson J, Wilson M, Menzies D et al. Postoperative adhesions: Ten-year follow-up of 12,584 patients undergoing lower abdominal surgery. *Dis Colon Rectum* 2001;44(6):822–29.

21. Dowson H, Bong J, Lovell D, Worthington T, Karanjia N, Rockall T. Reduced adhesion formation following laparoscopic versus open colorectal surgery. *Br J Surg* 2008;95(7):909–14.

22. Rosin D, Zmora O, Hoffman A, Khaikin M, Zakai B, Munz Y, Shabtai M, Ayalon A. Low incidence of adhesion-related bowel obstruction after laparoscopic colorectal surgery. *J Laparoendosc Adv Surg Tech* 2007;17(5):604–7.

23. Taylor G, Jayne D, Brown S, Thorpe H, Brown J, Dewberry S, Parker M, Guillou P. Adhesions and incisional hernias following laparoscopic versus open surgery for colorectal cancer in the CLASICC trial. *Br J Surg* 2010;97(1):70–8.

24. Vennix S, Pelzers L, Bouvy N, Beets GL, Pierie JP, Wiggers T, Breukink S. Laparoscopic versus open total mesorectal excision for rectal cancer. *Cochrane Database of Systematic Reviews* 2014, Issue 4. Art. No.: CD005200. DOI: 10.1002/14651858.CD005200.pub3.

25. Green BL, Marshall HC, Collinson F, Quirke P, Guillou P, Jayne DG, Brown JM. Long-term follow-up of the Medical Research Council CLASICC trial of conventional versus laparoscopically assisted resection in colorectal cancer. *Br J Surg* 2013;100:75–82.

26. Maeda T, Tan K, Konishi F, Tsujinaka S, Mizokami K, Sasaki J, Kawamura Y. Trainee surgeons do not cause more conversions in laparoscopic colorectal surgery if they are well supervised. *World J Surg* 2009;33(11):2439–43.

27. Richardson M, Bell G, Fullarton G. Incidence and nature of bile duct injuries following laparoscopic cholecystectomy: An audit of 5913 cases. West of Scotland Laparoscopic Cholecystectomy Audit Group. *Br J Surg* 1996;83(10):1356–60.

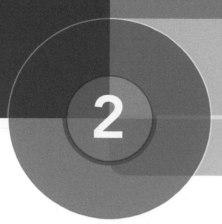

2

Design and development of a national training programme

MARK COLEMAN AND LAURA LANGSFORD

LEARNING OBJECTIVES

- Understand the development and structure of a laparoscopic colorectal training programme in the United Kingdom.

INTRODUCTION

Image-based medical interventions have revolutionised health care over the last decades. These are therapies conducted with a television screen and minimal access incisions in order to reduce the trauma of the treatment for the patient. There are challenges to safely learning these new techniques. The following chapter describes how these were addressed in the National Training Programme for Laparoscopic Colorectal Surgery in England.

BACKGROUND

Advanced laparoscopic surgery is now globally well established since its advent 25 years ago. During this time technological advances and the accumulation of surgical experience have led to increased benefits for patients. The laparoscopic approach for resection of the colon and rectum has gained in popularity, though not as quickly as certain other complex laparoscopic procedures. This can be attributed to oncological concerns over port site metastases and a lengthy predicted learning curve accompanied by worse outcomes.

In parallel over the last 25 years, many developed countries have moved from 'apprentice'-style surgical training to competence-based training accompanied by formative and summative assessment. This allows a more objective means to confirm the acquisition of surgical skills.

At the same time surgeons' performance has been placed under unprecedented scrutiny by patients, the public, politicians, and the media. The consequence is that it is no longer acceptable for surgeons to either learn a new technique or practice without confirmation of acceptable levels of surgical skills and safety for their patients. Moreover it is becoming the norm for surgeons to be required to objectively confirm their professional standing and for this to be 'revalidated' on a recurring basis. Publication of surgeon outcomes in the United Kingdom is now required by an increasing number of specialties including colorectal.

THE NATIONAL HEALTH SERVICE (NHS)

In the United Kingdom, general surgery has become progressively more specialised over the last 30 years since the Calman-Hine reforms of the UK NHS. Top-down reforms have resulted in a system where surgeons train, certificate, and practice within distinct areas of general surgery such as colorectal. Additional structures have also been created to improve, implement, and standardise evidence-based practice. These include multidisciplinary teams, peer review, and the National Institute for Health and Care Excellence (NICE).

FORMATION OF A NATIONAL TRAINING PROGRAMME

Evidence promoting the benefits of laparoscopic versus open surgery for colorectal cancer and other benign colorectal conditions is now well established in the global peer-reviewed surgical literature (see Chapter 1). In 2006, NICE, which issues evidence-based and legally binding guidance on novel therapies and techniques, evaluated laparoscopic colorectal surgery (LCS) and recommended that suitable patients should be offered the technique by appropriately trained surgeons. At this time in the United Kingdom, around 5% of colorectal resections were performed by the laparoscopic approach, and there was recognition that insufficient numbers of surgeons were competent in LCS for the NICE guidance to be introduced into practice. As a result, in 2007, the National Cancer Action Team, part of NHS-E, decided to institute a national training programme (NTP) for LCS in England, the aim of which was to safely increase the adoption of LCS to satisfy the NICE guidance. The programme was designed to provide hands-on training in LCS by experts to existing colorectal specialists (consultants).

NTP DEVELOPMENT

A hub-and-spoke system was devised with central organisation and 11 training centres located around England (see 'Background' section). Almost 70 experts were eventually recruited, and an initial scoping exercise established that up to 150 consultants in England wished to take advantage of the offers of training provided by the NTP. The scoping exercise comprised a questionnaire to all members of the Association of Coloproctology of Great Britain and Ireland (ACPGBI) in England to ascertain how many surgeons were undertaking little or no LCS and how many of these wished to be trained.

Although evidence from the global literature suggested that the learning curve was up to 150 cases with self-taught adoption, the NTP estimated that, due to the colorectal and laparoscopic experience of its delegates, and the presence of an expert mentor in the operating room, that competence in LCS could be obtained within 20–25 cases.

Mentorship is the term used in the NTP to define the relationship between the consultant delegate or 'trainee' and the expert or 'trainer'. Mentorship is defined differently for other purposes and in other contexts. For the NTP it embraced concepts that included the agreement between the trainee and trainer with respect to the objectives, structure, duration, and location of training; the commitment of both to assessment; and the audit of educational and clinical outcomes. Most importantly, the NTP mentorship was centred on the delivery of hands-on competence-based training in the operating room. No other form of training or simulation was accepted as a replacement that could guarantee satisfactory completion of training in LCS.

The NTP also decided to incorporate a full system of educational and clinical assessment to provide quality assurance for the effectiveness and efficiency of the NTP. This aspect of the NTP was conducted by the Academic Department of Surgery at Imperial College, London, led by Professor George Hanna (see Chapter 3).

LAPCO

The structure of the NTP was developed through 2008, during which time national leadership passed from John Monson from the Hull training centre, to Mark Coleman, from Plymouth Hospitals NHS Trust, the lead for the South West training centre. This led to the renaming of the NTP under the 'Lapco' banner centred on a web-based coordination of all the training methodologies, training centres, and educational tools.

The Lapco programme with the National Clinical Lead Mark Coleman and the Education and Research Lead George Hanna developed a steering group, which met regularly throughout the programme to create a consensus decision-making process. The Lapco Steering Group comprised both leads, the Lapco programme manager, representatives of each of the Lapco training centres, and a trainee representative. Invited members also came from the ACPGBI and the Association of Laparoscopic Surgeons of Great Britain and Ireland, and invited surgical representatives came from Wales and Scotland. The Steering Group Terms of Reference were as follows:

- Agree on the training methods.
- Agree on educational materials and the operative techniques to be employed.
- Agree on development of course educational material (DVD and written material) with advice from clinical leads.
- Agree on design and implementation of a 2 to 3 day course for the multiprofessional team.
- Agree on guidance as to what constitutes mandatory elements of training.
- Oversee the design and agree on the mechanism to assess surgeons to undertake independent laparoscopic colorectal surgery.
- Oversee the progress of the programme to ensure it is delivered on time and within budget.
- Develop methods to assess 'Sign Off' for completion of the National Training Programme, along with a follow-up procedure post sign-off.

A full-time programme manager (Laura Langsford) was appointed to support the national clinical lead and to performance manage the training centres.

The role included

- Facilitating registration of consultants for training and confirmation of eligibility
- Pairing consultant trainers and trainees

- Monitoring training progression
- Coordinating training centres
- Distributing programme finances to training centres
- Managing the website
- Ensuring steering group organisation
- Ensuring masterclass organisation

Training took place between January 2009 and March 2013. New registrations to Lapco were drawn to a close in October 2011 to ensure that all registered trainees were able to complete their training before the programme end in March 2013.

All colorectal consultants in substantive posts in England were eligible to apply to Lapco as trainees. Trainees were accepted onto the NTP by personal application through the website (http://www.lapco.nhs.uk). Each trainee obtained a username and password to access his or her own account within the site. Applicants were required to be consultant colorectal surgeons in a substantive post and to obtain the explicit support of their NHS employer, usually by a letter from their medical director or chief executive of their own NHS Hospital Trust. Each application was reviewed by the National Coordination Office and the applicant was written to by the national clinical lead, and offered a tailored package of preclinical and clinical training opportunities.

A Lapco training centre and trainer was allocated according to trainee preference, training capacity, and geographical location. A training centre manager or administrator contact who was the local coordination link for arranging training sessions was provided to each trainee in the trainee's appointment letter.

Once an application to Lapco had been accepted and a trainer appointed, the period of hands-on training could begin.

TRAINER APPOINTMENTS

To be appointed as a Lapco trainer, each applicant had to

- Be a substantive colorectal consultant post at a hospital in England.
- Be recommended to the national clinical lead by an existing Lapco trainer.
- Complete at least 100 colorectal resections prior to appointment.

Upon confirmation of the above, all trainer appointments to the programme were made formally in writing by the national clinical lead. All Lapco-appointed trainers were encouraged to attend the 2-day Lapco Train the Trainer TT Course (Lapco TT, see Chapter 5). By the end of the Lapco programme, over 90% of trainers had attended this course.

TRAINING PORTFOLIO

After application, each programme participant had his or her own web portfolio, accessed by username and password through the Lapco website. Information in each portfolio was also accessible by the National Coordination Office, the Educational Assessment Group, and the training centre responsible for that participant. All information was held in confidence. Lapco participants were able to download their own training portfolio in a usable (.csv) format for use in audit and appraisal, and could view their progress through their own proficiency gain curve or 'Learning Curve'.

LAPCO PROGRAMME STRUCTURE

Lapco offered a number of preclinical and clinical methods of training. The programme recognised that it needed to be flexible to the needs of surgeons and their varying levels of experience. It was expected that the trainees should have seen at least 10 live laparoscopic colorectal cases. Many had already attended masterclasses, cadaver courses, or wetlabs and also had extensive experience of laparoscopic procedures such as cholecystectomy. Therefore, the programme needed to offer different entry points accounting for level of skill. The NTP placed strong emphasis on team training throughout. It was funded to provide equipment for training centres, to fund places on preclinical courses, and to enable backfill of trainers' clinical sessions while engaged in Lapco activity.

PRECLINICAL TRAINING

The preclinical training opportunities and courses for consultants and their teams were made available throughout the country, including Lapco Funded Cadaveric Courses at Newcastle, Nottingham, and Bristol; Immersion Courses at Basingstoke (4-day courses) and Bradford (3-day courses); and Enhanced Recovery Courses at Bristol and St Marks, London. Lapco emphasised and encouraged team training as it was recognised that this hastens the ascent up the learning curve. Strong emphasis was placed on Enhanced Recovery Courses as data suggest a further reduction in hospital stays in patients undergoing bowel resection (see Chapter 11).

Lapco also ran 1-day laparoscopic colorectal education masterclasses for trainees and their teams for up to 100 delegates encompassing sessions on surgical presentations, techniques and approaches, and live theatre cases led by NTP trainers. In addition, further emphasis was placed on support and education for teams, and Lapco ran a number of Theatre Practitioner Courses.

Wetlab Courses also took place at two locations in Europe (ESI, Hamburg and Elancourt, Paris). These courses were sponsored and run by Ethicon (Hamburg) and Covidien (Paris). They were of a similar format covering 2 days. Each comprised lectures on the evidence for laparoscopic colorectal surgery, establishing a practice in LCS, theatre setup, and extensive material on how to perform LCS. Each also gave excellent hands-on experience in the wetlab. There were also opportunities for theatre teams to accompany surgeons on these trips.

CLINICAL TRAINING

It was generally envisaged that around a minimum of 20 mentored cases performed by the trainee would be required to reach a level of competence with variation in either direction depending on the skill and experience of the individual. A form of assessment of competence was incorporated into Lapco to provide surgeons in the programme a means of objectively determining that their training has been assessed and recorded. This information was also intended for use by consultants as part of their appraisal and revalidation.

All training centres offered ongoing opportunities for live observation of LCS cases, and Lapco encouraged theatre team involvement in such visits, which took place prior to hands-on clinical training.

TRAINING METHODS

In-reach training involved consultant trainees operating in the trainer's hospital with an honorary contract under the direct supervision of the trainer. The trainee attends the trainer's hospital to perform a case with a patient from the trainers trust.

In-reach with travelling patient involved the tariff to fund the patient's procedure and care traveling with the patient to the training centre. Follow-up of patients then returned to the responsibility of the trainee after discharge.

Approximately 65% of all NTP training sessions were carried out on an in-reach basis.

Outreach involved the trainer attending the trainee's hospital with the trainee operating in his or her own theatre on his or her own patient. An Honorary Contract was required to be in place for the visiting trainer. Approximately 35% of all NTP training sessions are carried out on an outreach basis.

Trainers and training centre managers were required to schedule a timetable of training cases to ensure where possible that they are performed over as short a period of time as to ensure rapid ascent up the learning curve. The NTP funded the trainers trust for both in-reach and outreach cases including travelling expenses.

In addition to individual clinical theatre training sessions, Lapco supported the delivery of clinical immersion courses in two of its training centres. These were particularly useful for trainees in the early stages of training, or as a refresher to provide increased intensity of training over a 3- or 4-day period, or as they moved towards the sign-off submission at the end of the training period.

Immersion courses comprised a 4-day course with eight consultant Lapco delegates and two laparoscopic colorectal procedures per day. Each delegate directly observed each case, held the camera for one, and performed one case under supervision observed by the other trainees. As before, the trainee obtained an honorary contract and occupational health clearance from the training centre.

ASSESSMENT

The process of assessment was devised and managed by the Education Department at Imperial College. Each training case during the clinical phase was accompanied by the use of an online Global Assessment Score (GAS) form. The GAS forms contain essential information on each case without the patient's name to protect confidentiality. On completion of the form, it is submitted via the website to the National Coordination Office, the Education Department, and the training centre responsible for that trainee. The information is locked out to prevent the scores being changed, but the data are then available for the trainee to download for his or her own purposes. The Education Department also devised a research programme to observe unedited videos and to determine if it is possible to define a proficiency gain curve for laparoscopic colorectal surgery. The trainer is also required to complete a Trainer GAS form after each case which once completed can be viewed by the trainee through their online account. The Trainer GAS form was also the 'currency' to demonstrate a training episode had taken place to allow payment to the training centre.

SIGN-OFF (LAPCO EXIT)

Successful exit from Lapco was triggered by agreement between trainer and trainee. The number of cases required to reach this point was determined between the trainer and trainee as it was recognised this figure would vary. The predicted figure was around 20 cases. For final assessment, two unedited videos were submitted for examination by two different Lapco trainers. Following successful examination of the videos, the Training Centre and Lapco National Lead Clinician wrote to the trainee to indicate completion of the programme and gave advice for future practice.

AUDIT AND REFLECTIVE PRACTICE

Both during and after training Lapco encouraged ongoing prospective audit of cases to observe operative and post-operative outcomes. Through the online Global Assessment Forms, data were accumulated and stored for each participant trainee to provide a useful archive for personal use, presentation, appraisal, and revalidation. Lapco also encouraged the creation and subsequent observation of operative videos as a useful means of reflective practice.

POST SIGN-OFF

Lapco requested that trainees signed off the programme submit post-sign-off data for a period of 12 months after the date of sign-off. This was submitted to the Education Team at Imperial College.

LAPCO TRAINING CENTRES

There were 11 training centres in England:

- Newcastle
- Bradford
- Hull
- Nottingham
- Oxford
- London 1: St Marks, Colchester, and Guildford
- London 2: Kings, Guys, and St Thomas
- Portsmouth
- Basingstoke and Frimley Park
- South West: Plymouth, Bristol and Yeovil
- North West: Salford

Immersion Courses

- Basingstoke and Frimley Park
- Bradford

Cadaver Courses

- Bristol and Newcastle

Education and Research

- Imperial College, London

SUMMARY

The Lapco programme was instituted to increase the use of the laparoscopic approach for colorectal resection in England by existing specialists. The programme used hands-on training in the operating room provided by existing experts in laparoscopic surgery to ensure the best clinical outcomes for patients. Training was funded and rigorously evaluated through processes of formative and summative assessment. Clinical outcome data were also collected and analysed. All trainers participated in a Lapco 'Train the Trainers' course to elevate and standardise their training skills. Educational and clinical outcome data have been published in the surgical peer-reviewed literature and suggest that the Lapco programme was one of the most successful training programmes for specialists in the world.

KEY POINTS

- The Lapco programme showed that surgeons training in a new advanced laparoscopic procedure can do so safely and effectively in the presence and under the guidance of an expert in the operating room.
- The Lapco programme demonstrated that both formative and summative assessment can be used in surgical training.
- A performance managed training programme across a regional or national healthcare system is effective in transforming the safe adoption of a new technique such as laparoscopic colorectal surgery.

TAKE-HOME MESSAGE

- Mentorship works.

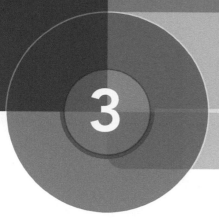

Educational tools and assessment for laparoscopic colorectal surgery

3

SUSANNAH M. WYLES AND DANILO MISKOVIC

LEARNING OBJECTIVES

- Understand the rationale behind the need for the development of educational assessment tools in surgery.
- Define the difference between formative and summative assessment.
- Determine how assessments can be used to measure trainee, and training programme, success.
- Understand how the assessment tools were developed and validated for use within the Lapco programme.

INTRODUCTION

In recent years there has been an increasing interest in the objective assessment of surgical performance and education. Simply passing post-graduate examinations and demonstration of an adequate case-log is no longer thought to be sufficient. In the United Kingdom, North America, and as well in other countries, trainees are required to provide a portfolio of evidence of detailed competencies. This attitudinal shift is not just true for trainees, but it has also begun to affect those already trained and in independent practice. For example, the adoption of new complex operative procedures used to occur simply after attendance at a course, whereas now fellowships, and government-funded initiatives have been developed to allow for careful mentoring prior to independent practice. The reasons for these changes are multifactorial. These include an increased awareness of patient safety and the impact of the surgical learning curve that is pertained to be avoidable and no longer acceptable. There is an increased trend in patients seeking legal compensation should complications occur, and hence, objective evidence of competency becomes an existential tool on behalf of the surgeon's defense team. There has been a complete alteration in the training structure for surgeons, meaning that they have reduced number of hours in the operating room, potentially reduced exposure to cases, and subspecialisation has changed the breadth of operations observed. There has been a tendency for more cases to become more technically advanced with the introduction of robotic and laparoscopic surgery. Cases traditionally performed by junior surgeons, for example an open inguinal hernia repair, may now be performed by a senior surgeon who is learning or perfecting the more challenging laparoscopic technique. Increased staff turnover and modern shift structures often lead to a less intimate and trusting relationship between senior and junior team members compared to more traditional apprenticeship models. Finally, the introduction of revalidation and relicensing will increasingly depend on objective assessment of surgical performance.

How can this necessary assessment be delivered? Assessment can be divided classically into formative and summative assessment. Formative assessment provides feedback to learners about their progress. Summative assessment measures the achievement of learning goals at the end of a course or programme of study (1). Assessments can be used to measure a trainee's learning and to grade the trainee against a standard or a comparative group; they can indicate a trainee's readiness to progress; motivate trainees to learn, focus, and direct their learning; summarise their achievement; inform the teaching programme; and contribute to education quality assurance, and hence, their popularity in modern training programmes.

In the context of Lapco (see Chapter 2), assessment was a fundamental part of the programme. Given that it was government funded, it was necessary to monitor the programme to determine its outcomes and demonstrate cost-effectiveness. Furthermore, it was designed to train surgeons with the ability to do a specific operation that was being recommended to be performed laparoscopically by the National Institute for Health and Care Excellence (NICE). Therefore it was essential that the surgeons' progress in technical ability was tracked effectively, throughout their time in the programme and beyond. Thus there was a need for both formative and summative assessments of the surgeons. Furthermore, the trainers within the programme needed to be monitored to ensure that a consistent standard of teaching was being delivered in all of the 11 training centres. It was therefore necessary for assessments for both the trainers and trainees to be put in place.

In this chapter we summarise the development, validation, and outcomes of the assessment methods employed in the Lapco programme.

ASSESSING THE TRAINEE

The obvious way to assess the progress and quality of training surgeons is to analyse their results and compare them directly with expert surgeons. This can be and has been done in various ways and a most recent analysis, performed by the authors, reveals a learning curve of up to 150 procedures for laparoscopic colorectal surgery, when self-taught (Figure 3.1).

Although auditing clinical results is important, it creates ethical, methodological, and practical dilemmas when using them to analyse training progress and competence. The retrospective nature of analysis is not practical for the live monitoring of training progression. It is also difficult to compare results of different patients, and risk adjustment, however fancy it may be, is always inadequate at an individual patient level. After analysing the literature on supervised (or mentored) training, it also becomes apparent that clinical outcomes do not vary between trainees and experts, as long as the trainees are supervised. Hence it becomes a serious ethical issue as to whether learning should be performed unsupervised if it leads to preventable negative clinical outcomes (3).

Based on these findings it became apparent that new ways of formative and summative assessment tools were required for Lapco.

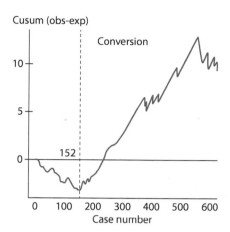

Figure 3.1 Learning curve for self-taught laparoscopic colorectal surgery. (From Miskovic D et al. *Dis Colon Rectum* 2012;55(12):1300 10. With permission.)

FORMATIVE ASSESSMENT

In an ideal world a good formative assessment tool should be objective, depict the reality in its entirety, provide detailed feedback, and be practical and quick to complete. Ideal worlds do not exist and neither do ideal assessment tools. For Lapco, the feasibility and user friendliness for a formative assessment tool were paramount, as it was expected that senior surgeons, stereotypically with a limited attention span and a cramped diary, would not use any form of time-consuming and cumbersome tool. The provision of a workable tool was required in a short time span due to the start date of the training programme, and a quick workable solution was needed.

The development of the tool was guided by the Lapco steering group (see Chapter 2) and other published work on technical steps for laparoscopic surgery. A task list that was applicable for most laparoscopic colorectal resections was established, and a generic, user-friendly rating system was introduced (see Table 3.1).

After validation of the tool, and directly linking the completion of the form for each training case with funding for the Lapco training centre, the success and impact of this simple assessment tool was quite dramatic. Despite the generic nature, not only details on the training progression for different steps of the procedure, but also differences between individual or defined groups of training surgeons became apparent and very useful for the analysis of the programme (Figure 3.2). The tool was generally liked by trainers and trainees as it provided a good framework for a more detailed and individual feedback session after an operative training case.

SUMMATIVE ASSESSMENT

The success of the programme was to a degree dependent on developing a validated summative competency assessment tool for use at the end of training. This would ensure not only the clinical quality of trainees exiting the programme but also reflect on the quality of training provided throughout the programme.

Due to the importance and potential impact for trainees, trainers, and patients of this kind of assessment, the development and validation process was more complex and more sophisticated than for the Global Assessment Score (GAS) tool.

Table 3.1 Global Assessment Score (GAS) for the formative assessment in Lapco

Generic Task List

A. Exposure
  A1. Operating room setup (position of surgeons, scrub nurse, drapes, etc.)
  A2. Patient positioning
  A3. Laparoscopic access (open, Veress needle or other techniques, and insertion of ports)
  A4. Exposure of operating field (moving of omentum, small bowel, etc.)

B. Dissection of vascular pedicle
  B1. Dissection of vascular pedicle (incision of peritoneum, creation of window below and
        above, and dissection with stapler, clips, ultrasound dissection tool or other techniques)
  B2. Retrocolic dissection of mesentry (right side towards hepatic flexure, left side towards
        splenic flexure)
  B3. Identification of landmark (right side: duodenum, left side: left ureter)

C. Mobilisation
  C1. Dissection of flexure (right side: hepatic, left side: splenic)
  C2. Mesorectal dissection (including total mesorectal excision [TME], only for rectal resections)
  C3. Dissection of bowel (transection, using stapler or other similar device)

D. Anastomosis
  D1. Extraction of specimen (creation of incision, bringing out specimen, completion of resection)
  D2. Anastomosis (intra- or extracorporeal)

Each task is rated from 1 to 6:
  1: Not performed, step had to be done by trainer
  2: Partly performed, step had to be partly done by trainer
  3: Performed, with substantial verbal support
  4: Performed with minor verbal support
  5: Competent performance, safe (without guidance)
  6: Proficient performance, could not be better

The Laparoscopic Competency Assessment Tool (L-CAT) was developed in several stages. These involved detailed analysis of semi-structured interviews of expert surgeons, a Delphi-type consensus process, and face validation. The result of this process was a single-page assessment framework (Figure 3.3).

The agreed objective and independent process involved the trainees, once agreed with their individual trainer as indicated by the progression on GAS scores, to submit unedited videos of two cases to the central office. The videos had to be fully performed by the trainees, they had to be complete (i.e. from port insertion to resection) and from two different anatomical areas (right hemicolectomy and left-sided resection). The videos were de-identified upon receipt by the educational central office and randomly distributed to two independent assessors across the country who received training in using the L-CAT forms. The scores from the L-CAT forms, together with some free comments, would then decide if the trainee would pass the assessment or fail. In case of failure, detailed feedback was given to the surgeon and the re-submission of two more cases requested. If the assessors disagreed about the outcome, the videos were sent to a third assessor.

This process, although not perfect, was thought to lead to an objective and very detailed assessment of competency. More recently it could be shown that the L-CAT scores directly correlate with clinical outcomes. It is the first time that the immediate impact of an educational assessment tool on individual patient results could be shown (Table 3.2).

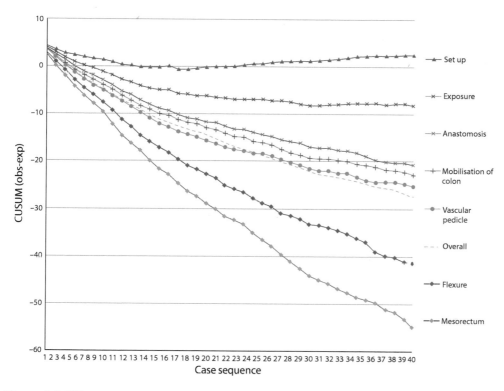

Figure 3.2 Different tasks of the procedure are learnt at different speeds. (With kind permission from Springer Science+Business Media: *Surg Endosc*, Clinical and educational proficiency gain of supervised laparoscopic colorectal surgical trainees, 27(8), 2013, 2704–11, Mackenzie H et al.)

ASSESSING THE TRAINER

The programme was highly dependent on high-quality training provided by expert laparoscopic surgeons all over England. It was therefore of crucial interest not only to assess the training surgeons but also the quality of training provided throughout the programme.

On review of the literature there were certain assessment tools already available for assessing the medical teacher. The majority tended to be opinion questionnaires, with Likert-scale scoring systems to be completed by medical students, trainees, fellows, or peers. Some tools combine the opinion of different raters, and those opinions given in different medical settings such as inpatient or outpatient teaching. The tools available to Lapco are summarised in Table 3.3. Only three existed for the assessment of surgical teachers, and these were all for use by residents rather than peers. The only peer evaluation for inpatient teaching was the Mayo Teaching Evaluation Form (MTEF), which was designed for assessing teaching on ward rounds in internal medicine, rather than any procedural or surgical teaching. It was therefore deemed necessary to create a new teaching assessment, specifically for surgery.

THE MINI-STTAR

Through semi-structured interviews, experts gave their opinion on what was thought to be necessary to enable good surgical teaching. These different points were extracted and the

L-CAT
Laparoscopic Competency Assessment Tool
City of Hearts Imperial College London

Trainee ID ☐☐☐☐☐ Assessor ID ☐☐☐☐☐☐ Case No. ☐☐ Date ☐☐☐☐☐☐

© 2010 Imperial College London

TASK	EXPOSURE	PEDICLE CONTROL	MOBILISATION	RESECTION/ANASTOMOSIS
	Ports are safely inserted in an ergonomically ideal position, operating field is exposed	Vascular pedicle is identified and vessels dissected out at an appropriate level	Mobilisation following anatomical planes, landmarks adequately defined and protected	Adequate and appropriate resection and safe performance of anastomosis

INSTRUMENT USE — Safe use of instruments

EXPOSURE — Port insertion/placement:	PEDICLE CONTROL — Use of haemostatic tool (clip applier / diathermy/stapler):	MOBILISATION — Use of graspers/dissection tools:	RESECTION/ANASTOMOSIS — Use of intestinal stapler (straight, circular):
1 Dangerous technique (not visualised), hazardous or wrong position	1 Dangerous (uncontrolled moves/views, wrong instrument)	1 Dangerous (traumatic grasping, hazardous use of dissection tool)	1 Dangerous (uncontrolled movements/views, wrong cartridge)
2 Incompetent (several attempts) or ergonomically poor position	2 Incompetent (awkward, repeated attempts, impaired views)	2 Incompetent (awkward and inefficient grasping, use of dissection tool)	2 Incompetent (awkward, repeated attempts, impaired views)
3 Safe insertion and ergonomically good position	3 Safe (instrument accurately placed and engaged)	3 Safe (safe grasping, safe use of dissection tool)	3 Safe (instrument visualised, good position and safely engaged)
4 Masterful insertion, ideal positioning	4 Efficient (minimal attempts, ideal position and safety)	4 Masterful (safe, ideal and efficient use of graspers, dissection tools)	4 Efficient (minimal attempts, ideal position and safety)
x Not applicable	x Not applicable	x Not applicable	x Not applicable

TISSUE HANDLING — Meaningful, precise and fluent hand movements

EXPOSURE — Manipulating small bowel:	PEDICLE CONTROL — Dissection around pedicle and division of blood vessels:	MOBILISATION — Anatomical dissection technique:	RESECTION/ANASTOMOSIS — Preparation of bowel for resection, division of mesentery
1 Traumatic grasping, uncontrolled and forceful movements, insufficient view	1 Dangerous (views, uncontrolled movements, energy device)	1 Wrong tissue plane, unable to correct quickly	1 Dangerous (forceful grasping, dangerous use of energy device)
2 Laborious and repeated attempts, ineffective patient positioning	2 Ineffective (several, hesitant cuts, jerky movements)	2 Repeatedly wrong tissue plane, able to correct	2 Ineffective dissection technique, safe tissue handling
3 Safe and effective handling of bowel, effective patient positioning	3 Safe dissection technique, slightly laborious	3 Rarely wrong plane, able to correct quickly	3 Safe dissection technique, slightly laborious
4 Safe and expeditious handling of bowel, effective patient positioning	4 Safe and expeditious dissection technique	4 Constantly stays in correct tissue plane	4 Safe and expeditious dissection technique
x Not applicable	x Not applicable	x Not applicable	x Not applicable

ERRORS — Completes the procedure without making any avoidable errors

EXPOSURE — This task was performed with:	PEDICLE CONTROL — This task was performed with:	MOBILISATION — This task was performed with:	RESECTION/ANASTOMOSIS — This task was performed with:
1 Bleeding, regular tissue avulsion, potential perforation of bowel	1 Uncontrolled bleeding, tissue avulsion, potential perforation	1 Uncontrolled bleeding, potential perforation, gross injuries to planes	1 Uncontrolled bleeding, tissue avulsion, potential perforation
2 Minor bleeding/occasional tissue avulsion, no perforation	2 Minor, controlled bleeding, occasional t. avulsion, no perforation	2 Minor, controlled bleeding, perforation, repeated injuries to planes	2 Minor, controlled bleeding, occasional tissue avulsion, no perforation
3 Minimal bleeding, no tissue avulsion, no perforation	3 Minimal bleeding, no perforation	3 Minimal bleeding, no perforation, planes mainly preserved	3 Minimal bleeding, no avulsion, no perforation
4 No bleeding, no tissue avulsion, no perforation	4 No bleeding, no avulsion, no perforation	4 No bleeding, no perforation, planes completely preserved	4 No bleeding, no avulsion, no perforation
x Not applicable	x Not applicable	x Not applicable	x Not applicable

END-PRODUCT — Reaches standards of quality for each task-area

EXPOSURE — Was the operating field sufficiently exposed?	PEDICLE CONTROL — How was the management of the vascular pedicle?	MOBILISATION — Was the large bowel safely mobilised and were the landmarks identified?	RESECTION/ANASTOMOSIS — How is the quality of the stump/anastomosis?
1 Small bowel not removed, vascular pedicle not exposed	1 Vascular pedicle not secured or grossly at wrong level	1 Inadequate mobilisation, landmarks not identified (ureter, duodenum)	1 Likely to compromise integrity of anastomosis
2 Small bowel loops partially obscure view for dissection, pedicle exposed	2 Secured, but divided to distally/proximally	2 Inadequate mobilisation, landmarks identified, but incorrect correct plane	2 Too short, mesentry inadequately dissected, safe anastomosis
3 Safe and adequate exposure, occasional fall back of small bowel	3 Vessels safely secured, correct level of division	3 Adequate mobilisation, landmarks correctly identified	3 Adequate resection level, safe anastomosis
4 Expeditious and safe exposure, no fall back of small bowel	4 Vessels efficiently secured, ideal level of division	4 Ideal mobilisation, landmarks clearly demonstrated	4 Ideal stump management, ideal anastomosis
x Not applicable	x Not applicable	x Not applicable	x Not applicable

Figure 3.3 L-CAT summative assessment form. Scores represent different levels of competency (novice, advanced beginner, competent, proficient).

Table 3.2 Impact of an average CAT score >2.7 (pass grade) on clinical outcomes

	HR/OR	95%CI	p-Value
Complications	0.19	0.06–0.65	0.008
Lymph node yield	6.85	3.45–10.25	<0.001
Distal resection margin	1.07	1.01–1.141	0.027

Source: From MacKenzie H et al. *Br J Surg* 2015;102(8):991–7.

importance of each item determined through a Delphi consensus process. The teaching assessment, the mini-STTAR (Structured Training Trainer Assessment Report), was developed using the items deemed the most important (20). This has 21 statements for the trainee to rate the degree to which he or she thought the item occurred during the teaching session, using a 5-point Likert scale. The mini-STTAR focuses on the training structure, the teaching behavior and attributes, and role modeling (Figure 3.4). The mini-STTAR became mandatory for the Lapco delegates to complete, and in this way Lapco trainers could be monitored for their teaching skills.

DEVELOPMENT OF THE LAPCO TRAIN THE TRAINER (LAPCO TT)

A course, run over 2 days and based on the 'Train the trainer for colonoscopy' was designed and developed under the guidance of Dr. Roland Valori and Dr. John Anderson. The purpose of this course was to train up the trainers within Lapco, to ensure that their teaching abilities met a gold standard. During day one, course delegates take part in small group discussions, role-play, and practice using a specific teaching structure. On day two, the course delegates actually train a trainee during an operation. They are observed and assessed during this session and provided with feedback to improve their surgical teaching. This course is described in greater detail in Chapter 5.

SUMMARY

The GAS, LCAT, and mini-STTAR assessment forms proved to be pivotal in analysing the success of Lapco. Through the combination of formative and summative assessment, all aspects of training were monitored. This set a new standard for surgical training programmes, which should become the norm. Given the academically rigorous way the forms were developed, they are generic enough to be applicable to other subspecialties of surgical or procedural teaching.

KEY POINTS

- Assessment can be divided into formative and summative assessment.
- The Lapco trainee was assessed using the GAS form and the LCAT form.
- The Lapco trainer was assessed using the mini-STTAR form.
- These assessment forms were developed and validated through rigorous qualitative research methods.
- A specific Lapco train the trainer course was developed to maintain a gold standard for the quality and teaching skill of Lapco trainers.

Table 3.3 Available clinical assessment tools rated by residents or peers

Instrument	Teaching area	Setting	Teachers (n)	Evaluators (n)	Evaluators
Beckman, Lee, Rohren, et al. (6)	MTEF	Internal medicine	I	10	3	P
Copeland and Hewson (7)	CTEI	All faculties	I, O	711	–	S, R, F
Donner-Banzhoff, Merle, Baum, et al. (8)	–	GP trainers	–	–	80	R
Guyatt, Nishikawa, Willan, et al. (9)	–	Internal medicine	I	41	–	R
Litzelman, Westmoreland, Skeff, et al. (10)	SFDP	Internal medicine, paediatrics	I, O	38	36	R
Ramsbottom-Lucier, Gillmore, Irby, et al. (11)	CTAF	Medicine	I, O	29	–	R
McLeod, James, and Abrahamowicz (12)	CTEQ	–	I, O	37(S), 15(R)	–	S, R
Risucci, Lutsky, Rosati, et al. (13)	–	Surgery	–	62	23	R
Tortolani, Risucci, and Rosati (14)	–	Surgery	–	62	23	R
Steiner, Franc-Law, Kelly, et al. (15)	ERS	Emergency room	ED	29	18	R
Williams, Litzelman, Babbott, et al. (16)	GRS	Internal medicine	I, O	96	98	R
Cassar (17)	STEEM	Learning environment in the operating theatre	I	?	25	R
Beckman and Mandrekar (18)	–	Internal medicine	I	60	1000	R
Cox and Swanson (19)	–	Surgery	I, O	16	753	R

Source: From Beckman TJ et al. *J Gen Intern Med* 2004;19(9):971–7.

Notes: MTEF, Mayo Teaching Evaluation Form; CTEI, Clinical Teaching Effectiveness Instrument; SFDP, Stanford Faculty Development Program; CTAF, Clinical Teaching Assessment Form; CTEQ, Clinical Tutor Evaluation Questionnaire; ERS, Emergency Rotation Scale; GRS, Global Rating Scale; STEEM, Surgical Theatre Educational Environment Measure.

Mini-STTAR: Trainee evaluation of trainer

Trainer:	Trainee:	Level:
Procedure:	Previous number of specific procedure:	
Total number of cases with this trainer:		Hospital:

This trainer:

	Strongly Disagree	Disagree	Neutral	Agree	Strongly Agree	N/A
Had a structured approach to the training	☐	☐	☐	☐	☐	☐
Agreed clear aims for this training episode	☐	☐	☐	☐	☐	☐
Adjusted training appropriately to level of trainee	☐	☐	☐	☐	☐	☐
Was encouraging	☐	☐	☐	☐	☐	☐
Was non-threatening	☐	☐	☐	☐	☐	☐
Was patient	☐	☐	☐	☐	☐	☐
Provided opportunities to ask questions	☐	☐	☐	☐	☐	☐
Communicated well	☐	☐	☐	☐	☐	☐
Took over procedure when appropriate	☐	☐	☐	☐	☐	☐
Provided too much verbal input (e.g. difficult to concentrate on procedure)	☐	☐	☐	☐	☐	☐
Provided too little verbal input (e.g. didn't always give guidance when required)	☐	☐	☐	☐	☐	☐
Provided too much physical input (e.g. didn't stretch trainee's abilities)	☐	☐	☐	☐	☐	☐
Provided too little physical input (e.g. trainee's abilities over-stretched)	☐	☐	☐	☐	☐	☐
Provided corrective critique during procedure (e.g. criticised but with explanation)	☐	☐	☐	☐	☐	☐
Provided positive critique during procedure (e.g. praised but with explanation)	☐	☐	☐	☐	☐	☐
Encouraged team awareness	☐	☐	☐	☐	☐	☐
Was patient-focused	☐	☐	☐	☐	☐	☐
Encouraged self-reflection on performance	☐	☐	☐	☐	☐	☐
Derived and agreed learning points from the case	☐	☐	☐	☐	☐	☐
Is a good role model with respect to their attitude and behaviour (for trainees in general)	☐	☐	☐	☐	☐	☐
Overall is an excellent teacher	☐	☐	☐	☐	☐	☐

Overall, please indicate the extent to which the training met your expectations: Below ☐   Met ☐   Exceeded ☐

Further comments about trainer and/or specific details about case:

	Extremely relevant	Relevant	Neutral	Irrelevant	Extremely irrelevant
Overall, how relevant did you find this form?	☐	☐	☐	☐	☐

How long did it take you to complete it?   ☐☐ Minutes

Figure 3.4 Mini-STTAR: Trainee evaluation of trainer. (From Wyles SM et al. *Surg Endosc.* 2016;30(3):993–1003. With permission.)

TAKE-HOME MESSAGE

Educational assessment tools can be invaluable in providing a '360°' evaluation of a training programme, and their inclusion should be considered in all future surgical or procedural training curricula.

REFERENCES

1. Swanwick T. *Understanding medical education, evidence, theory and practice*. Wiley-Blackwell, 2010 Oxford. Chapter 18: Formative assessment, Diana Wood. P 259–270.
2. Miskovic D, Ni M, Wyles SM, Tekkis P, Hanna GB. Learning curve and case selection in laparoscopic colorectal surgery: Systematic review and international multicenter analysis of 4852 cases. *Dis Colon Rectum* 2012;55(12):1300–10.
3. Miskovic D, Wyles SM, Ni M, Darzi AW, Hanna GB. Systematic review on mentoring and simulation in laparoscopic colorectal surgery. *Ann Surg* 2010;252(6):943–51.
4. MacKenzie H, Ni M, Miskovic D, Motson RW, Gudgeon M, Khan Z, Longman R, Coleman MG, Hanna GB. Clinical validity of consultant technical skills assessment in the English National Training Programme for Laparoscopic Colorectal Surgery. *Br J Surg* 2015;102(8):991–7.
5. Beckman TJ, Ghosh AK, Cook DA, Erwin PJ, Mandrekar JN. How reliable are assessments of clinical teaching? A review of the published instruments. *J Gen Intern Med* 2004;19(9):971–7.
6. Beckman TJ, Lee MC, Rohren CH, Pankratz VS. Evaluating an instrument for the peer review of inpatient teaching. *Med Teach* 2003;25(2):131–5.
7. Copeland HL, Hewson MG. Developing and testing an instrument to measure the effectiveness of clinical teaching in an academic medical center. *Acad Med* 2000;75(2):161–6.
8. Donner-Banzhoff N, Merle H, Baum E, Basler HD. Feedback for general practice trainers: Developing and testing a standardized instrument using the importance-quality-score method. *Med Educ* 2003;37(9):772–7.
9. Guyatt GH, Nishikawa J, Willan A, et al. A measurement process for evaluating clinical teachers in internal medicine. *CMAJ* 1993;149(8):1097–102.
10. Litzelman DK, Westmoreland GR, Skeff KM, Stratos GA. Student and resident evaluations of faculty—How dependable are they? *Acad Med* 1999;74(10 (S)):S25–7.
11. Ramsbottom-Lucier MT, Gillmore GM, Irby DM, Ramsey PG. Evaluation of clinical teaching by general internal medicine faculty in outpatient and inpatient settings. *Acad Med* 1994;69(2):152–4.
12. McLeod PJ, James CA, Abrahamowicz M. Clinical tutor evaluation: A 5-year study by students on an in-patient service and residents in an ambulatory care clinic. *Med Educ* 1993;27(1):48–54.
13. Risucci DA, Lutsky L, Rosati RJ, Tortolani AJ. Reliability and accuracy of resident evaluations of surgical faculty. *Eval Health Prof* 1992;15(3):313–24.
14. Tortolani AJ, Risucci DA, Rosati RJ. Resident evaluation of surgical faculty. *J Surg Res* 1991;51(3):186–91.
15. Steiner IP, Franc-Law J, Kelly KD, Rowe BH. Faculty evaluation by residents in an emergency medicine program: A new evaluation instrument. *Acad Emerg Med* 2000;7(9):1015–21.

16. Williams BC, Litzelman DK, Babbott SF, Lubitz RM, Hofer TP. Validation of a global measure of faculty's clinical teaching performance. *Acad Med* 2002;77(2):177–80.

17. Cassar K. Development of an instrument to measure the surgical operating theatre learning environment as perceived by basic surgical trainees. *Med Teach* 2004;26(3):260–4.

18. Beckman TJ, Mandrekar JN. The interpersonal, cognitive and efficiency domains of clinical teaching: Construct validity of a multi-dimensional scale. *Med Educ* 2005;39(12):1221–9.

19. Cox SS, Swanson MS. Identification of teaching excellence in operation room and clinic settings. *Am J Surg* 2002;183(3):251–5.

20. Wyles SM, Miskovic D, Ni Z, Darzi AW, Valori RM, Coleman MG, Hanna GB. Development and implementation of the Structured Training Trainer Assessment Report (STTAR) in the English National Training Programme for laparoscopic colorectal surgery. *Surg Endosc* 2016;30(3):993–1003.

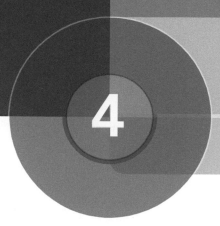

Outcomes of a national training programme

4

HUGH MACKENZIE AND GEORGE HANNA

LEARNING OBJECTIVES

- Understand and define the self-taught learning curve for laparoscopic colorectal surgery.
- Appreciate the influence of expert supervision on clinical outcomes.
- Determine the impact of case selection on clinical outcomes and training benefit.
- Identify the mechanisms within Lapco to ensure clinical safety and efficacy.
- Examine the efficacy, safety, and clinical impact of the Lapco programme.

INTRODUCTION

The first laparoscopic colorectal resection was performed in 1991; however, following this, the technique was very slow to disseminate (1). There were two primary reasons for this: oncological concerns including port-site metastases and the protracted learning curve associated with the technique. A number of large randomised controlled trials (RCTs) confirmed that both the short-term clinical and long-term oncological outcomes of laparoscopic colorectal surgery (LCS) were equivalent to open surgery (2–10). However, there remains the concern regarding the learning curve (11).

THE LEARNING CURVE

Initial attempts to describe the learning curve in LCS used single surgeon or institution data, split sample methodology, and relied on operative time (11–15). The estimated number of cases was thought to be between 15 and 30 cases; however, this appeared to be an underestimate. More robust methods were later used and aimed more specifically at different resection types, although still relied on single institution data. The learning curve for sigmoid colectomy was derived for operative time and intra- and post-operative complications using moving average and cumulative sum (CUSUM), respectively (16). From a two surgeons case series the learning curve was calculated to be between 70 and 110 cases (16). Tekkis et al. were the first to use case mix adjustment in their analysis of the learning curve of left- and right-sided colorectal resections, though their data was still reliant on a single institution experience (17). They used both efficiency (operative time and conversion) and quality (complications and re-admission) metrics and found that the learning curve of 62 cases for left-sided resections was slightly longer than that for right-sided resections, which was 55 cases (17). Miskovic et al. were the first to combine multi-institutional data to discern the learning curve, again using risk-adjusted CUSUM methodology (18). They collated raw data of 4852 cases from published series; for operative time the inflection point was at 96 cases compared to around 150 cases for complication and conversion (18). There is also now evidence that the introduction of LCS in England was actually associated with a learning curve for mortality. There was a significant reduction in 30-day and 90-day mortality after 20 cases in rectal and 3 cases in colonic surgery (19).

As supervision may negate the adverse clinical results, it significantly restricts estimation of the learning curve. Studies thus far have shown a reduction in operative time and found the curve to be 25 cases (20,21). No research as yet has robustly defined the learning curve for supervised surgeons across multiple institutions. In addition there is a paucity of evidence on the impact on clinical outcomes once the supervised surgeons enter independent practice. Once a surgeon is self-reliant there may be a concomitant increase in complications and mortality, signifying they are still on the learning curve. Research on this topic is extremely limited; there is currently one single surgeon case series that demonstrates no decline in performance once in independent practice (22). Comparison is made between 70 supervised cases and 73 independent cases – operative time, blood loss, intra- and post-operative complication, and conversion in the two groups (22).

EVIDENCE THAT MENTORED TRAINING IMPROVES CLINICAL SAFETY

Although intra-operative training is the cornerstone of mastering LCS, achieving competency at the patients' expense is unacceptable. The adverse outcomes in the early part of the learning curve seen in self-taught training should not occur; therefore, intra-operative training has evolved to expert supervision. Even within mentored training, patient safety must remain the priority. Lin et al. described the first study investigating whether mentored trainees achieved acceptable outcomes; in 1999 they integrated a structured training programme including animal laboratory sessions, preoperative tutorials and post-operative debriefing in conjunction with intra-operative supervision (23). Unfortunately they only compared measures of efficiency, length of stay, operating time, and conversion; however, these metrics remained at their baseline rate (23). There have been a number of further single centre studies that all demonstrate similar efficiency between the trainees and trainers in terms of operative time and conversion (24,25). The first study to compare quality metrics between trainees and consultants revealed increased operating time (decreased efficiency) but comparable safety; there was no significant difference in complication, blood loss, and re-operation between the two groups (26). Further studies have replicated the findings of equivalent quality between supervised trainees and their trainers, with comparable complications, blood loss, and lymph node harvest (27,28).

The only multi-institutional study was a systematic review performed to identify the impact of a mentor on training in LCS; a total of 751 mentored cases were combined and compared with 5313 expert cases and 695 non-mentored training cases (29). It found no difference between the mentored and expert cases in conversions, complications, anastomotic leak, and mortality. In contrast the conversion rate was significantly lower in the mentored cases than in the non-mentored; data were insufficient to compare the other outcomes. Overall the evidence suggests that well-supervised LCS training is safe for patients, although this conclusion must be tempered by the quality of the currently available data.

IMPACT OF CASE SELECTION

The complexity of the case has been shown to have significant impact on clinical outcomes when performing LCS (18). This impact is particularly seen during the learning curve. A previous study assessing the self-taught learning curve demonstrated that the factors that influenced patient outcome were body mass index (BMI), resection type, male gender, and also tumour characteristics (18). These findings are consistent with other studies assessing the impact of case complexity in LCS (30–32). The presence of an expert mentor may reduce the negative impact of inappropriate case selection during the learning curve, but to date there are no studies assessing this issue.

Selection of appropriate cases during the learning curve may be particularly important because it may not only influence patient outcome but also the educational benefit achieved. Task complexity has been shown to influence the rate of learning in other areas, but again there is no evidence for its impact on technical skills learning in surgery (33,34).

CLINICAL IMPACT OF LAPCO

Based on the rationale of the clinical safety of mentored training, Lapco used a model of one-on-one expert intra-operative training. The aim was to disseminate LCS throughout England while avoiding the steep early learning curve and therefore optimising patient safety. To ensure this was achieved certain safeguards were put into place.

CONTINUOUS AUDIT OF CLINICAL OUTCOMES

Prospectively collected clinical data were submitted during the period of supervised training; patient and case demographics and short-term clinical outcomes were completed on each GAS form (see Chapter 3). Furthermore, once the delegates were in independent practice they were required to submit the clinical outcomes of their laparoscopic cases for 12 months.

An initial analysis of the submitted clinical outcomes from Lapco training cases reveals good clinical outcomes. Analysis of approximately the first 800 cases revealed an in-hospital mortality rate of 0.5%, an overall complication rate was 14.3% including an anastomotic leak rate of 2.6%, a conversion rate of 5%, and a median length of stay of 5 days (35). These results are roughly equivalent to those published on expert performance, and they also compare favourably to those derived from Hospital Episode Statistics (HES) data for elective LCS resections in England over the last 10 years (19,29).

SUMMATIVE ASSESSMENT PROCESS PRIOR TO INDEPENDENT PRACTICE

Once both delegate and trainer agreed that they had reached competency, the delegate underwent a summative assessment, the sign-off process. They submitted two recordings of two independently performed cases. Two independent blinded assessors using the objective Competency Assessment Tool (CAT) then scored these videos (more detail in Chapter 3). The CAT form assesses 16 skill areas; these are scored on a scale from 1 (hazardous) to 4 (proficient) (36). Each case was awarded a pass (safe), insufficient evidence, or needs further training. This assessment was designed to ensure that a high operative standard was achieved before delegates embarked on independent practice.

The results from the mentored Lapco cases show that this model of training is safe for patients. To identify whether this model is able to train surgeons technically competent in LCS, the CAT results and clinical outcomes from the sign-off cases were analysed. There were some interesting relationships found; first the number of training cases performed correlated with the technical performance in the 'sign-off' process (37). However, there was no correlation with the total experience in LCS. These facts support the theory of deliberate practice—that it is not overall volume of experience that determines expertise but the amount of time spent on specific training (38). Second the technical performance in the 'sign-off' videos correlated with the patients' clinical outcomes.

When CUSUM curves were plotted for training volume and complications against average CAT score, there were three levels of technical performance demarcated by the changes in the curves at a score of 2.69 and 3.09 (Figure 4.1) (37). There were significant improvements in complication rate above a score of 2.69 and again at 3.09 (25% vs. 12.9% vs. 3.5%, $p = .049$ and $p = .031$). These improvements were also associated with a significant increase in the number of Lapco training cases (9 vs. 15 vs. 20, $p = .002$ and $p = .012$) (37). There were also improvements seen in the markers of oncological parameters seen with improved technical performance; there was a stepwise increase in lymph node number and length of distal resection margin (Table 4.1) (37).

The results from this study provide strong evidence that the mentored training was effective at improving technical performance. The improvement in tehnical skill resulted in improved clinical and oncological results for the patients.

DEVELOPMENT OF A CASE SELECTION TOOL TO ENHANCE SAFETY

To guide appropriate case selection, a risk prediction tool was developed. A logistic regression model was created to identify risk factors for conversion using the prospectively collected data on clinical outcomes (39). These included male gender, high BMI, high American Society of Anesthesiologists (ASA) grade, prior abdominal surgery, and resection type. The odds ratios were adjusted to create a simple risk prediction score out of 10 (Table 4.2).

There was a steady rise in conversion rate with the increase in risk prediction score; however, there was a significant increase above a score of 6 in complication rate (13% vs. 21.5% for scores ≤6 and >6, respectively, $p = .001$) and the dependency of the trainees on trainers' input (low GAS score [1–3]) (19.9% vs. 32.2% for scores ≤6 and >6, respectively, $p < .001$) (Figure 4.2) (39). Therefore, the cases were dichotomised by splitting the cases into low risk (risk prediction

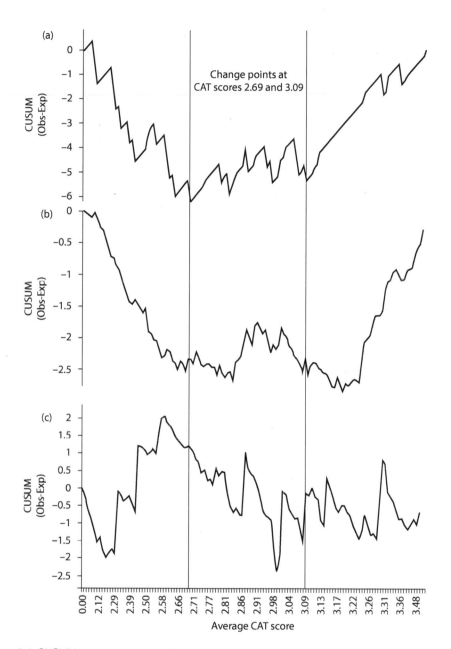

Figure 4.1 CUSUM curves demonstrating improved clinical outcomes and increased training volume associated with improved technical skill (average CAT score). (a) Post-operative complications, (b) Number of NTP training cases, (c) Total number of LCS cases. (From Mackenzie H et al. *Ann Surg* 2015;261(2):338–44.)

score ≤6) and high risk (risk prediction score >6). High-risk cases had a significantly longer hospital stay, higher mortality, more post-operative complications, and increased re-operation rates (Table 4.3) (39). In addition the high-risk cases had an adverse impact on training benefit; they increased dependency of trainees on their trainers' input for the majority of tasks (Table 4.4) (39).

Table 4.1 Improved clinical and oncological outcomes associated with higher CAT scores (superior technical proficiency) and concomitant increase in training volume

	CAT score <2.69	p-Value	CAT score 2.69–3.09	p-Value	CAT score >3.09
Number of cases	44		70		57
Complications	11 (25.0%)	.049	9 (12.9%)	.031	2 (3.5%)
Surgical complication	8 (18.2%)	.104	7 (10.0%)	.029	1 (1.8%)
Medical complication	3 (6.8%)	.160	2 (2.9%)	.667	1 (1.8%)
Lymph node count	13 (8–20)	.101	15 (11–22)	.001	20 (16–25)
Distal resection margin (cm) (left-sided cases only)	3.0 (1.0–4.5)	.036	3.0 (2.0–6.0)	.346	3.5 (3.0–5.0)
Number of NTP cases	9 (2–13)	.002	15 (6–23)	.012	20 (13–28)
Total number of laparoscopic colorectal cases	40 (27–60)	.261	37 (26–48)	.492	34 (27–54)

Source: From Mackenzie H et al. *Br J Surg* 2015;102(8):991–7.
Note: There was no link with overall LCS volume.

These results demonstrate that appropriate case selection is imperative not only to ensuring patient safety but also in optimising the training benefit. The risk prediction score can be used for selection of low-risk cases for training. The score is widely available using a newly developed software application for mobile phones and tablet computer devices. This will facilitate a practical calculation of the score in a day-to-day clinical environment, selection of cases, and discussion of increasing risks with patient.

Table 4.2 Significant risk factors for conversion in logistic regression model and their value in the risk prediction score

Risk factor	Categories	Odds ratio (OR)	p-Value	Points in risk prediction score
Gender	Female	Intercept	<.001	0
	Male	2.686		2
BMI	<25	Intercept	<.003	0
	25–27.5	1.289		1
	27.5–30	1.338		1
	>30	2.349		2
ASA grade	1/2	Intercept	.018	0
	3/4	1.642		1
Prior abdominal surgery	No	Intercept	<.001	0
	Yes	2.109		2
Resection	Right	Intercept	<.001	0
	Left	2.405		2
	High AR	2.223		2
	Low AR	2.827		3
	Other	3.607		3

Source: From Mackenzie H et al. *Ann Surg* 2015;261(2):338–44.

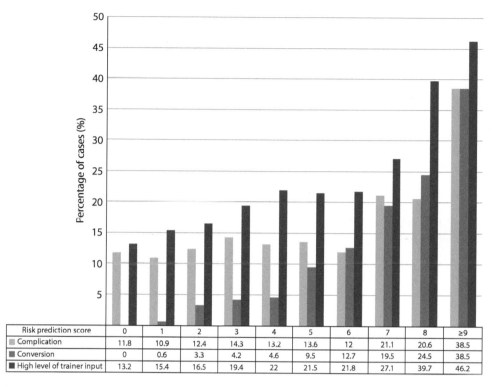

Risk prediction score	0	1	2	3	4	5	6	7	8	≥9
▒ Complication	11.8	10.9	12.4	14.3	13.2	13.6	12	21.1	20.6	38.5
▒ Conversion	0	0.6	3.3	4.2	4.6	9.5	12.7	19.5	24.5	38.5
▮ High level of trainer input	13.2	15.4	16.5	19.4	22	21.5	21.8	27.1	39.7	46.2

Figure 4.2 Histogram showing conversion, overall complication, and high level of trainer input rates according to the risk prediction score.

Table 4.3 Comparisons of the post-operative clinical outcomes in high- and low-risk cases

Clinical outcome	Low risk (≤6) (number of cases)	High risk (>6) (number of cases)	p-Value
Number of cases	2132	209	
Complications			
Overall	278 (13.0%)	45 (21.5%)	0.001
Overall surgical	240 (11.3%)	41 (19.6%)	<0.001
Leak	30 (1.4%)	9 (4.3%)	0.002
Bleeding	33 (1.5%)	4 (1.9%)	0.159
Abdominal collection	28 (1.3%)	4 (1.9%)	0.475
Ileus	88 (4.1%)	12 (5.7%)	0.271
Obstruction	11 (0.5%)	4 (1.9%)	0.016
Wound infection	63 (3.0%)	15 (7.2%)	0.001
Overall medical	54 (2.4%)	13 (6.2%)	0.001
Chest sepsis	25 (1.2%)	7 (3.3%)	0.010
Re-operation	62 (2.9%)	19 (9.1%)	<0.001
Re-admission	45 (2.1%)	4 (1.9%)	0.850
Mean hospital stay	6.2 days	10.0 days	<0.001
Mortality	10 (0.5%)	6 (2.9%)	<0.001

Source: From Mackenzie H et al. *Ann Surg* 2015;261(2):338–44.

Table 4.4 Comparison of GAS scores in high- and low-risk cases

GAS form item	Mean GAS score, low risk (≤6)	Mean GAS score, high risk (>6)	Difference (Δ)	p-Value
High level of trainer input	19.9%	32.2%	12.3%	<0.001
Theatre setup	4.78	4.69	0.09 (1.9%)	0.149
Patient positioning	4.82	4.73	0.09 (1.9%)	0.132
Access technique	4.75	4.62	0.13 (2.7%)	0.162
Exposure	4.49	4.19	0.30 (6.7%)	0.011
Dissection of pedicle	4.17	3.85	0.32 (7.7%)	0.025
Dissection of mesentery	4.20	3.90	0.30 (7.1%)	0.008
Identification of anatomy	4.32	3.93	0.39 (9.0%)	0.001
Mobilisation of flexure	3.87	3.27	0.60 (15.5%)	<0.001
Dissection of mesorectum	3.52	3.06	0.46 (13.1%)	0.001
Resection of bowel	4.29	4.02	0.27 (6.3%)	0.044
Retrieval of specimen	4.46	4.25	0.21 (4.7%)	0.145
Anastomosis	4.42	4.17	0.25 (5.7%)	0.040
Overall	4.15	3.82	0.33 (8.0%)	<0.001

Source: From Mackenzie H et al. *Ann Surg* 2015;261(2):338–44.

NATIONAL INCREASE IN LCS

In 2006 National Institute for Health and Care Excellence (NICE) guidance stated that all suitable patients should be offered a laparoscopic resection for colorectal cancer. However, at that time it was estimated that only 5% of surgeons were trained in LCS (35). Therefore, the guidance was waived and Lapco instigated to make this possible; it aimed to have a LCS-trained surgeon in each multidisciplinary team throughout the country. By the end of the programme it had achieved this aim, and 40% of elective colorectal resections were performed laparoscopically (Figure 4.3).

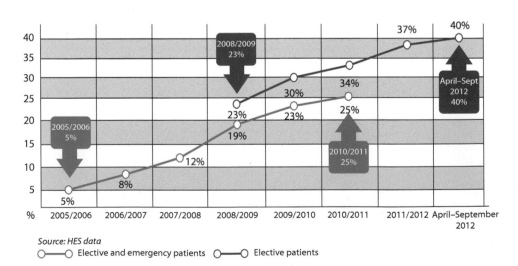

Source: HES data

○——○ Elective and emergency patients   ○——○ Elective patients

Figure 4.3 HES data demonstrating an increasing volume of LCS resections in England.

KEY POINTS

- The self-taught learning curve for laparoscopic colorectal surgery is long and is associated with adverse patient outcomes.
- Adverse clinical outcomes in the learning curve can be negated by expert supervision.
- Appropriate case selection is important to optimise patient outcomes and maximise training benefit.
- Supervised training in Lapco was safe, improved technical proficiency, and in turn improved post-operative results.
- Since the inception of Lapco there has been an increase in the rate of laparoscopic colorectal surgery to world leading levels.

TAKE-HOME MESSAGE

Expert supervised training negates the adverse outcomes seen in self-taught learning and improves technical proficiency and post-operative results. This should be the standard model for the safe introduction and dissemination of new surgical procedures.

REFERENCES

1. Jacobs M, Verdeja JC, Goldstein HS. Minimally invasive colon resection (laparoscopic colectomy). *Surg Laparosc Endosc* 1991;1(3):144–50.
2. Guillou PJ, Quirke P, Thorpe H et al. Short-term endpoints of conventional versus laparoscopic-assisted surgery in patients with colorectal cancer (MRC CLASICC trial): Multicentre, randomised controlled trial. *Lancet* 2005;365(9472):1718–26.
3. Jayne DG, Thorpe HC, Copeland J et al. Five-year follow-up of the Medical Research Council CLASICC trial of laparoscopically assisted versus open surgery for colorectal cancer. *Br J Surg* 2010;97(11):1638–45.
4. Green BL, Marshall HC, Collinson F et al. Long-term follow-up of the Medical Research Council CLASICC trial of conventional versus laparoscopically assisted resection in colorectal cancer. *Br J Surg* 2013;100(1):75–82.
5. Group COOSTS. A comparison of laparoscopically assisted and open colectomy for colon cancer. *N Engl J Med* 2004;350(20):2050–9.
6. Fleshman J, Sargent DJ, Green E et al. Laparoscopic colectomy for cancer is not inferior to open surgery based on 5-year data from the COST Study Group trial. *Ann Surg* 2007;246(4):655–62; discussion 62–4.
7. Veldkamp R, Kuhry E, Hop WC et al. Laparoscopic surgery versus open surgery for colon cancer: Short-term outcomes of a randomised trial. *Lancet Oncol* 2005;6(7):477–84.
8. Lacy AM, Garcia-Valdecasas JC, Delgado S et al. Laparoscopy-assisted colectomy versus open colectomy for treatment of non-metastatic colon cancer: A randomised trial. *Lancet* 2002;359(9325):2224–9.
9. Lacy AM, Delgado S, Castells A et al. The long-term results of a randomized clinical trial of laparoscopy-assisted versus open surgery for colon cancer. *Ann Surg* 2008;248(1):1–7.

10. Buunen M, Veldkamp R, Hop WC et al. Survival after laparoscopic surgery versus open surgery for colon cancer: Long-term outcome of a randomised clinical trial. *Lancet Oncol* 2009;10(1):44–52.

11. Reissman P, Cohen S, Weiss EG et al. Laparoscopic colorectal surgery: Ascending the learning curve. *World J Surg* 1996;20(3):277–81; discussion 82.

12. Simons AJ, Anthone GJ, Ortega AE et al. Laparoscopic-assisted colectomy learning curve. *Dis Colon Rectum* 1995;38(6):600–3.

13. Bennett CL, Stryker SJ, Ferreira MR et al. The learning curve for laparoscopic colorectal surgery. Preliminary results from a prospective analysis of 1194 laparoscopic-assisted colectomies. *Arch Surg* 1997;132(1):41–4; discussion 5.

14. Schlachta CM, Mamazza J, Seshadri PA et al. Defining a learning curve for laparoscopic colorectal resections. *Dis Colon Rectum* 2001;44(2):217–22.

15. Kang JC, Jao SW, Chung MH et al. The learning curve for hand-assisted laparoscopic colectomy: A single surgeon's experience. *Surg Endosc* 2007;21(2):234–7.

16. Dincler S, Koller MT, Steurer J et al. Multidimensional analysis of learning curves in laparoscopic sigmoid resection: Eight-year results. *Dis Colon Rectum* 2003;46(10):1371–8; discussion 8–9.

17. Tekkis PP, Senagore AJ, Delaney CP et al. Evaluation of the learning curve in laparoscopic colorectal surgery: Comparison of right-sided and left-sided resections. *Ann Surg* 2005;242(1):83–91.

18. Miskovic D, Ni M, Wyles SM et al. Learning curve and case selection in laparoscopic colorectal surgery: Systematic review and international multicenter analysis of 4852 cases. *Dis Colon Rectum* 2012;55(12):1300–10.

19. Mackenzie H, Markar SR, Askari A et al. National proficiency-gain curves for minimally invasive gastrointestinal cancer surgery. *Br J Surg* 2016;103(1):88–96.

20. Maeda T, Tan KY, Konishi F et al. Accelerated learning curve for colorectal resection, open versus laparoscopic approach, can be attained with expert supervision. *Surg Endosc* 2010;24(11):2850–4.

21. Chen G, Liu Z, Han P et al. The learning curve for the laparoscopic approach for colorectal cancer: A single institution's experience. *J Laparoendosc Adv Surg Tech A* 2013;23(1):17–21.

22. Kim JH, Lee IK, Kang WK et al. Initial experience of a surgical fellow in laparoscopic colorectal cancer surgery under training protocol and supervision: Comparison of short-term results for 70 early cases (under supervision) and 73 late cases (without supervision). *Surg Endosc* 2013;27(8):2900–6.

23. Lin E, Szomstein S, Addasi T et al. Model for teaching laparoscopic colectomy to surgical residents. *Am J Surg* 2003;186(1):45–8.

24. Maeda T, Tan KY, Konishi F et al. Trainee surgeons do not cause more conversions in laparoscopic colorectal surgery if they are well supervised. *World J Surg* 2009;33(11):2439–43.

25. Chikkappa MG, Jagger S, Griffith JP et al. In-house colorectal laparoscopic preceptorship: A model for changing a unit's practice safely and efficiently. *Int J Colorectal Dis* 2009;24(7):771–6.

26. Mehall JR, Shroff S, Fassler SA et al. Comparing results of residents and attending surgeons to determine whether laparoscopic colectomy is safe. *Am J Surg* 2005;189(6):738–41.

27. Costantino F, Mutter D, D'agostino J et al. Mentored trainees obtain comparable operative results to experts in complex laparoscopic colorectal surgery. *Int J Colorectal Dis* 2012;27(1):65–9.

28. Li JC, Mak TW, Hon SS et al. Laparoscopic colorectal fellowship training programme: A 6-year experience in a university colorectal unit. *Int J Colorectal Dis* 2013;28(6):823–8.

29. Miskovic D, Wyles SM, Ni M et al. Systematic review on mentoring and simulation in laparoscopic colorectal surgery. *Ann Surg* 2010;252(6):943–51.

30. Schlachta CM, Mamazza J, Seshadri PA et al. Predicting conversion to open surgery in laparoscopic colorectal resections. A simple clinical model. *Surg Endosc* 2000;14(12):1114–7.

31. Schwandner O, Schiedeck TH, Bruch H. The role of conversion in laparoscopic colorectal surgery: Do predictive factors exist? *Surg Endosc* 1999;13(2):151–6.

32. Tekkis PP, Senagore AJ, Delaney CP. Conversion rates in laparoscopic colorectal surgery: A predictive model with 1253 patients. *Surg Endosc* 2005;19(1):47–54.

33. Nembhard D. The effects of task complexity and experience on learning and forgetting: A field study. *Hum Factors* 2000;42(2):272–86.

34. Nembhard D, Osothsilp N. Task complexity effects on between-individual learning/forgetting variability. *Int J Ind Ergon* 2002;29(5):297–306.

35. Coleman MG, Hanna GB, Kennedy R et al. The national training programme for laparoscopic colorectal surgery in England: A new training paradigm. *Colorectal Dis* 2011;13(6):614–6.

36. Miskovic D, Ni M, Wyles SM et al. Is competency assessment at the specialist level achievable? A study for the national training programme in laparoscopic colorectal surgery in England. *Ann Surg* 2013;257(3):476–82.

37. Mackenzie H, Ni M, Miskovic D et al. Clinical validity of consultant technical skills assessment in the English national training programme for laparoscopic colorectal surgery. *Br J Surg* 2015;102(8):991–7.

38. Dreyfus H, Dreyfus S. Expertise in real world contexts. *Organ Stud* 2005;26(5):779–92.

39. Mackenzie H, Miskovic D, Ni M et al. Risk prediction score in laparoscopic colorectal surgery training: Experience from the English National Training Program. *Ann Surg* 2015;261(2):338–44.

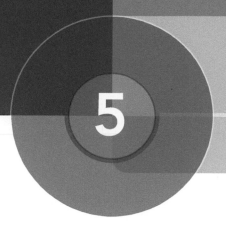

Training the trainer in minimal access surgery

5

NADER FRANCIS AND JOHN GRIFFITH

LEARNING OBJECTIVES

- Describe how a surgeon can become a teacher.
- Understand a training framework of teaching technical skills and other factors including psychological, leadership, and human factors that underpin a successful trainer in minimal access surgery (MAS).
- Explore the concept of conscious competence as a surgeon and a trainer and how this can be applied in teaching advanced laparoscopic skills with lessons learned from the Laparoscopic Colorectal National Training Programme Training the Trainer (LAPCO TT) curriculum that can be applied to other surgical specialities.

INTRODUCTION

Surgery used to be a cognitive apprenticeship that comprised the gradual acquisition of knowledge, skills, and behaviours under the supervision of an expert trainer. Never before has the effectiveness of surgery and safety been more closely scrutinised by the public (1,2). It is no longer acceptable for trainee surgeons to learn unsupervised; confirmation of competence is a vital prerequisite to independent performance.

Enhancing the quality of surgical training to achieve competency has received much more attention recently, particularly within minimal access surgery (MAS), due to its known prolonged long performance-gain curve and the shortening of training time available in this technically challenging field (3–6).

MAS, however, affords the best opportunity for both direct and retrospective observation of surgical performance compared to traditional open surgery. It also provides an accurate means to objectively scrutinise the contribution of a trainer to the performance of a surgical procedure.

Optimum surgical performance requires a combination of knowledge, technical skills, and behaviour (7). For index procedures and parts of procedures, within the subspecialty of MAS, the performance of trainees can be observed by using a structured predetermined assessment format to assess the acquisition of skills (8). Beyond the process of learning the technical skills themselves are the less tangible elements of the enhancement of knowledge and behaviours essential to the development of a surgeon. Surgical training has changed from a craft apprenticeship, where skills were acquired gradually by observation and practice, to a more structured competency-based approach (9–11).

This chapter explores the process of becoming a trainer in MAS in terms of understanding the technical and non-technical skills that underpin optimum teaching, the best structure for training, and the most efficient way to improve teaching in MAS.

WHAT MAKES 'A GREAT TRAINER'?

Not all surgeons make good trainers. Some great surgeons are poor performers when it comes to the transference of their own knowledge, skills, and behaviour to junior colleagues.

In recent years, there has been an increased awareness and better understanding of the importance of communication, teamwork, and the effect of 'non-technical' skills on clinical outcome, as opposed to simply learning the practical skills (12–14). For an adult to learn a practical skill effectively, the trainer needs to be aware of the trainee's needs. This involves the amount of new information that is imparted to ensure that the trainee maintains motivation, continues to progress, and does not suffer from cognitive overload, while remaining mindful that the training episode does not affect patient safety.

Nevertheless, within MAS a high level of technical skill is required for optimum surgical performance. Often in MAS, a long performance-gain curve prohibits a self-taught approach, with evidence that supervised teaching promotes a better patient outcome (15). It is well known that, in general, there is a lack of uniformity in operative approach among surgeons and surgical faculty. Although there are essential steps in the performance of MAS, some surgeons execute certain tasks in different ways, often due to being self-taught. Little is known about whether there is a consensus about the 'right' way to structure the training of MAS. The provision of high-quality teaching is imperative to maximise the chance of trainees acquiring proficiency in new skills and procedures, and different trainers have been shown to impact on trainees' performance, even in basic skills.

With prior experience in teaching and education in MAS, we can summarise that the basic general characteristics of a good trainer can include competency in the task, enthusiasm, confidence, clear and well-organised presentation of instructional material, and skill in interaction with students/residents individually or in group settings. It is also important to involve the trainee in the teaching process, have a humanistic or empathic orientation, have a good knowledge of the subject, and most importantly, be learner-focused, inspiring, and a role model.

THE TRAINING THE TRAINER CURRICULUM

Teaching methods have been evaluated within some specialties of medicine, but none of these have been designed for use with peers or senior surgical trainees teaching (16). In endoscopy, however, a highly regarded Training the Colonoscopy Trainers (TCT) was developed by the UK National Joint Advisory Group for Gastrointestinal Endoscopy (JAG) to provide a training framework for teaching endoscopy (17). In MAS, an adapted model was developed based on the TCT and modified to be applied and validated in laparoscopic colorectal surgery for over 70 national trainers within the Lapco National Training programme in England (18).

This course was set out to explore the means whereby a more structured, reflective, and cognitive approach to training is likely to improve the training process. Although the course is bespoke to laparoscopic colorectal surgery, it is highly applicable to other specialties in MAS. The basis for Lapco TT is to provide a framework of training in order to maximise every opportunity from before, during, and after training occurs. This starts with preoperative preparation, which is termed 'Set', the process that occurs during the MAS procedure itself termed 'Dialogue', and the period after the procedure termed 'Closure'.

PREOPERATIVE PREPARATION: THE 'SET'

PHYSICAL SET

The physical set in laparoscopy is defined here as the layout of the operating room (OR) and the function of all the manpower and equipment therein. Although no two ORs are alike, the position and function of all its human and non-human resources are vital to the safe, effective, and efficient performance of MAS. Moreover, MAS is arguably more dependent on such factors than open surgery. An effective trainer needs to be highly skilled to make the OR environment more conducive to training. In MAS, trainees are often more drawn into the technical details of the procedure itself, without checking the optimum physical set and ergonomics and how these factors can be crucial to their performance and learning.

The factors that are keys to the physical set are as follows:

- Laparoscopic stack placement
- Appropriate settings for gas insufflation, energy devices, and camera/light controls and all ergonomics of laparoscopic instruments
- Patient and table positioning
- Personnel placement in the OR relative to the patient, each other, and the equipment

By leading the physical set, the trainer not only demonstrates to and involves the trainee in optimal OR setup, but also makes sure the procedure runs smoothly and acts as a good role model for the whole team prior to the start of the procedure. Modern ORs often have integrated equipment that can facilitate the physical set. The position of the trainer in the OR is also worthy of consideration. The level, confidence, and expectations of the trainer and trainee will determine whether the trainer is scrubbed or unscrubbed in the OR.

ALIGNMENT OF AGENDAS

This is the process whereby trainer and trainee integrate a common understanding for a planned training episode. The training episode might include a placement or prolonged period, an operating list, or an individual case. Both trainer and trainee need to have a constructive dialogue about the trainee's prior experience, capabilities, confidence, and expectations. This discussion can be used to form an agreement as to how the subsequent training episode will proceed. It should include consideration by the trainer and trainee as to what the trainee can reasonably expect to be able to do, taking into account prior experience. The objective of alignment of agendas is to obtain a clear common understanding, and the benefit is that both avoid disappointment when undisclosed expectations are not achieved.

Alignment of agendas includes the following:

- Review trainee's prior experience.
- Review trainee's most recent learning objective and take-home message from the previous training episode.
- Agree to a training plan for the placement, operating list, or individual case.
- Set ground rules.

Prior to the start of a training episode it is vital that the trainer and trainee have a clear understanding of the language of training. This is not only necessary for patient safety, but vital so that there is unequivocal communication between the trainee and trainer. Simple commands such as 'stop' need prior discussion to avoid disappointment in the trainee, who might misunderstand that the training opportunity is over. In MAS, directions from the trainer to the trainee with regard to MAS instrument path and directions need prior explanation and agreement to avoid confusion. Examples include as discussed the word 'Stop' and whether directional commands such as up, down, left, and right refer to hand movements or screen movements. In MAS there is potential for confusion due to the fulcrum effect of the instruments, and to avoid confusion instructions should be referred to the monitor view, rather than focusing on hand movements. The setting of ground rules can also include the camera assistant.

It is crucial in training to adhere to the process of the preparation or 'Set' prior to commencing the actual coaching. Although this process can take a long time at the initial phase between trainers and their new trainees, it can take only a few minutes especially between trainers and trainees who are familiar with each other. Alignment of agendas should take place before each case to agree on clear mutual objectives, no matter how long the trainer and trainee have been working together.

THE PROCEDURE: THE 'DIALOGUE'

The 'Dialogue' is the process of clinical coaching in the OR that occurs during a procedure. It should only occur after all aspects of the 'Set' are complete. The dialogue involves whether the trainer is scrubbed or not, where the trainer is positioned, and whether the trainer plays a physical role in the procedure or not. Clear, concise, common language is required to avoid confusion.

Effective clinical coaching in advanced laparoscopic surgery requires three important key teaching skills:

1. Conscious competence as a trainer
2. Performance-enhancing instruction
3. A structured approach to avoid taking over

CONSCIOUS COMPETENCE

Competence (Figure 5.1) is defined as performing the task safely and within a reasonable time frame (19). The concept of conscious competence has been noted in medical education where learners move from conscious competence, where they can perform a technique but have to think about it, to unconscious competence where they have acquired mastery of the technique

Unconscious incompetence UI	Conscious incompetence CI
Junior trainee Experienced surgeon making an error such as inadvertent ureteric injury	More experienced trainee or fellow performing difficult task Experienced surgeon asking for help from a different speciality
Unconscious competence UC	Conscious competence CC
Experienced surgeon Perform tasks automatically without thinking	Consciously able to deconstruct the procedure to trainee The trainer needs to be in this box to be a good trainer

Figure 5.1 Stages of learning.

and no longer have to think about it (20). However, it is worth saying here that trainees without adequate insight might have 'unconscious incompetence', a lack of awareness that they are unable to perform a procedure satisfactorily. That insight should be provided by the trainer. Through a process of training by the acquisition and application of skills and knowledge, the trainees become 'consciously competent'; they are aware that they can perform the procedure and each of the key steps therein. As they progress further they can develop the skill to perform the procedure, which is to say, they can perform the procedure without deconstruction – 'unconscious competence'. All competent surgeons will have a limit to their competency and will be conscious of that limit – the boundary where they go from competence to incompetence. In most cases they have the insight and situational awareness to know the limit and seek help. A good example would be a situation that requires a different surgical expertise.

CONSCIOUS COMPETENCE AS A TRAINER

The same model of conscious competence can be applied to the ability of a trainer. Most trainers are accomplished surgical experts who can perform MAS procedures without thought; they are 'unconsciously competent' for most cases they perform. This is not a useful realm to be in as a trainer. A good trainer is one who can deconstruct each task and train by explanation and demonstration, in other words be a 'consciously competent trainer'. The more a trainer remains consciously competent, the greater the chances trainees have to acquire skills. Of course, as a trainee progresses to conscious competence himself or herself, the trainer, though still present, no longer needs to explain and deconstruct. Equally if a trainee cannot perform a part of a procedure, the trainer may not be able to proceed with the training episode without taking over temporarily: this can be defined as conscious incompetence as a trainer. Hopefully by deconstruction and/or taking over, conscious competence as a trainer can be restored such that control can be handed back to the trainee to allow the training to proceed. We explore taking over in theatre in the next section.

PERFORMANCE-ENHANCING INSTRUCTION

This section explores examples of the effects of different levels of verbal instruction from a trainer to a trainee during a surgical procedure. During the process of training, different types of verbal instruction are used. It is necessary for trainers to have a good understanding of the effects of differing instruction on the trainee's ability. This can be divided into five levels (Figure 5.2). Level 1 is where no comment or instruction is provided by the trainer to the trainee. Although this might be completely appropriate where a trainee is competent to proceed, level 1 instruction will be unlikely to obtain any learning benefit. Level 2 is negative criticism (e.g. 'that's rubbish!' or 'that's not how I do it'). Other than in a light-hearted context, level 2 is likely to be detrimental to both morale and performance and can impact negatively on the trainee's confidence. Although, it is understandable that in certain occasions, criticism may be required, this needs to be carried out in a constructive way, rather than in a patronising and insulting manner. Level 3 is positive but non-specific (e.g. 'that's great, well done!' or 'you're the best!'). This level might help morale but is also unlikely to result in an improvement, as it lacks clarity on what exactly the trainee has achieved well. Level 4 is instruction that is directive but not specific or focused, which entails providing some instructions but perhaps vague and non-specific (e.g. 'up a bit, down a bit, left, right'). Finally, level 5 is directive, specific, focused, and achieved by asking the trainee for feedback: 'what do you need to know?' or 'are you happy with my instructions?' By using level 5 instruction, the coaching would be trainee focused, and the performance of the trainee is more likely to be optimal.

STRATEGY TO AVOID TAKING OVER

One of the main challenges in surgical training is to avoid a situation where the trainer takes over the procedure from the trainee, thereby depriving the latter of a valuable training opportunity. This section explores the moment where the performance of an operation is interrupted by the trainer whose temptation is to take over. The aim of this session is to promote the adoption of a framework whereby this might be avoided.

Lack of progress during surgical training usually occurs when a trainee cannot proceed safely. This might be identified by either the trainer or trainee. The trainee might be aware of the reasons for inability to proceed or the trainer might halt the procedure. In MAS this is most often due to anatomical uncertainty, an inadequate view, or a lack of ability to interpret the anatomy from the screen. In many instances the trainer will take over, often for the remainder of the procedure, thus losing a valuable training opportunity. If the reason for failure to progress can be identified and resolved without taking over, the training episode can proceed.

Level	Faculty comments
Level 1	No comment
Level 2	Critic without explanation, negative non-specific (That was rubbish!)
Level 3	No directions – positive, non-specific (Well done!)
Level 4	Some directions, but not specific (bit more left or right)
Level 5	Directive, specific, and focused by asking the trainee of what they want to know

Figure 5.2 Levels of instructions during coaching.

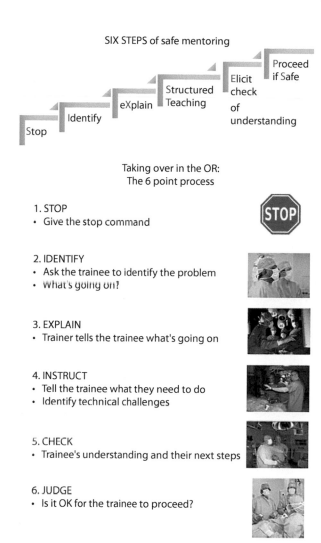

Figure 5.3 Six-point process to avoid taking over in operating room.

The first step (see Figure 5.3) is to stop the procedure. Stopping or rather pausing the procedure should be agreed on during the 'Set' phase as an opportunity to explain the causes of the lack of progress. Trainees need to understand that when the trainer is asking them to stop it is not offending them, but rather to discuss progress or the lack of it. The second step is to ask the trainee to identify the reason that this part of the procedure is not going as planned. The third step is for the trainer to explain the reason for the problem if the trainee failed to identify the reason(s) and develop a matched understanding. The fourth is for the trainer to instruct the trainee how to proceed in such a way as to rectify the problem. The fifth is for the trainee to explain how they plan to proceed and for the trainer to check that their explanation in steps three and four has been understood. Finally in step 6 the trainee recommences the procedure and the trainer judges the trainee's capability to proceed. It might be necessary to repeat the six-point plan more than once if progress remains hesitant.

By using this six-point plan accompanied by good preparation in the 'Set', the trainer is less likely to take over and the trainee more likely to benefit from the training episode.

POST-OPERATIVE: THE 'CLOSURE' OR FEEDBACK

Feedback is a vital part of training (21). The main priorities are to reflect on the procedure just completed and develop learning objectives that are likely to result in improvements in future performance.

For psycho-motor skills acquisition, feedback is the foundation of effective training and is considered one of the most important variables, aside from practice (21).

There are two types of feedback (22):

- Concurrent feedback: which is referred to the feedback received during the performance and is covered in the previous section (performance-enhancing instructions).
- Terminal feedback, which is referred to the feedback provided after the completion of the task. The potential use of terminal feedback as a learning tool in simulation-based surgical training is significant and results in better learning when compared to concurrent feedback. The downfall of terminal feedback in clinical settings is that errors cannot be allowed to progress due to patient safety.

FEEDBACK MODEL IN LAPCO TT

There are a number of ways to provide feedback, but we examine here the model that was adopted for the LAPCO TT Programme. Feedback can take place after a single procedure, operating list, or training placement. Often service pressures result in feedback being overlooked, but it is a vital opportunity to summarise and crystallise a training episode in such a way that is likely to result in performance improvement.

The means whereby this can be achieved is to start by shared reflection between the trainer and trainee to gain an understanding of how the procedure went. Usually this takes the form of a question from trainer to trainee: 'how do you think that went?' This allows the trainee to reflect on his or her performance and allows the trainer to see whether the trainee's perspective matches his or her own. This is often followed by an exploration of the trainer's perspective: 'yes, I agree that went well'. Then, the trainer asks the trainee to reflect on the areas of difficulty, analyse and identify the reasons for them, come up with learning objectives, and develop a take-home message. Ideally there should be only one main point that the trainee needs to focus on for the next case.

For feedback to be effective there are several considerations to take into account:

- The physical environment where feedback takes place. Ideally this should be quiet and confidential, so the trainer and trainee can engage in a frank discussion without being overheard.
- The feedback session should be a two-way process, whereby both the trainer and trainee discuss the training episode openly. The session should start with a question from the trainer: for example, 'how do you think that went?' This allows the trainer and trainee to align agendas and gain a common understanding.

- Video feedback may be used to analyse the performance. A critical aspect in the video feedback involves directing the attention of the trainee to specific aspects of the performance that require modification or correction to improve focus.
- Feedback should have the objective of delivering a simple understandable message or learning objective for the trainee to improve subsequent performance.

OTHER TRAINING ISSUES IN MAS

DUAL TASK INTERFERENCE

All humans have a variable but limited capacity to perform manual tasks (23). The more familiar the task and the more practiced the individual, the better is the ability to maintain performance in the presence of additional sensory stimuli. It is expected, therefore, that novices to MAS will be more susceptible to reduced performance in the presence of interference. The presence of interference that is not in itself required in the OR is likely to reduce the performance of the trainee. Examples of interference are most often auditory, including music, conversation, radio pagers, and telephones, or visual including movement of people or objects in the field of vision of the trainee, or even in front of the laparoscopic television monitor. The trainer will most often have a higher level of authority and situational awareness than the trainee, and a good trainer will effectively control the OR to reduce interference with the trainee.

ASSESSMENT AND ACCREDITATION

There are two types of assessment tools, which were both used in the LAPCO programme: formative and summative tools.

FORMATIVE ASSESSMENT

Within LAPCO, a bespoke assessment tool was created to monitor progression and proficiency gain in laparoscopic colorectal surgery – the Global Assessment Scale (GAS) (24). This is a formative tool, which divides laparoscopic colorectal operations into twelve steps, which are rated by both the trainee and the trainer immediately after the case, using an objective scoring scale. The scale differs from many assessment tools in that it uses statements describing the degree of independence with which the step was performed by the trainee, rather than more subjective judgmental descriptors of how well it was performed such as 'good' or 'poor performance'. The form was used after every training case to structure feedback, and it allows areas of weakness and strength to be identified and a trainee's progress to be tracked. The GAS tool has since been adopted by surgical trainees in the United Kingdom outside the LAPCO programme, in particular those undertaking fellowship and residency training in laparoscopic colorectal surgery (25).

SUMMATIVE ASSESSMENT

A summative assessment tool was developed for sign-off of surgeons from the LAPCO programme. Trainees were required to submit two DVDs showing a right- and a left-sided colon resection. The Laparoscopic Competency Assessment Tool (L-CAT) was designed to provide a framework of objective criteria to facilitate objective evaluation of the DVD by blinded expert assessors (26). Construct validity at the specialist level has been demonstrated, with the tool capable of differentiating between experts and trainees, and also between those trainees who the experts felt should pass the assessment versus those who did not pass.

HUMAN FACTORS AND TRAINING

Within the context of training the trainer, 'Human factors' is the process of learning where we try to understand and improve the roles of individuals and teams involved in health care with the objective of trying to reduce the incidence of harmful incidents. The contributions of surgical trainers as individuals and the teams they work in are complex and multifactorial. All individuals have their own innate personalities, developed at an early age. These personalities have a key impact on the way a team works. Day-to-day behaviour might be different from how individuals like to behave naturally and is influenced by a number of factors. Selecting and maintaining appropriate behaviours are essential to the effective discharge of individual and collective professional responsibilities. Key to the function of a team is effective leadership in MAS and equally effective followership.

The human factors that influence the functional effectiveness of a team are as follows (14):

- Communication: Managing professional-to-professional communication in a safety-critical environment
- Situation awareness: The often flawed process of understanding what is 'going on'
- Risk management: How we can discharge our responsibility to reduce risk and harm
- Personality: Personality and its impact on performance and team working
- Human factors feedback: Regulating those behaviours as an everyday process
- Managing overload and using the tools: Staying in control in stressful situations or extremely risky environments and making briefings, debriefings, handovers, and checklists work effectively
- Leading, following, and motivating: Our professional responsibilities to everyone else in the team

SUMMARY

Training in MAS presents unique challenges compared to training in open surgery: loss of tactile sense, lack of 3D visuo-spatial awareness, greater reliance on the non-dominant hand and reduced ability for the trainer to facilitate the procedure by traction and counter-traction. Yet there are also distinct advantages: magnified and high-definition views of the operative field, the potential to train without being scrubbed, and the ability to video record procedures easily for subsequent reflection and independent review. As with all surgical training, the key elements should not be forgotten: conscious competence as a surgeon and a trainer, empathy, patience, communication skills, leadership, organisation, situational awareness, and emotional intelligence. Structured, validated, and reliable forms of formative and summative assessment enable performance-enhancing feedback and allow high-fidelity observation of the proficiency-gain curve for individual trainees and groups of trainees.

The lessons learned from LAPCO, a performance-managed transformational national training programme for laparoscopic colorectal surgery, can be applied in any healthcare system or region and can be reproduced in all specialties of MAS.

KEY POINTS

- The endoscopy model of 'Set', 'Dialogue', and 'Closure' can be applied effectively in MAS to provide a structured training framework.
- An effective trainer needs to be highly skilled to make the OR environment more conducive to training in the physical set.
- Alignment of agenda is an essential component of the verbal set prior to undergoing training in MAS.
- Effective clinical coaching in MAS requires conscious competence as a trainer, performance-enhancing instruction, and a structured approach to avoid taking over in OR.
- Constructive and structured feedback is essential to close any training episode with a clear take-home message after every training episode.
- Assessment is essential to promote learning and in LAPCO, a formative assessment model has been successfully used in the programme.
- There are key human factors that can influence learning and must be considered during MAS training including communication skills, situation awareness, and leadership.

TAKE-HOME MESSAGE

We need to be trained as trainers as well as surgeons to be effective teachers.

REFERENCES

1. Kligman M. Training considerations for laparoscopic bariatric surgery. In *Minimally Invasive Surgery Training: Theories, Models, Outcomes*. [Online]. National Institutes of Health, National Library of Medicine, Washington, DC. http://www.doc896. yuanmengying.com/laparoscopic-bariatric-surgery–P-g0lu6.pdf. Accessed April 28, 2015.
2. Bristol Royal Infirmary Inquiry [Internet]. Learning from Bristol: The report of the public inquiry into children's heart surgery at the Bristol Royal Infirmary 1984 to 1995. Command paper: CM 5207, BRII; 2001. http://webarchive. nationalarchives.gov.uk/+/www.dh.gov.uk/en/Publicationsandstatistics/Publications/ PublicationsPolicyAndGuidance/DH_4005620. Accessed September 13, 2016.
3. Deziel DJ, Millikan KW, Economou SG, Doolas A, Ko ST, Airan MC. Complications of laparoscopic cholecystectomy: A national survey of 4,292 hospitals and an analysis of 77,604 cases. *Am J Surg* 1993;165:9–14.
4. Moore MJ, Bennett CL. The learning curve for laparoscopic cholecystectomy: The Southern Surgeons Club. *Am J Surg* 1995;170:55–9.
5. Kumar U, Gill IS. Learning curve in human laparoscopic surgery. *Curr Urol Rep* 2006;7:120–4.
6. Secin FP, Savage C, Abbou C, de La Taille A, Salomon L, Rassweiler J et al. The learning curve for laparoscopic radical prostatectomy: An international multicenter study. *J Urol* 2010;184:2291–6.
7. Gowande AA. Creating the educated surgeon in the twenty-first century. *Am J Surg* 2001;181:551–6.
8. van Sickle KR, Gallagher AG, Smith CD. The effect of escalating feedback on the acquisition of psychomotor skills for laparoscopy. *Surg Endosc* 2007;21:220–4.

9. American Board of Surgery. Available at: http://www.absurgery.org/default.jsp?certgsqe_resassess. Last accessed 14 July 2014.
10. Larson JL, Williams RG, Ketchum J, Boehler ML, Dunnington GL. Feasibility, reliability and validity of an operative performance rating system for evaluating surgery residents. *Surgery* 2005;138(4):640–7.
11. Intercollegiate Surgical Curriculum Project. Available at: http://www.iscp.ac.uk. Last accessed 14 July 2014.
12. Siu J, Maran N, Paterson-Brown S. Observation of behavioural markers of non-technical skills in the operating room and their relationship to intra-operative incidents. *Surgeon* 2016;14(3):119–28.
13. McCrory B, LaGrange CA, Hallbeck M. Quality and safety of minimally invasive surgery: Past, present, and future. *Biomed Eng Comput Biol* 2014;6:1–11.
14. Flin R, O'Connor P, Crichton M. *Safety at the Sharp End: A Guide to Non-Technical Skills.* Boca Raton, FL: CRC Press/Ashgate, 2008.
15. Miskovic D, Wyles SM, Ni M, Darzi AW, Hanna GB. Systematic review on mentoring and simulation in laparoscopic colorectal surgery. *Ann Surg.* 2010;252(6):943–51.
16. Steinert Y, Mann K, Centeno A et al. A systematic review of faculty development initiatives designed to improve teaching effectiveness in medical education: BEME Guide No. 8. *Medical Teacher* 2006;28(6):497–526, doi: 10.1080/01421590600902976.
17. Joint Advisory Group on GI Endoscopy. Secondary Joint Advisory Group on GI Endoscopy JAG Endoscopy Training System. http://www.jets.nhs.uk/.
18. Mackenzie H, Cuming T, Miskovic D, Wyles S, Langsford L, Valori R, Hanna GB, Coleman MG, Francis N. Design, delivery and validation of a training the trainer curriculum of the English National Laparoscopic Colorectal Training Program in England. *Ann Surg* 2013;261(1):149–56.
19. Barnes RW. Surgical handcraft: Teaching and learning surgical skills. *Am J Surg* 1987;157:422–7.
20. Peyton J. The learning cycle. In J. Peyton J (Ed.) *Teaching and Learning in Medical Practice.* First edition. Guildford: Manticore Europe Limited, 1998, pp. 1–12.
21. Ende J. Feedback in clinical medical education. *JAMA* 1983:250,777–81.
22. Swinnen SP. Information feedback for motor skill learning: A review. In N. Zelaznik (Ed.) *Advances in Motor Learning and Control.* Champaign, IL: Human Kinetics Press, 1996, pp. 37–66.
23. Coderre S, Anderson J, Rostom A, Mclaughlin K. Training the endoscopy trainer: From general principles to specific concepts. *Can J Gastroenterol* 2010;24(12):700–4.
24. Miskovic D, Wyles SM, Carter F, Coleman MG, Hanna GB. Development, validation and implementation of a monitoring tool for training in laparoscopic colorectal surgery in the English National Training Program. *Surg Endosc* 2011;25(4):1136–42.
25. Mackenzie H, Miskovic D, Ni M, Parvaiz A, Acheson AG, Jenkins JT, Griffith J, Coleman MG, Hanna GB. Clinical and educational proficiency gain of supervised laparoscopic colorectal surgical trainees. *Surg Endosc* 2013;27(8):2704–11.
26. Miskovic D, Ni M, Wyles SM, Kennedy RH, Francis NK, Parvaiz A et al. National training programme in laparoscopic colorectal surgery in England. Is competency assessment at the specialist level achievable? A study for the national training programme in laparoscopic colorectal surgery in England. *Ann Surg* 2013;257(3):476–82.

PART 2

DIALOGUE

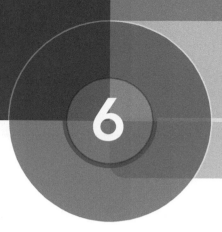

Laparoscopic right hemicolectomy

6

GARY NICHOLSON, ROEL HOMPES,
AND CHRIS CUNNINGHAM

LEARNING OBJECTIVES

- Understand the indications and contraindications to laparoscopic right hemicolectomy.
- Develop a stepwise modular approach to the procedure.
- Develop a systematic approach to decision making in complex advanced cases.

BACKGROUND AND INDICATIONS

Right-sided cancer represents 15% of all colorectal cancers (1). The benefits of laparoscopic colorectal surgery have been demonstrated in randomised trials (2).

Consequently the laparoscopic approach for right-sided lesions has changed from being the preserve of a few enthusiasts in a limited number of patients to becoming the preferred approach of the majority of practicing colorectal surgeons in the United Kingdom.

There are two main groups of patients to whom laparoscopic right hemicolectomy applies. First, those with neoplasia affecting the right colon or appendix, and second those with symptomatic inflammatory bowel disease in whom medical management has failed or complications have developed requiring resection of the diseased bowel. In the vast majority of cases these are patients with Crohn's disease (see Chapter 13).

These two groups of patients require different types of resection, namely an oncological approach to surgery in the former and a limited resection in the latter. This chapter focuses on resection for cancer or suspected malignancy of the right colon.

CAUTIONS AND RELATIVE CONTRAINDICATIONS

Tumours identified as large on preoperative imaging or seen to be invading adjacent structures are more difficult to manage laparoscopically and in most surgeons' hands benefit from an open procedure. Significant obstruction of the bowel may also make laparoscopic approach difficult or hazardous. However, locally advanced cancers may be dealt with laparoscopically in experienced hands (3). A pragmatic balance of risks and benefits for the patient should be considered in the context of the surgeon's experience and laparoscopic skills. The Conventional versus Laparoscopic-Assisted Surgery in Colorectal Cancer (CLASICC) trial reported poorer outcomes in those patients who had conversion to open surgery (4). In the authors' experience early conversion following laparoscopic assessment of the tumour does not compromise patients, but late conversion after prolonged attempt at laparoscopic mobilisation is best avoided. Even in the presence of locally advanced disease most experienced laparoscopic colorectal surgeons would consider an initial laparoscopic assessment as a trial, with a low threshold for converting to open surgery. This approach may gain more traction in the future with accumulating evidence that locally advanced cancers with peritoneal involvement may benefit from more radical peritonectomy and hyperthermic intra-operative chemotherapy. Thus, the presence of unexpected peritoneal spread on laparoscopic assessment may, in the future, prompt rescheduling the patient for more extensive surgery and treatment. These approaches will also be influenced by trials exploring the use of neoadjuvant chemotherapy in advanced cancer.

Patient-related factors include a history of previous abdominal surgery and thus a prediction of a higher possibility of adhesions, potentially compromising the abdomen or mobilisation of the colon and mesentery (5). Patients suffering from severe or debilitating cardiopulmonary comorbidity have a relative contraindication for laparoscopic surgery due to their inability to tolerate pneumoperitoneum, extreme positioning, and prolonged anaesthesia that may be associated with laparoscopic surgery. However, in general, laparoscopic surgery is tolerated in older patients with comorbidity, and this group should not be deprived the advantages of a minimally invasive approach (6). If there is any doubt regarding patients' fitness for pneumoperitoneum, a short trial of laparoscopy may be undertaken with early conversion to open surgery if cardiopulmonary compromise is noted.

GENERAL SURGICAL PRINCIPLES FOR RIGHT HEMICOLECTOMY

The surgical and anatomical principles pertaining to laparoscopic right hemicolectomy are outlined below. We refer to resection with curative intent.

A radical procedure requires that the tumour be removed with an adequate margin of normal colon together with the associated vascular pedicle with high vascular ligation. This also ensures removal of the draining lymph nodes. Adequate proximal and distal margins must accompany the specimen along with a margin of mesentery, in order to satisfy current national standards outlined in the minimum dataset of the Royal College of Pathologists. These standards are invaluable in optimising the staging process and thus decision making regarding further treatment (7). They are based on the knowledge that superior oncological quality results from a radical approach (8). The focus is therefore directed to obtaining an intact specimen in the mesocolic plane. This shares the principles of good total meso-rectal excision (TME) surgery directed by anatomical planes using precise dissection (see Chapter 10).

The gold standard approach for neoplasms of the right colon applies the principles of TME to colonic resection. They are based on the embryological, bloodless planes of gut development and ensure that the entire lymph drainage from the right colon is included in the resection specimen. The key lies in finding the correct plane of dissection. Doing this means the fascial envelope surrounding the tumour will be intact, hence minimising local dissemination of the disease. It is termed *complete mesocolic excision* (CME).

A more radical approach has been suggested by Hohenberger but there remain concerns about the level of technical ability and extensive dissection involved to adopt this as a gold standard approach worldwide (9).

It is therefore generally accepted that a compromise between the radical Hohenberger approach and a laparoscopic approach is required as the radical resection can really only be performed as an open procedure and has increased morbidity. Whereas it could offer an advantage in those with stage III disease, it could be considered as overtreatment for those with earlier disease. Indeed, in their recent systematic review on this topic, Killeen et al. caution against universal adoption of the technique until such times as contemporary controlled study results are available for scrutiny (9).

Finally, a no-touch technique should be observed to avoid disruption of the tumour and local dissemination. Care must also be taken to avoid trauma to the mesentery through instrument manipulation. The loss of tactile sensation may predispose to this, particularly in the hands of a less experienced surgeon. Care should always be taken at the time of extraction as this can both damage the specimen and cause traction injury to the mesentery.

STEPS INVOLVED IN LAPAROSCOPIC RIGHT HEMICOLECTOMY

CORRECT THEATRE SETUP AND PREPARATION

Preoperative staging by computed tomography (CT) of the chest, abdomen, and pelvis is mandatory. This not only confirms tumour position but defines adjacent structures that may pose technical challenges or effect a change of plan to a palliative procedure. It also identifies those patients with metastatic disease. Multidisciplinary team discussion is also mandatory for all patients with a diagnosis of colorectal cancer requiring right hemicolectomy.

Tattooing at the time of endoscopic tumour assessment aids intra-operative laparoscopic identification of colonic polyps and early neoplasms. Quality Assurance Guidelines for Colonoscopy from the National Health Service (NHS) Bowel Cancer Screening Programme (BCSP) advise that local agreement between screening centres and their colorectal multidisciplinary team (MDT) will aid in refining policy on tattooing (10).

The authors' protocol is to tattoo all lesions proximal to the rectum. The tattoos are placed approximately 5 centimetres distal to the lesion, at three equidistant points on the circumference of the mucosa. Normal saline is injected first to raise a submucosal bleb. Tattoo medium is then injected. We currently use Black Eye (The Standard Co., Ltd) composed of water, glycerol, polysorbate 80, benzyl alcohol, simethicone, and high-purity carbon black. This, along with injecting at an acute angle rather than perpendicular to the mucosa, reduces the chances of transmural injection, which produces dramatic spread of ink through the tissues and peritoneal surface impairing vision and dissection at time of surgery. This is also known as 'sooting'.

All patients should have investigations comprising baseline blood tests: full blood count, clotting screen, urea, electrolytes, and liver function tests. Carcinoembryonic antigen (CEA) may also be checked if it forms part of the local colorectal cancer surveillance protocol.

Body mass index (BMI) and need for weight loss, need for cardiopulmonary exercise (CPEX) testing, timely correction of anaemia, achieving optimal nutritional status, and smoking cessation are all important considerations when aiming for optimising timing and patients' condition for elective surgery.

Antibiotic prophylaxis is required in accordance with either the evidence-based Scottish Intercollegiate Guidelines Network (SIGN) guidelines or local protocol (11). Similarly, prophylaxis for deep vein thrombosis (DVT) in the form of thromboembolic deterrent stockings (TEDS) and mechanical thromboprophylactic boots are mandatory unless contraindicated as per SIGN guidelines or local protocol.

Enhanced Recovery After Surgery (ERAS) is a further multimodal approach to patient care with an evidence base resulting in improved outcomes for patients. See Chapter 11 for further details.

APPROPRIATE PATIENT POSITIONING

Both supine and modified Lloyd-Davies positions are used routinely for laparoscopic right hemicolectomy according to surgeon preference. In the authors' practice supine position is preferred. Both arms are positioned at the patient's side.

The surgeon and assistant should stand on the patient's left side with screen(s) on the right of the patient. These should be positioned slightly lower than head height to avoid straining of the neck. The scrub nurse stands on the right of the patient (Photo 6.1).

The authors' preference is to use a 30° camera which, although more difficult to use, offers additional range of view which is beneficial in advanced laparoscopic surgery.

SAFE ACCESS TECHNIQUE

Our preferred placement of ports for a standard right hemicolectomy can be seen in Figure 6.1 and Photo 6.2. Deviations from this occur according to the habitus of the patient or if they have a relatively short distance from the symphysis pubis to the umbilicus.

1. A 12-mm midline umbilical port is used for camera placement. This is then extended both inferiorly and superiorly to act as the specimen extraction site.
2. 5-mm ports are placed in the suprapubic area, left iliac fossa, and left upper quadrants.

EXPOSURE OF THE OPERATING FIELD

Once safe laparoscopic access has been gained to the peritoneal cavity and a sufficient pneumoperitoneum achieved, a panoramic laparoscopy confirms the site and size of tumour as well as presence of peritoneal deposits or radiologically occult hepatic metastases. The omentum is placed in the supracolic compartment above the transverse colon. Small bowel should also

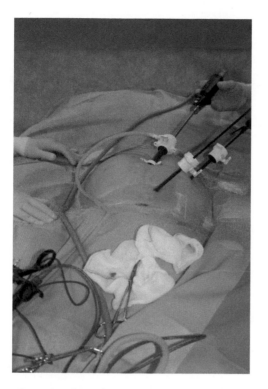

Photo 6.1 Position of surgeon and assistant for right hemicolectomy.

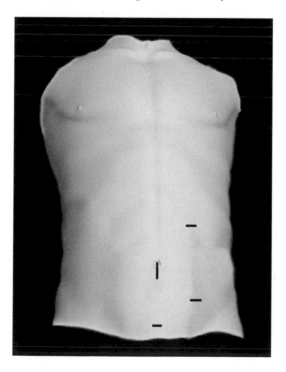

Figure 6.1 Oxford University Hospitals' port positions for right hemicolectomy.

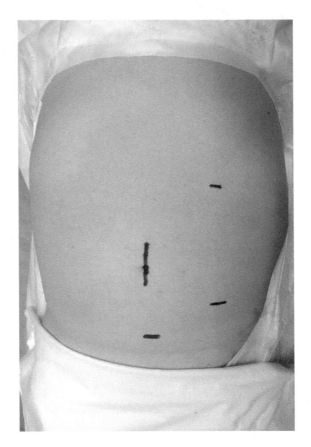

Photo 6.2 Port positions for right hemicolectomy.

be stacked safely away from the operating field. If difficulty is encountered at this stage a dry mastoid swab can aid retraction. Head-down tilt can also help.

VASCULAR DISSECTION

SAFE DISSECTION OF VASCULAR PEDICLE

Once the operative field is prepared the initial task is identification and exposure of the ileocolic vessels (Photo 6.3). An adequate window is then created both above and below the vessels (Photo 6.4). The duodenum is usually seen through the upper window. The mesenteric plane can then be identified after dissection along the length of the ileocolic vessels. The duodenum is then dissected free from the vessels prior to their division. These may be dissected individually (Photo 6.5) and clipped (e.g. Hem-o-lok) (Photo 6.6) or divided with a vascular stapler or energy source (e.g. LigaSure). The origin of the right colic vessel can be divided at this point (Photo 6.7). Alternatively, if the identification process is difficult it may be deferred pending more complete mobilisation away for the duodenum and pancreas.

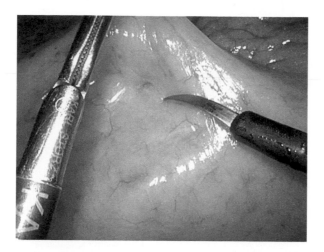

Photo 6.3 Exposure of ileocolic vessels.

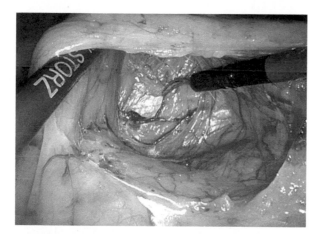

Photo 6.4 Window under ileocolic vessels.

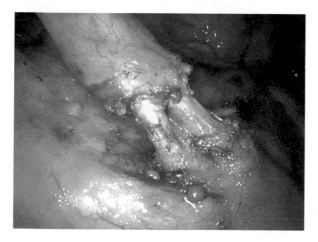

Photo 6.5 Dissection of individual ileocolic vessels.

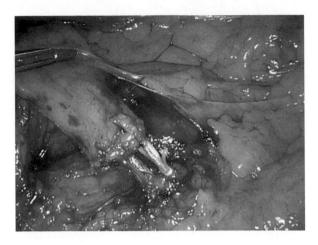

Photo 6.6 Hem-o-lok® clip on ileocolic vein.

DISSECTION OF MESENTERY AND IDENTIFICATION OF THE DUODENUM

The mobilisation of the right colon should be regarded as a dissection of the duodenum (Photo 6.8). We consider it in three phases as follows.

First, following division of the vessels, the approach should be from the medial aspect of the colon, aiming to dissect the D2-3 junction from the colon giving full exposure of D2, extending as far as possible to the peritoneal reflection superior to the hepatic flexure (Photo 6.9). This may be marked by placing a mastoid swab in the newly created space.

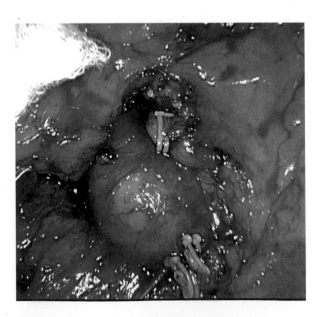

Photo 6.7 Hem-o-lok® clips on ileocolics and right colic vessels.

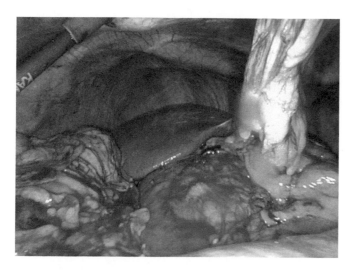

Photo 6.8 Exposed duodenum (after full mobilisation).

Second, the space laterally and inferiorly is enlarged (Photo 6.10), providing exposure and, cancer pathology allowing, completion of the mobilisation. Division of the peritoneum (Photo 6.11) then follows allowing connection with the space created. Traction on the colon reflecting it anteriorly allows mobilisation to continue as far as possible, usually to the caecum.

Third, complete right colon mobilisation is achieved by placing the patient in the Trendelenburg position and placing the small bowel in the upper abdomen. This allows for exposure of the inferior attachments of the caecum, appendix, and terminal ileum. These are divided giving access to the retroperitoneum and third part of the duodenum, connecting the space with the original medial dissection below the ileocolic vessels (Photo 6.12). The right colon is then completely mobilised.

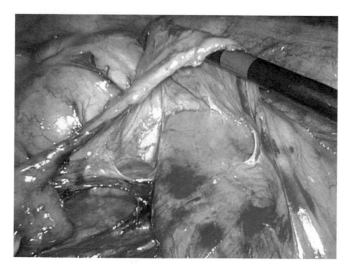

Photo 6.9 Dissection of duodenum.

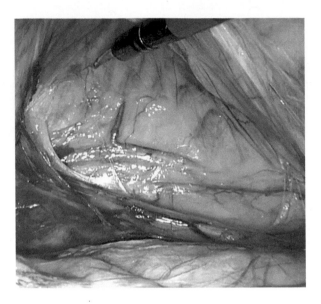

Photo 6.10 Medial to lateral dissection.

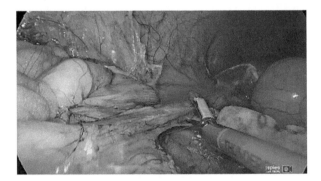

Photo 6.11 Division of the peritoneum of the hepatic flexure.

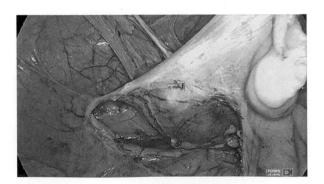

Photo 6.12 Division of the attachments of the caecum, appendix and terminal ileum.

MOBILISATION

DISSECTION OF HEPATIC FLEXURE

Cancers at (or distal to) the hepatic flexure require division of the right branch of the middle colic artery (Photo 6.13), or the middle colic artery with subsequent entry into the lesser sac. This requires division of the gastrocolic omentum and is best done at its thinnest point, more commonly to the left of the falciform ligament. Dividing the gastrocolic omentum ensures that the approach is directly on to the transverse mesocolon. The required artery can then be identified and divided.

The surgeon should remain cognizant of both the considerable variation in the vascular anatomy of this region, and that the right gastroepiploic vessels consistently lie intimately related to the posterior aspect of the middle colic vessels. The right colic artery is usually a branch of the middle colic vessel. Its division allows further dissection of the transverse mesocolon from the pancreas (see Chapter 7).

The length of colonic resection is determined by the viability of the remaining bowel. The latter will vary from case to case. For tumours of the hepatic flexure, the middle colic artery is divided, together with the right colic artery, but the ileocolic artery is retained. Details on extended right hemicolectomy are found in Chapter 7.

Deviation from the approach outlined above is not uncommon. This usually comes down to surgeon preference or to specific anatomical and pathological considerations (e.g. desmoplastic process, fatty or involved mesentery in neuroendocrine tumours) that may make one approach easier than the other. The medial to lateral approach, though, has been demonstrated to provide acceptable short-term oncologic results and shorter operating time compared to the lateral to medial approach. This was in the context of a phase 2 clinical trial (12).

SAFE DISSECTION OF BOWEL

The ileum can be divided either intra-peritoneally with a stapling device or extracorporeally with a stapler, cutting diathermy, or scalpel. If an end-to-end anastomosis is planned, the division is performed obliquely to ensure as wide an anastomotic lumen as possible.

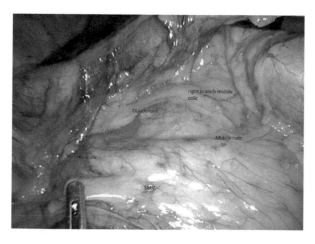

Photo 6.13 Middle colic anatomy.

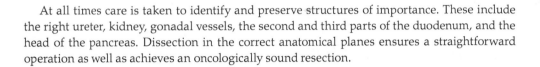

At all times care is taken to identify and preserve structures of importance. These include the right ureter, kidney, gonadal vessels, the second and third parts of the duodenum, and the head of the pancreas. Dissection in the correct anatomical planes ensures a straightforward operation as well as achieves an oncologically sound resection.

ANASTOMOSIS

SAFE EXTRACTION OF SPECIMEN

Extraction of the specimen can be undertaken in a variety of ways via a number of sites. If mobilisation is definitely complete, our favoured extraction site is transverse via the Alexis wound protector device (http://www.appliedmedical.com/Products/Alexis.aspx). If there is uncertainty regarding adequacy of mobilisation, a midline extraction site can be chosen as it affords the benefit of being easily extended in a cranial direction. Other centres favour removal of the specimen in a bag via sites including epigastric, lower transverse, or right iliac fossa.

Following extraction of specimen and completion of anastomosis, there is the option of closing the mesenteric defect although this is not our practice. The wound protector can be left in place while a final check of the peritoneal cavity is made for haemostasis and removal of the ports under vision. Port sites larger than 5 mm are closed in layers. No drains are left in the abdomen.

ANASTOMOSIS

Following excision of the tumour along with adequate margins and sufficient draining lymph nodes, conduit continuity is restored by anastomosis. Care is always taken to avoid spillage of bowel contents.

The main decision with regard to anastomosis is whether to perform a totally laparoscopic (intra-corporeal) or laparoscopic-assisted (extracorporeal) join. A recent systematic review and meta-analysis found no randomised controlled trials on this topic (13). Despite this it was concluded that better outcomes seem to be associated with totally laparoscopic right colectomy, especially in terms of return of bowel function, length of hospital stay, and cosmetic results. However, the meta-analysis did not show a significant difference between the two techniques in terms of anastomotic leak rate or short-term overall morbidity. A further advantage of intra-corporeal anastomosis is the reduced tension on the mesentery exerted during extracorporeal anastomosis creation. Facy et al. have confirmed these advantages, even in obese patients (14). These findings have to be weighed against the recognition of intra-corporeal anastomosis being the less common form of anastomosis owing to its more challenging technical nature and resultant longer operating time.

We generally perform an extracorporeal end-to-end stapled anastomosis. This is accomplished with two firings of a linear cutting stapler (GIA 80 by Autosuture by Covidien).

The mesenteric fat around the colon and the terminal ileum are removed for a distance of approximately 1.5 cm. Transverse incisions about 1-cm long are then made with cutting diathermy on the specimen side of these cleared areas on the antimesenteric borders of ileum and colon, respectively. Each limb of the linear cutting stapler is then inserted into the bowel lumen, first in the small bowel (smaller limb) and then in the colon (larger limb). The jaws are then closed, approximating the small bowel to the colon along their antimesenteric borders. Once a final check is then made to ensure that the bowel rests in a good orientation and there is no mesentery caught in the stapler, the stapler is fired.

We then use two pairs of Babcock clamps to grasp opposite sides of the new, single enterotomy. This is done in such a way as to offset the anterior and posterior staple lines from being directly opposite one another in the anastomosis. Then the same stapler with reload is placed across the ileum and transverse colon perpendicular to the previous staple line. With retraction of the previous enterotomy, the stapler is fired thus completing the surgical resection and anastomosis. This second staple line can be reinforced with interrupted 4/0 monofilament sutures. A further 'good night' suture is also placed at the crotch of the anastomosis, as this could be a site of leak.

The mesenteric defect can be closed or left open, depending on the surgeon's preference. It is not our current practice to close the defect. The omentum can also be placed over the anastomosis to provide further protection against post-operative anastomotic leakage.

OVERALL PERFORMANCE

ALTERNATIVE APPROACHES

The approach to laparoscopic right hemicolectomy can also be lateral to medial, inferior to superior, or superior to inferior. The medial to lateral mobilisation has become the main approach of choice. In our opinion it represents a logical, reproducible, easily taught, and above all safe procedure. Other methods bring with them difficulties with adequacy of view, exposure of key anatomical structures, and challenging retraction of the colon thus breaching the tenet of no touch. Port placement necessarily differs according to approach. The inferior to superior approach may be employed in patients with Crohn's disease in whom there is thickening and inflammation of the mesentery. This approach offers a potentially less traumatic technique for ileocolic vessel identification at the expense of being able to identify the ureter and gonadal vessels less easily.

A lateral approach may be beneficial in obese patients or those with some small bowel obstruction where control over the small bowel and intra-abdominal compartment can be difficult. This aids high ligation of vessels in patients who normally have thick mesentery with a high degree of adiposity where vessels can often be difficult to approach and secure in a medial to lateral approach.

APPROACHES IN ADVANCED DISEASE

In cancers identified as locally advanced on preoperative imaging, a more radical resection is required. This may include resection of the parietal peritoneum, perinephric fat, or abdominal wall. The principles are shared with basic mobilisation, but in the authors' experience, final mobilisation of the invasive component should be deferred until the entire colon is mobilised. This is likely to require a combination of both medial and lateral mobilisation. To ensure that the point of invasion is adequately isolated all major structures including ureter, kidney, and duodenum are identified and protected. These advanced resections can be challenging so a conversion to open surgery should be considered if patient safety is brought into question. In all cases the surgeon should ask a number of questions:

- Is the tumour relatively localised and mobile?
- Is there gross peritoneal disease?

- Is there evidence of adherence or fistulation to the sigmoid colon or to loops of small bowel?
- Is there infiltration of the retroperitoneum?
- Is there fixity to the bladder?

The answers to these will determine whether the standard approach is likely to be successful or if an alternative strategy needs to be adopted remembering the importance of planned early conversion.

SUMMARY

Right hemicolectomy is a common laparoscopic surgical procedure owing to the incidence of right-sided colonic cancers diagnosed at a resectable stage. We have outlined current practice with regard to our approach to this operation. We feel that in order to achieve the best outcomes a right hemicolectomy should be addressed in a logical manner. We also advocate a medial to lateral strategy for the aforementioned reasons.

KEY POINTS

- Good preparation and setup.
- Modular stepwise approach.
- In complex or advanced disease a systematic initial assessment may allow a laparoscopic approach or planned early conversion.

TAKE-HOME MESSAGE

The key to laparoscopic right hemicolectomy is the dissection of the duodenum.

REFERENCES

1. Roscio F, Bertoglio C, De Luca A, Frattini P, Scandroglio I. Totally laparoscopic versus laparoscopic assisted right colectomy for cancer. *Int J Surg* 2012;10(6):290–5.
2. The Colon Cancer Laparoscopic or Open Resection Study Group. Survival after laparoscopic surgery versus open surgery for colon cancer: Long-term outcome of a randomised clinical trial. *Lancet Oncol* 2009;10(1):44–52.
3. Ng DCK, Co CS, Cheung HYS, Chung CC, Li MKW. The outcome of laparoscopic colorectal resection in T4 cancer. *Colorectal Dis* 2011;13(10):e349–52.
4. Green BL, Marshall HC, Collinson F, Quirke P, Guillou P, Jayne DG et al. Long-term follow-up of the Medical Research Council CLASICC trial of conventional versus laparoscopically assisted resection in colorectal cancer. *Br J Surg* 2013;100(1):75–82.
5. Franko J, O'Connell BG, Mehall JR, Harper SG, Nejman JH, Zebley DM et al. The influence of prior abdominal operations on conversion and complication rates in laparoscopic colorectal surgery. *JSLS* 2006;10(2):169–75.
6. Mutch MG. Laparoscopic colectomy in the elderly: When is too old? *Clin Colon Rectal Surg* 2006;19(1):33–9.

7. Loughrey MB, Quirke P, Shepherd NA. *Dataset for Colorectal Cancer Histopathology Reports*. Document G049. Version 3. The Royal College of Pathologists, London, 2014.

8. West NP, Hohenberger W, Weber K, Perrakis A, Finan PJ, Quirke P. Complete mesocolic excision with central vascular ligation produces an oncologically superior specimen compared with standard surgery for carcinoma of the colon. *J Clin Oncol* 2010;28(2):272–8.

9. Killeen S, Mannion M, Devaney A, Winter DC. Complete mesocolic resection and extended lymphadenectomy for colon cancer: A systematic review. *Colorectal Dis* 2014;16(8):577–94.

10. NHS BCSP. *Quality Assurance Guidelines for Colonoscopy*, 2011. Available at: http://www.cancerscreening.nhs.uk/bowel/publications/nhsbcsp06.pdf. Accessed February 3, 2015.

11. Scottish Intercollegiate Guidelines Network (SIGN). *Diagnosis and Management of Colorectal Cancer*. Publication no. 126. SIGN, Edinburgh, December 2011.

12. Liang J, Lai H, Lee P. Laparoscopic medial-to-lateral approach for the curative resection of right-sided colon cancer. *Ann Surg Oncol* 2007;14(6):1878–9.

13. Carnuccio P, Jimeno J, Parés D. Laparoscopic right colectomy: A systematic review and meta-analysis of observational studies comparing two types of anastomosis. *Tech Coloproctol* 2014;18(1):5–12.

14. Facy O, De Magistris L, Poulain V, Goergen M, Orlando G, Azagra JS. Right colectomy: Value of the totally laparoscopic approach. *J Visc Surg* 2013;150(3):207–12.

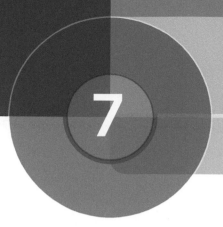

7

Laparoscopic extended right hemicolectomy and transverse colectomy

IRSHAD SHAIKH AND JOHN T. JENKINS

LEARNING OBJECTIVES

- Understand variations in vascular anatomy during extended right hemicolectomy and transverse colectomy.
- Obtain adequate exposure for colonic mobilisation.
- Understand the technical steps in medial to lateral complete mesocolic dissection and central vascular ligation.
- Adopt a standardised approach to flexure mobilisation.

BACKGROUND AND INDICATIONS

Right hemicolectomy includes resection of part of the terminal ileum, caecum, ascending colon, and proximal transverse colon with the associated mesenteric vasculature. Where the resection is extended to excise the distal transverse colon including the splenic flexure and its associated blood supply, it is defined as an extended right hemicolectomy. Transverse colectomy is a segmental resection of transverse colon and the associated middle colic vasculature.

In many studies assessing the role of laparoscopy in colorectal disease management, surgery for transverse colonic tumours has been regarded as a contraindication owing to perceived technical difficulties. This chapter aims to simplify and standardise the approach to this anatomically difficult area for the laparoscopic colorectal surgeon.

INDICATIONS

The most common indications for right hemicolectomy in Western countries are right colon cancers and large benign polyps that are otherwise regarded as irresectable by therapeutic endoscopy. Other indications include complicated ileocaecal Crohn disease, right colonic diverticulitis, caecal volvulus, appendiceal malignancies, and complicated ileocaecal tuberculosis. On occasions, after appendicectomy, a right hemicolectomy may be required for incidental prognostically high-risk neuroendocrine tumours (NETs). An emergency right hemicolectomy may be required for an obstructing right colonic cancer, right colon ischaemia, or traumatic perforation.

Extended right hemicolectomy is performed for cancers or large precancerous or endoscopically irresectable polyps located in mid-transverse colon to splenic flexure or in the emergency setting with an obstructing distal transverse/splenic flexure lesion. A segmental transverse colectomy has been performed for cancers/large polyps of the transverse colon. An alternative to the resection of distal transverse and splenic flexure lesions remains segmental left hemicolectomy.

Due to technical and anatomical complexities, tumours of the transverse colon have been omitted from large, randomised controlled trials that compare laparoscopic colon cancer resection to open resection (e.g. Clinical Outcomes of Surgical Therapy [COST], Colon Carcinoma Laparoscopic or Open Resection [COLOR], and Conventional versus Laparoscopic-Assisted Surgery in Colorectal Cancer [CLASICC] trials) (1–4). The results of these trials are therefore not directly applicable to transverse colon tumours, and there remains doubt regarding the best approach from the available evidence. Because cancer of the transverse colon is rare (10% of all colon cancer cases), it is unlikely that separate trials will resolve this issue. However, in the literature, single institution non-randomised cohort studies and quantitative comparisons strongly suggest that laparoscopic surgery for transverse colon cancer is as safe and feasible as any other laparoscopic surgery for colon cancer.

With any colonic cancer resection, the proximal and distal colonic resection margins are dictated by the associated vascular dissection that will also be dependent on the tumour location and the predicted route of nodal spread while adhering to the principles of complete mesocolic excision. Tumours in the transverse colon pose several challenges for the surgeon. They may receive their blood supply from the right colic, middle colic, as well as left colic arteries; hence, the lymph-bearing area can be wide. A segmental resection of the transverse colon alone can result in tension on the anastomosis secondary to the fixity of the ascending and descending colon in the retroperitoneum, unless they are fully mobilised. In addition, there is a potentially increased risk of anastomotic leak when performing colon-to-colon anastomosis compared to ileocolic anastomosis. To avoid this, and make sure that all the lymph-bearing area of the tumour has been removed, it has become common practice to perform an extended right or left hemicolectomy rather than a segmental resection of the transverse colon. An extended right hemicolectomy requires division of the middle colic vessels, and this can be challenging laparoscopically, particularly near their origins, requiring advanced laparoscopic skills. We aim to simplify these challenges below. The role of laparoscopy in replicating the specimen results from open complete mesocolic excision with central vascular ligation has been supported in recent studies (5). It is our view that the standardised approach to laparoscopic colonic surgery below can be replicated with the use of educational adjuncts including videos and a multimodality approach to training (6).

ANATOMY

Particular to colonic cancer surgery, a clear understanding of both arterial and venous anatomy is crucial to permit a standardised technical approach and obtain safe central vascular ligation while adhering to anatomical planes to maintain a complete mesocolic excision. Standard teaching has been that the right colon derives its blood supply from the superior mesenteric artery (SMA) from which arises the ileocolic artery (ICA), [true] right colic artery (RCA), and right-sided branches of middle colic artery (MCA) (7). The transverse colon is supplied by the MCA up to the distal transverse colon, and the rest of the distal colon is supplied by branches of the inferior mesenteric artery (IMA). A marginal artery runs along the mesenteric colonic border that is formed by anastomoses between branches of MCA and IMA. Vasa recta, branches of marginal artery, then supply the bowel wall. In reality, the arterial and venous anatomy of the right and transverse colon is highly variable, and understanding this variability becomes even more important with laparoscopic resection, not only to optimise safety and obtain suitable proximal vessel ligation with a colonic cancer but also to minimise the size of the retrieval incision and avoid extracorporeal vascular ligation – a technical aspect that we regard as a 'conversion' to open surgery (8). The ICA is the most constant branch of SMA. ICA provides blood supply to the ileum, appendix, and caecum. RCA supplies the ascending colon, hepatic flexure. MCA branches supply the proximal and distal transverse colon. The MCA is absent in about 25% (9). A true right colic artery arising from the SMA is a rare entity. Figures 7.1 to 7.3 indicate the potential vascular anatomical variations that may be encountered. For simplicity, we refer to these highly variable vessels generically as the MCA.

For colonic cancer, an appropriate clearance of the associated lymphatics, particularly where pretreatment staging suggests mesenteric nodal disease, will be achievable by dissecting and ligating the relevant vessels close to their origin (10,11). For an oncologically radical laparoscopic right hemicolectomy, the following vessels are ligated close to their origin (accepting the variation in arterial anatomy): ICA, RCA, and right branch of MCA including their accompanying veins. In this circumstance, the left and right branches are identified with the MCA origin. For extended right hemicolectomy, the main trunk of MCA is ligated near its origin from the SMA without the necessity to skeletonise the left- and right-sided branches. In more challenging cases, however, the left and right branches can be used to facilitate dissection proximally

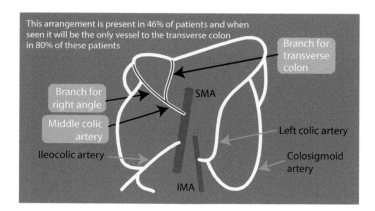

Figure 7.1 Blood Supply 1.

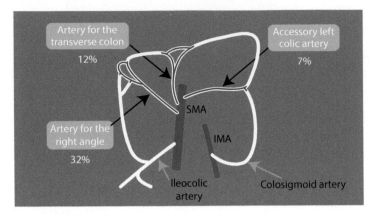

Figure 7.2 Blood Supply 2.

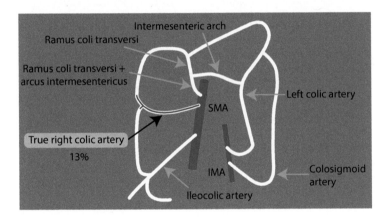

Figure 7.3 Blood Supply 3.

towards the MCA and its origin. An extended right hemicolectomy should be used for colon cancers arising between the two flexures with an anastomosis between the ileum and descending colon. We do not regard T4 extension into adjacent organs as a contraindication to laparoscopic resection (e.g. omentum, greater curve of stomach, adjacent colon, or small bowel loops).

PREOPERATIVE CONDITIONING AND PREPARATION

Managing a patient's understanding and expectations remains a key part of all preoperative preparation as embodied by Enhanced Recovery After Surgery (ERAS) principles. The specifics of ERAS programmes are beyond the scope of this chapter (see Chapter 11). Any concurrent medical conditions are optimised preoperatively. Treatment options must be discussed with the patient. The patient's questions should be answered to the patient's satisfaction and informed consent obtained.

All patients will receive preoperative carbohydrate drinks up to 2 hours prior to surgery (12,13). Bowel preparation for right, extended right hemicolectomy and transverse colectomy is regarded as unnecessary. All patients will receive preoperative deep venous thrombosis prophylaxis and a single dose of antibiotic prophylaxis at the time of induction according to the hospital protocol and antimicrobial guidelines.

STEPS IN EXTENDED RIGHT HEMICOLECTOMY OR TRANSVERSE COLECTOMY

CORRECT THEATRE SETUP

The preoperative management, surgical interventions, and processes are standardised for all elective colorectal resections in our practice. This facilitates understanding by the surgical team and allied healthcare workers.

Intra-operative bowel manipulation is minimised not only by employing a laparoscopic approach but also with the appropriate use of gravitational retraction. This is made possible by using an appropriate operating table that permits and supports patients in extreme positions. Our preference is to use a Maquet Magnus table (Maquet Holding B.V. & Co. KG, Germany) that is versatile for such requirements. Similarly, a 30° laparoscopic camera is regarded as helpful by most laparoscopic colorectal surgeons; however, we routinely employ a zero-degree, flexible-tipped, high-definition laparoscope (Endoeye flexible laparoscopic camera [Olympus, KeyMed House, Southend-on-Sea, UK]) that provides adjustable flexibility in multiple angles. We regard this as particularly useful around the hepatic and splenic flexures and with deep pelvic dissection.

APPROPRIATE PATIENT POSITIONING

The patient is placed in a modified Lloyd-Davies position with the lower limbs in Yellowfin stirrups. This position is used for all laparoscopic resections to minimise variation and avoid any confusion for the operating team. Shoulder supports are used to secure the patient to the table to permit the safe use of an unrestricted Trendelenburg position and lateral tilt where needed. Shoulder supports are used above and lateral to each shoulder. Inappropriate shoulder support may produce injury to the brachial plexus, and placement is therefore carefully performed. We secure the supports in a position adjacent to the acromion of the scapula and high on the upper arms, as proximally as possible, to avoid compression injury to the radial nerve. The patient's arms are wrapped at each side to minimise clashing with the surgical team. All pressure points are checked prior to starting skin preparation and draping. It remains the responsibility of both the surgeon and anaesthetist to ensure the patient is safely secured before the start of surgery.

The operating team is positioned in such a way to avoid collision and permit the smooth transfer of instruments. For right and extended right hemicolectomy, the operating surgeon stands between the legs, with the assistant standing on the patient's left side, and the scrub nurse also on the left side. The surgeon operates caudocranially from between the legs and will not move position until completion of mobilisation and vascular ligation for specimen retrieval. We prefer to use two monitor screens. The main operating screen is placed directly above the patient's head.

SAFE ACCESS TECHNIQUE

Pneumoperitoneum may be induced by using either an open access or Veress needle approach. Our preference is to use a Veress needle technique as we believe the eventual seal between

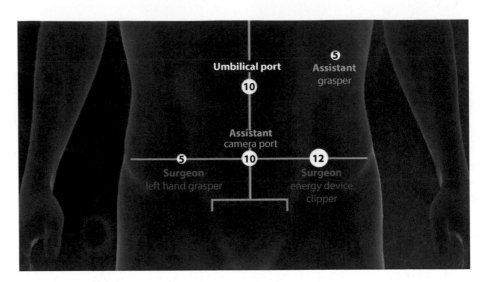

Figure 7.4 Lap port sites.

port and skin is better, which helps in avoiding a nuisance gas leak around the port during the operation. Where there is a previous laparotomy wound, the initial insertion site is changed to a more lateral position either using a Veress needle after cut down onto the fascia with two or three retaining fascial sutures being inserted to elevate the fascia ('remote insertion'); an open access technique; or using a transparent port (e.g. Optiview port [Endopath XCEL, Ethicon, Johnson & Johnson Medical Limited, Livingston, UK) into which the laparoscope is inserted, again using fascial elevation sutures for port insertion.

Port placement and extraction sites differ between surgeons but our standard port placement is as follows (Figure 7.4):

Umbilical 10-mm port; hypogastric 10-mm port (two-thirds between umbilicus and pubis) – will be the working camera port; right iliac fossa 12-mm port (for intra-corporeal bowel transection); left iliac fossa 5-mm port; a further 5-mm port about 2–3 cm above the trans-umbilical line in the left flank; to assist splenic flexure mobilisation an additional 5-mm port may be inserted in the subxiphoid area; to further facilitate dissection by optimising the view, an additional 10-mm camera port may be placed in the epigastrium around five fingerbreadths below the subxiphoid 5-mm port.

EXPOSURE OF OPERATING FIELD

The operating surgeon stands in between the patient's legs operating in a caudocranial direction with full visualisation of the MCA, ICA, RCA, and transverse colon from this point. The camera port is in the hypogastric position. The table is tilted to a 5° head up and left shoulder down position. With gravity and gentle manipulation with a few sweeps of the small bowel mesentery from the duodenum to the ileocaecal area, the small bowel will position itself in the left lower quadrant, exposing the ileocolic pedicle.

The operating surgeon works using the ports in both iliac fossae. If required, the umbilical port can also be used to aid dissection. The assistant can augment triangulation by using the 5-mm left flank port, with the apex of the dissection triangle being the vessel targeted for ligation.

The ICA and ileocolic vein (ICV) are exposed initially, and the skeletonised vessels are then used to guide the dissection proximally on the SMA/SMV to reach the MCA vessels that are then ligated near their origin for an extended right hemicolectomy.

VASCULAR DISSECTION

SAFE DISSECTION OF VASCULAR PEDICLE

For an extended right hemicolectomy, we routinely mobilise the right colon first, the transverse colon, and then the splenic flexure and descending colon. Using atraumatic graspers (Microfrance/Medtronic, Minneapolis, Minnesota), the ICA pedicle is grasped near its distal end and elevated from the retroperitoneum. The overlying peritoneum is incised with an energy device; our preference is Thunderbeat (Olympus, KeyMed House, Southend-on-Sea, UK) as this permits not only fine-controlled dissection around important structures but also rapidly cuts tissues and safely seals visceral blood vessels.

The peritoneum is cut along its medial aspect under the ICA towards its origin on the SMA. As dissection proceeds towards ICA origin, the surgeon's left hand moves progressively medially and cranially to provide appropriate traction. Opening the peritoneum permits gas infiltration along the ICA and facilitates dissection with gentle stroking of the avascular plane towards the duodenum. If bleeding is encountered during this dissection, then it is likely to signify an incorrect plane. The proximal ileocolic pedicle will then be encountered and comprises both ICA and ICV. Keeping the dissection directly on the vessel and into the surrounding adventitia will allow precise exposure of both artery and vein for complete individual vessel ligation and sealing using the energy device.

On occasion, titanium or locking clips may be required if vessels are larger in diameter or significantly atherosclerotic. Often, an apparently 'large'-diameter visceral vessel will be found to be of much smaller calibre with precise dissection through the perivascular tissues. Bleeding from the vessel can be easily controlled with gentle traction along the pedicle before an energy device is used to seal the bleeding point.

After ICA/ ICV ligation, dissection continues along the SMA/SMV to open the peritoneal fold at the base of the transverse mesocolon and expose the MCA (Photo 7.1). For this manoeuvre the surgeon's grasper is placed on the transverse colon mesentery on the patient's right

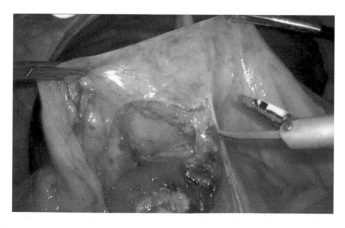

Photo 7.1 Middle colic dissection.

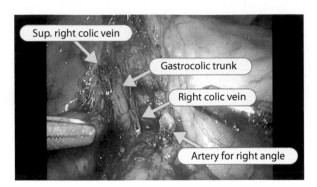

Sup. right colic vein

Gastrocolic trunk

Right colic vein

Artery for right angle

Photo 7.2 Lap vascular view.

side of the MCA pedicle. The assistant's grasper is placed on the left side of the mesentery. This manoeuvre allows optimal exposure in even the most obese of patients. In many patients it may be difficult to immediately visualise the MCA pedicle through extensive visceral fat or owing to adhesions to the proximal small bowel mesentery. In such situations a progressive dissection through the mesentery with reference to the underlying SMA will eventually expose the MCA. The accompanying middle colic veins (MCV) lie posterior to the MCA. Care must be taken to skeletonise the vessels above and below the points of their transection. Division of the MCA will allow exposure of the gastrocolic trunk (Photo 7.2). Division of the MCA/MCV will then encounter a further peritoneal layer that must be breached to allow access to the lesser sac. Should dissection be taken to the patient's right side within the lesser sac, then the gastroepiploic artery and vein will be eventually encountered, and this will be visible, in most patients, arising through the pancreas.

IDENTIFICATION OF DUODENUM

Duodenal 'tunnel': Following ICA/ICV division, a subperitoneal avascular layer is dissected caudocranially and from medial to lateral to expose the duodenum to at least its second part. Often the gallbladder will be seen easily through the transparent peritoneum. The operating surgeon will use the left-hand instrument to elevate the tissues and the right-hand energy device to delicately separate the peritoneum and duodenum. On the medial aspect of this dissection multiple small vessels are present in the groove between duodenum and pancreatic head. These vessels should be avoided where possible and a more lateral approach to the duodenum will ensure this. This dissection will join the previous MCA/MCV dissection, leaving only a small bridge of peritoneum in addition to the gastroepiploic vessels arising through the pancreas.

MOBILISATION

Supra-colic dissection: The transverse colon is then pulled towards the pelvis, and the omentum is elevated by an assistant to permit freeing of the colon from the omentum. For this manoeuvre to be successful, the assistant's grasper elevates the omentum and the surgeon's grasper pulls the transverse colon via an appendix epiploica inferiorly, to otherwise avoid tearing on the colonic serosa or mesentery. For extended right hemicolectomy, the omentum will be dissected entirely free from the colon between the flexures unless it is directly involved with malignancy. The gastrocolic ligament is identified and is retracted by the assistant inferior to the gastroepiploic artery, as it meets the greater curve of the stomach. The assistant's grasper protects the gastroepiploic artery by providing traction adjacent to the vessel. The surgeon then enters the lesser sac and the previous infracolic dissection will become apparent. This plane is further developed on either side, and dissection to the patient's left in this plane facilitates eventual splenic flexure mobilisation.

Hepatic flexure dissection: Hepatic flexure mobilisation follows supra-colic dissection. Upon joining both the supra-colic dissection with the prior infra-colic mobilisation, the peritoneal planes around the hepatic flexure then become evident. Direct traction on the hepatic flexure by the operating surgeon allows the duodenum to be seen from above, and the visceral peritoneum around the flexure can be safely incised to allow the hepatic flexure to be mobilised completely. Once the plane has been established, simple traction will often free the hepatic flexure. A full view of the distal duodenum after this manoeuvre indicates sufficient hepatic flexure mobilisation.

Caecal mobilisation: For this manoeuvre, following hepatic flexure mobilisation, the operating table is moved to a 5° to 10° Trendelenburg tilt with lateral rotation from right to left of 5° to 10°. Using gravity, the small bowel can be lifted from the pelvis allowing a view of the pelvic brim to allow identification of the right ureter and gonadal vessels. On occasion, adhesions will bind the caecum or distal ileum into the pelvis, and sharp dissection with scissors is required to free the adherent bowel before caecal mobilisation is attempted. The assistant grasps and lifts the ileocaecal fat pad and lifts the caecum from the retroperitoneal structures in a lateral direction. This will reveal the medial aspect of the distal ileal mesentery and with slight lateral tension will delineate a line of peritoneal incision from the ileocolic area to the duodenum. Incising the peritoneum will take the dissection onto a plane anterior to Toldt fascia and hence anterior to the ureter and gonadal vessels and allow the operating surgeon to use the left hand to elevate the right colon as dissection proceeds cranially, leaving only a section of peritoneum on the medial aspect of the specimen that is attached to the distal duodenum. This may be divided from a lateral or medial approach to complete mobilisation.

Splenic flexure mobilisation: Following completion of a full right colonic and middle colic vascular ligation, our preference is to then perform splenic flexure mobilisation in a medial to lateral fashion. To maintain the existing port positions, we rely on the flexible-tipped laparoscope to optimise the view around the splenic flexure. Alternatively, two additional 'splenic flexure ports' may be inserted in the epigastrium to facilitate mobilisation in more difficult cases. The table is placed in a 5° reverse Trendelenburg position with 5° to 10° left to right rotation. The cut edge of the root of the transverse mesocolon from prior MCA/MCV division is identified, and the operating surgeon's left hand passes into the lesser sac to elevate the transverse mesocolon. The pancreas will be identifiable from this manoeuvre and will guide peritoneal division of the root of the transverse mesocolon near its inferior border that will lift the mesocolon from the retroperitoneum. The IMV is routinely preserved for mobilisation of the splenic flexure with an extended right hemicolectomy, meaning that peritoneal divisions skirt around the IMV at the pancreas. This is in contrast to splenic flexure mobilisation for total mesorectal excision where a high ligation of the IMV at the pancreas is routinely performed. Leaving the IMV intact will mean that it will not be easy to fully mobilise the transverse mesocolon at its lateral end without inappropriately cutting across the mesocolon; hence, to completely free the splenic flexure, a return to the supra-colic approach is required. Nevertheless, staying close to the pancreatic surface will make progress and very few small vessels will be encountered if the correct plane is maintained.

Returning to the supra-colic dissection identifies the previously mobilised omentum and with its elevation by the assistant, the operating surgeon can re-enter the lesser sac from above. The flexible-tipped laparoscope permits a down-facing view over the colon into the lesser sac. The omentum is freed from the splenic flexure with cranial retraction of the omentum by the assistant and caudal retraction on an appendix epiploica of the transverse colon by the operating surgeon. Once the omentum has been freed, then the residual peritoneal attachments from the inferior pancreatic border to the transverse mesocolon come into view and can then be divided to free the flexure completely. To ensure adequate colonic length for ileocolic anastomosis, the descending colon needs to be mobilised from its peritoneal attachments, and this is performed in a lateral to medial fashion from the flexure downward to at least the proximal sigmoid colon/flexure, maintaining an intact descending and sigmoid mesocolon.

ANASTOMOSIS

SAFE EXTRACTION OF SPECIMEN

In preparation for specimen retrieval, the patient is returned to the original operating position, and the extent of colonic and ileal mobilisation is confirmed, and there should be no residual attachments to the specimen from the retroperitoneum. Once confirmed, the ileal mesentery is divided using the energy device, and this is facilitated by the assistant putting traction on the specimen side of the divided ileocolic artery and the operating surgeon retracting near the fold of Treves. The ileal mesentery is then divided to the bowel edge around 10 cm from the ileocaecal valve. A laparoscopic stapler is then used through the 12-mm right lower quadrant port to transect the ileum. Attention is then directed towards the descending colonic end of the specimen and the mesentery is divided towards the colonic wall, sealing the adjacent marginal vessel with the energy device. A laparoscopic stapler is then used to transect the colon.

The specimen is placed in the right upper quadrant of the abdomen, and the mobilised ileal and colonic ends are identified. The ileal mesentery is orientated with the transected ileum lying across the small bowel and its mesentery. The ileum and colon are orientated in a side-to-side position that is antiperistaltic, and two absorbable sutures are placed proximally and distally by laparoscopy to maintain the position and orientation. This manoeuvre ensures that there is no torsion on the small bowel or colon at the time of exteriorisation for anastomosis that might produce post-operative obstruction.

ANASTOMOSIS

More recently, we have adopted an intra-corporeal ileocolic stapled anastomosis technique, but our predominant practice, to date, has been to lift the sutured ileum and colonic ends to the surface and perform an extracorporal stapled side-to-side anastomosis, with stapling of the ileal and colonic ends through the specimen retrieval site. However, prior to anastomosis, the specimen is grasped at the ileal end and brought up to the peritoneal aspect of the retrieval site. The retrieval site will be dictated, in part, by the mobilised length of descending colon but will usually be suitable to be extracted at the umbilicus, a transverse supra-umbilical wound or a left-sided transverse wound all with an approximate 5-cm length. The incision is muscle separating to enter the peritoneum. In all cases a disposable wound protector is used, and the specimen is delivered using gentle traction. If a tumour is large, we enlarge the fascial wound to accommodate its size to avoid tumour disruption.

The wound is closed in layers with polydioxanone (PDS), and pneumoperitoneum is re-established and relaparoscopy performed to confirm appropriate orientation of the anastomosis and intervening small bowel. The fascial layers of all 10-mm and 12-mm port sites are closed routinely with an absorbable suture. The skin is closed using an absorbable subcuticular suture, and glue is used as a wound dressing.

OVERALL PERFORMANCE

TRANSVERSE COLECTOMY

A colonic cancer situated in or near the mid-transverse colon may be suitable for transverse colectomy although, in our view, this is not oncologically sound for most patients. Alternative indications include adenomatous polyps that are not amenable to endoscopic resection and ischaemic strictures. Unless the transverse colon is particularly long, it will become necessary to mobilise both hepatic and splenic flexures to ensure adequate length for anastomosis and avoid tension.

The setup and approach are identical to that for extended right hemicolectomy described above. The operation will neither dissect nor ligate the ICA/ICV and will commence directly with MCA dissection. The setup and approach are identical to that defined above but will require a transverse peritoneal incision at the base of the transverse mesocolon that is dissected into the mesenteric fat to expose the MCA. Thereafter the dissection follows the steps described above.

The specimen may be transected at its proximal and distal ends using a laparoscopic stapler before the specimen and bowel ends are exteriorised for either stapled side-to-side or hand-sewn end-to-end colo-colonic anastomosis. Again, the exteriorisation process is identical for this operation although a transverse supra-umbilical incision may be the most appropriate retrieval site.

POST-OPERATIVE CARE

Post-operative care is based on ERAS principles. Nasogastric tubes are avoided, and short-acting anaesthetic agents are used. Post-operative analgesia is with opiate by patient-controlled analgesia (PCA) augmented by bilateral transverse abdominis plane (TAP) blocks with local anaesthetic at the triangle of Petit; these blocks are believed to act upon the anterior divisions of the segmental spinal nerves as they pass through the abdominal wall. This may be done using ultrasound guidance or the blind 'two-pop' technique. Inflammatory markers including C-reactive protein (CRP) are checked routinely for the first 5 days to identify any early signs of impending complications that might require further investigation or delay discharge (14,15). A median hospital stay of 3–5 days can be anticipated.

KEY POINTS

- For beginners, careful patient selection is imperative (e.g. avoid obese patients or those with previous laparotomies).
- A fully prepared team using a standardised approach to surgery and perioperative care is crucial to obtaining satisfactory outcomes.
- Understanding the potential vascular variations and their early intra-operative recognition may avoid any confusion and unsafe surgery.
- The dissection of MCA is performed by providing adequate traction upon the transverse mesocolon with continued reference to the pancreas and gastroepiploic vessels. It is feasible that the operating surgeon can inadvertently dissect under the pancreas, particularly in an obese patient without careful attention to these reference points.
- Veins arising around the gastrocolic trunk can be easily torn by excessive traction during dissection; hence, traction and countertraction need to be carefully balanced. Precise perivascular vascular dissection with a laparoscopic view close to the dissection will minimise the risk of inadvertent injury.
- Entry into the lesser sac from the infracolic compartment can be difficult in patients with visceral obesity, however to the patient's left of MCA, the plane is relatively thin and can easily be identified and entered. Entry to the lesser sac facilitates further anatomical certainty.
- If a particular component of the operation is difficult due to poor exposure or difficult anatomy, consider changing the patient position or working more productively in a different area of dissection and then returning. If adequate exposure is not obtained or anatomy remains unclear, considering conversion to an open procedure is wiser and sound judgement.
- Occasionally, omental adhesions are found attached to the anterior abdominal wall, pelvis, or the ascending or descending colon making right and transverse mesocolic dissection more difficult. Provided that a malignancy is not covered by the adjacent omentum, these adhesions must be carefully divided to restore the anatomy where feasible. A marginal artery will lie close to the flexures, and dissecting near the mesentery near these areas places it at risk; identifying 'normal' adjacent colon may permit safe dissection of the omental adhesion from the adjacent structures.
- Splenic flexure dissection is made more difficult where the IMV remains in continuity in an extended right hemicolectomy. Understanding the potential risk of cutting through the mesocolon rather than achieving elevation of the base of the transverse mesocolon as dissection moves laterally is important. Provided that a clear window has been opened from the infra-colic approach into the lesser sac, then dissection of the mesocolic base can be completed from a supra-colic approach. Where difficulties are encountered with achieving full mobilisation, it is suitable to perform high IMV ligation although there are concerns regarding venous congestion of the residual colon that may necessitate a more distal colonic resection.

TAKE-HOME MESSAGE

A significant variation exists in mesenteric vascular anatomy for the transverse and right colon. A standardised approach to right and transverse colonic laparoscopic mobilisation facilitates

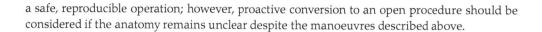

a safe, reproducible operation; however, proactive conversion to an open procedure should be considered if the anatomy remains unclear despite the manoeuvres described above.

REFERENCES

1. COLOR Study Group. COLOR: A randomized clinical trial comparing laparoscopic and open resection for colon cancer. *Dig Surg* 2000;17(6):617–22.
2. Clinical Outcomes of Surgical Therapy Study Group. A comparison of laparoscopically assisted and open colectomy for colon cancer. *N Engl J Med* 2004;350(20):2050–9.
3. Guillou PJ, Quirke P, Thorpe H et al. Short-term endpoints of conventional versus laparoscopic-assisted surgery in patients with colorectal cancer (MRC CLASICC trial): Multicentre, randomised controlled trial. *Lancet* 2005;365(9472):1718–26.
4. Veldkamp R, Kuhry E, Hop WC et al. Laparoscopic surgery versus open surgery for colon cancer: Short-term outcomes of a randomised trial. *Lancet Oncol* 2005;6(7):477–84.
5. West NP, Kennedy RH, Magro T et al. Morphometric analysis and lymph node yield in laparoscopic complete mesocolic excision performed by supervised trainees. *Br J Surg* 2014;101(11):1460–7.
6. Jenkins JT, Currie A, Sala S, Kennedy RH. A multi-modal approach to training in laparoscopic colorectal surgery accelerates proficiency gain. *Surg Endosc* 2016;30(7):3007–3014. [Epub ahead of print]
7. Acar HI, Comert A, Avsar A, Celik S, Kuzu MA. Dynamic article: Surgical anatomical planes for complete mesocolic excision and applied vascular anatomy of the right colon. *Dis Colon Rectum* 2014;57(10):1169–75.
8. Buchanan GN, Malik A, Parvaiz A, Sheffield JP, Kennedy RH. Laparoscopic resection for colorectal cancer. *Br J Surg* 2008;95(7):893–902.
9. Sakorafas GH, Zouros E, Peros G. Applied vascular anatomy of the colon and rectum: Clinical implications for the surgical oncologist. *Surg Oncol* 2006;15(4):243–55.
10. Hohenberger W, Weber K, Matzel K, Papadopoulos T, Merkel S. Standardized surgery for colonic cancer: Complete mesocolic excision and central ligation—Technical notes and outcome. *Colorectal Dis* 2009;11(4):354–64; discussion 364–5.
11. West NP, Hohenberger W, Weber K, Perrakis A, Finan PJ, Quirke P. Complete mesocolic excision with central vascular ligation produces an oncologically superior specimen compared with standard surgery for carcinoma of the colon. *J Clin Oncol* 2010;28(2):272–8.
12. Nygren J, Thacker J, Carli F et al. Guidelines for perioperative care in elective rectal/pelvic surgery: Enhanced recovery after surgery (ERAS®) society recommendations. *Clin Nutr* 2012;31(6):801–16.
13. Nygren J, Thacker J, Carli F et al. Guidelines for perioperative care in elective rectal/pelvic surgery: Enhanced recovery after surgery (ERAS®) society recommendations. *World J Surg* 2013;37(2):285–305.
14. Platt JJ, Ramanathan ML, Crosbie RA et al. C-reactive protein as a predictor of postoperative infective complications after curative resection in patients with colorectal cancer. *Ann Surg Oncol* 2012;19(13):4168–77.
15. Lane JC, Wright S, Burch J, Kennedy RH, Jenkins JT. Early prediction of adverse events in enhanced recovery based on the host's systemic inflammatory response. *Colorectal Dis* 2013;15(2):224–30.

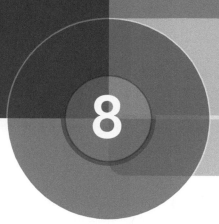

8

Splenic flexure and left hemicolectomy

KATHRYN THOMAS, CHARLES MAXWELL-ARMSTRONG, AND AUSTIN ACHESON

LEARNING OBJECTIVES

- Recognise indications for and challenges of splenic flexure mobilisation.
- Know variations in positioning and setup for the procedure.
- Understand different approaches to mobilising the splenic flexure.

BACKGROUND AND INDICATIONS

Splenic flexure mobilisation is a frequently performed procedure, and the methods of performing it are varied. A number of contributing factors are used to identify the particular operative technique adopted in each case.

The indication for splenic flexure mobilisation is critical in planning surgery. When mobilising for length in a low anterior resection, one needs to preserve the marginal vessel assiduously. When dealing with higher tumours splenic flexure mobilisation may not be essential. Undertaking mobilisation of a splenic flexure tumour has oncological implications and concerns regarding local adhesions and invasion risk. A subtotal colectomy, particularly for benign disease, has utmost focus on protection of local structures such as spleen and pancreas.

Pure left hemicolectomies are rarely performed. This is not an oncological procedure; however, it may be carried out in benign disease, including diverticular disease and polyps. In this procedure, the inferior mesenteric artery (IMA) would be preserved, and just the left colic branch or individual perforating branches divided near the colonic wall. Studies have suggested that preservation of the IMA can reduce sympathetic denervation of the distal colon and rectum, improving post-operative anorectal function (1,2).

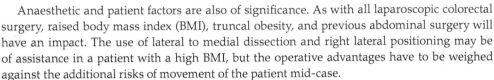

Anaesthetic and patient factors are also of significance. As with all laparoscopic colorectal surgery, raised body mass index (BMI), truncal obesity, and previous abdominal surgery will have an impact. The use of lateral to medial dissection and right lateral positioning may be of assistance in a patient with a high BMI, but the operative advantages have to be weighed against the additional risks of movement of the patient mid-case.

There remains controversy regarding the necessity for routine splenic flexure mobilisation in colorectal cancer surgery. This debate has been ongoing since before the laparoscopic era and is not necessarily evidence based. Benign disease is generally simpler. The Association of Coloproctology of Great Britain and Ireland (ACPGBI) recommends that the splenic flexure should be routinely mobilised for diverticular disease resections, to 'facilitate the anastomosis being made from soft, compliant bowel being brought down to the rectum' (3, p7).

Some surgeons advocate that mobilisation of the splenic flexure in an anterior resection must be undertaken to ensure a tension-free, well-vascularised anastomosis (4). This is done to avoid using the often thickened, sigmoid colon with a more tenuous blood supply. However, this procedure is often time consuming, technically challenging, and not without risks, so is it essential? Splenic flexure mobilisation has been suggested to be the most difficult step to learn in laparoscopic colorectal surgery (5), ahead of rectal mobilisation.

The debate was succinctly summarised by Kennedy et al. (6), discussing oncological and operative outcomes as well as technical issues. Oncological outcome is generally accepted to not be compromised when the left colic artery is preserved (i.e. splenic flexure is not mobilised). Leak rate related to this is more contentious, but studies comparing the two techniques (7,8), although small, do not appear to show a significant difference. Overall, outside of diverticular disease surgery, a selective approach would appear the most reasonable, with employment of other techniques for obtaining adequate length where necessary.

PATIENT SETUP AND APPROACHES FOR SPLENIC FLEXURE AND LEFT HEMICOLECTOMY

In all laparoscopic procedures, there are many individual approaches and variations. In this text, we describe the two main and contrasting methods of mobilising the splenic flexure with the patient either supine or positioned in the right lateral position. There will of course be other divergences and approaches available, depending on patient factors, anaesthetic considerations, as well as surgeon preference and experience.

For both described methods, the basic room setup is similar.

The laparoscopic stack should be placed to the left of the patient, with the energy source on this side towards the head and the scrub nurse towards the feet. The surgeon and assistant, once operating, stand on the right, with the second assistant, if available, on the left (Figure 8.1).

APPROACH WITH PATIENT SUPINE

EXPOSURE

Position the patient in low Lloyd-Davies, with the thighs almost horizontal to avoid obstruction of the instruments (Photo 8.1). Supports should be in place to minimise sliding in extreme

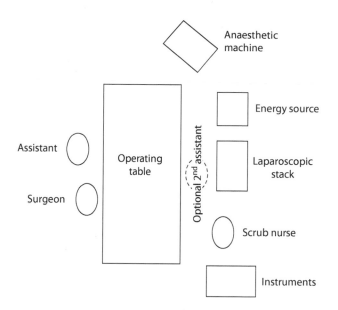

Figure 8.1 Room setup.

positions of the operating table and to protect pressure areas. The authors' unit would use a bean bag and gel mat, in combination with lateral supports on the right side. Prepare the skin and drape as per local practice.

The authors use an open insertion technique to place the first 10/12-mm port in the right abdominal wall, at the level of the umbilicus, lateral to the rectus muscle and establish a pneumoperitoneum with CO_2 and a pressure of 12–15 mm Hg. This off-centre port is used for the camera and gives a wide view of the whole left side of the abdomen (Figure 8.2). Under direct

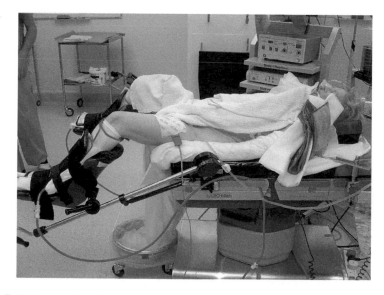

Photo 8.1 Patient in low Lloyd-Davies.

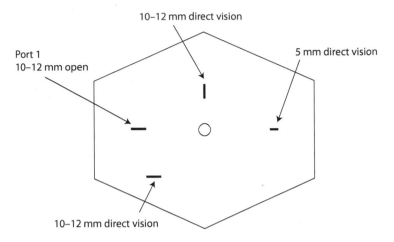

Figure 8.2 Ports for supine position for splenic flexure mobilisation.

vision, a further 10/12-mm port should be inserted in the right iliac fossa and a third in the right upper quadrant or epigastrium. A 5-mm port should be inserted in the left iliac fossa (LIF) or left of the umbilicus. If there is no second assistant available, this port may need to be placed more cranially, sometimes even in the left upper quadrant for the acceptable function and comfort of your assistant and camera operator from the right side of the patient. This may then have an effect on the specimen delivery side used.

There are clearly variations in insertion techniques and port positioning that will work for different surgeons, but what is described above are the authors' preferences. Some would advocate the use of an infra-umbilical port as the first, open port. This can make visualisation more challenging in some cases, but improve the access as a delivery site; therefore, this is preferred in some situations.

VASCULAR DISSECTION

VASCULAR PEDICLE

Place a 10-mm 30° laparoscope through the right middle port, and a 5-mm atraumatic grasper through the right upper port and energy device through the right lower port. Place the patient in steep head down with the right side tilted down to aid access by allowing the small bowel to be moved out of the operative field with the help of gravity. Initially the surgeon will stand on the patient's right and by dividing any tethering adhesions laterally on the sigmoid colon using scissor or energy device will allow the sigmoid colon to be lifted from the pelvis. Using a 5-mm atraumatic ratcheted grasper through the left-sided port, tissue adjacent to the sigmoid colon (appendicies epiplocae) are grasped and with appropriate tension and lifting of the sigmoid colon the IMA is tented so that it appears 45° to the horizon (Photo 8.2). This instrument is then handed to your assistant to maintain the tension.

Starting at the sacral promontory, score the sigmoid mesocolon along its medial aspect using the energy device of choice. This allows entry to the bloodless medial to lateral plane beneath the IMA (Photo 8.3).

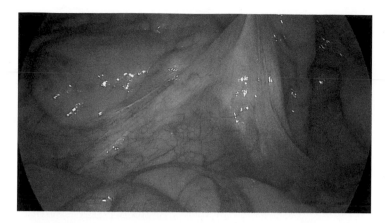

Photo 8.2 IMA tented at 45.

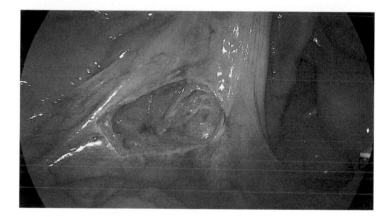

Photo 8.3 Bloodless plane at sacral promontory.

DISSECTION OF MESENTERY

Continue using a combination of pneumo-dissection and blunt dissection between the colonic mesentry and the retroperitoneum as far lateral and superior as possible. Use the 5-mm grasper in your left hand to retract the mesentery towards the anterior abdominal wall either by directly grasping it or by inserting it closed into the developing plane.

IDENTIFICATION OF THE URETER

Continue in this plane as far lateral and superior as possible identifying and protecting the left ureter and gonadal vessels along the way. The left colic branch of the IMA should be identified, and a mesenteric window created above the IMA, 2 to 4 cm from the origin, and another lateral to the vessel. Once the ureter is identified and protected (Photo 8.4), the left colic vessel can be prepared for division. Some surgeons would skeletonise the vessel using the energy source and then clip and divide; others prefer to use a vascular stapling device or energy device to divide the vessel in one movement.

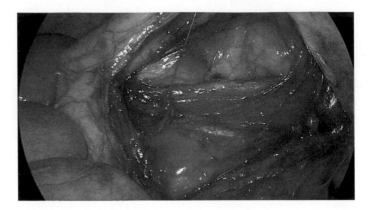

Photo 8.4 Medial to lateral with ureter in view.

Moving your assistant to retract the mesocolon cranially and laterally, continue blunt dissection as far as you can from the medial aspect separating the retroperitoneal structures including the pancreas and kidney surrounded by perinephric fat and Gerota fascias from the mesocolon and colon above. The lesser sac may be entered during this superior dissection. Once the limit of the dissection in the medial to lateral plane is reached, the surgeon needs to divert attention to the lateral mobilisation and position the patient with head up tilt to allow gravity to move the small bowel to the pelvis.

MOBILISATION OF SPLENIC FLEXURE

LATERAL APPROACH

Position the patient head up with the right side tilt maintained. Have your assistant retract the descending colon medially, remembering to protect the colon itself and the marginal vessel from any traumatic damage. Divide the lateral attachments of the descending colon as far towards the spleen as possible, with attention to avoid excessive traction of the spleen. Beware with this technique that you do not inadvertently dissect posterior to the kidney.

Proceed to dissect the omentum from the transverse colon by entering the lesser sac in the mid-transverse colon and follow this plane laterally towards the splenic flexure (Photo 8.5). At this

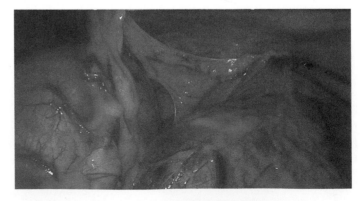

Photo 8.5 Entering lesser sac from above by dissecting omentum from transverse colon.

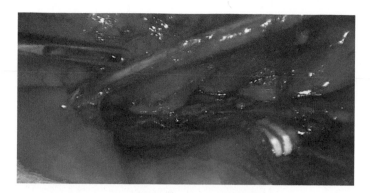

Photo 8.6 IMV at inferior border of pancreas clips on IMA.

stage, the camera can be re-positioned to the more cranial (RUQ) port. Your assistant should lift the greater omentum through the left upper quadrant port and gravity should assist retraction allowing the colon to fall away from you as it is released with dissection. Your left hand will also lift the greater omentum close to the colon, creating a screen of omentum to work with. This technique described preserves the omentum although at times it is necessary and important to remove the omentum for oncological reasons; therefore, this method can be modified in such cases.

Divide the inferior mesenteric vein (IMV) at the lower border of the pancreas to improve length either with clips, energy device, or staples (Photo 8.6).

MEDIAL APPROACH

Alternatively the splenic flexure can be mobilised first from medial to lateral by identifying and dividing the IMV first and then entering the lesser sac from below. The omentum is retracted cephalad above the liver and spleen. Some right tilt can be useful to encourage the small bowel mesentery to fall to the right to allow identification of the duodenal-jejunal flexure and inferior mesenteric vein (Photo 8.7). The inferior mesenteric vein is mobilised and divided above the

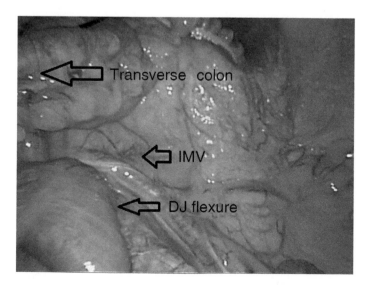

Photo 8.7 DJ flexure and IMV.

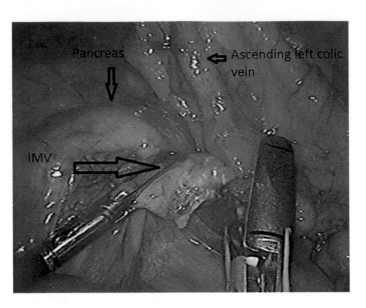

Photo 8.8 Ligasure bipolar diathermy to divide IMV.

ascending left colic vein as it dives below the pancreas. We use either clips, or LigaSure bipolar diathermy to divide the vein (Photo 8.8). The lesser sac is opened above the pancreas and lateral to the middle colic vessels (Photo 8.9). This allows the transverse mesocolon to be mobilised off the pancreas. The vein is then lifted and the two areas of dissection can be connected to allow a medial to lateral dissection out over Gerota fascia and the pancreas up to the splenic flexure. The omentum is then detached from the transverse colon which can usually be achieved by sharp dissection with scissors and diathermy. In obese patients it may be easier to divide the gastrocolic ligament with LigaSure, starting medially and entering the lesser sac from above and moving out laterally. Finally the lateral attachments of the descending colon and splenic flexure are divided to complete the mobilisation.

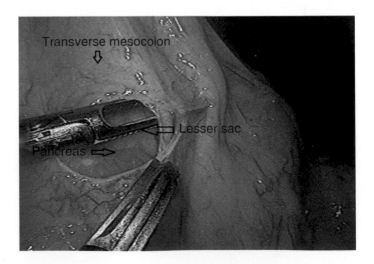

Photo 8.9 Lesser sac opened above the pancreas and lateral to the middle colic vessels.

Splenic flexure mobilisation can be challenging, and sometimes moving between a combination of medial, lateral, and superior approaches is required to continue to make progress.

SAFE DISSECTION OF BOWEL

To divide the lateral adhesions and descending colon, place the patient head down again, maintaining the right-sided tilt. Complete the division of the lateral adhesions of the remaining descending and sigmoid colon caudally. When undertaking this, your left hand grasper should retract the colon medially as well as lifting anteriorly with the assistant providing countertraction on the abdominal wall through the LIF 5-mm port.

MESORECTAL DISSECTION

The site for distal division should be selected at this stage, and undertaken intra-corporeally with the use of an appropriate energy device to divide the mesocolon and a stapling device for the colon. A ratcheted 5-mm atraumatic grasper via a right-sided port should be placed on the distal end of the specimen for delivery.

ANASTOMOSIS

SAFE EXTRACTION OF SPECIMEN

The extraction site can be varied, but we suggest a left iliac fossa transverse incision of sufficient size to allow atraumatic delivery of the specimen. A left-sided transverse incision has the advantage of simply extending one of the port sites, but a Pfannenstiel or umbilical incision is often advocated.

Use of a wound protector (9) is recommended to protect the abdominal wall from direct contamination risking possible port site metastases.

ANASTOMOSIS

The distal end of the specimen is delivered, with gentle traction to the following bowel. Situation-specific decisions will be made regarding formation of an anastomosis or stoma, ensuring appropriate tension-free, well-perfused and non-rotated colon is used. Re-establishment of pneumoperitoneum at the end of the procedure can ensure this is carefully assessed, and haemostasis confirmed.

All 10/12-mm port sites should have their fascia and peritoneum closed (10). The extraction site fascia requires careful wound repair, which can be continuous or interrupted as per surgeon preference.

APPROACH TO SPLENIC FLEXURE WITH PATIENT IN RIGHT LATERAL POSITION

EXPOSURE

This is undertaken initially in the right lateral position, using the advantages of gravity as an atraumatic retractor. Place the patient in the right lateral position (Photo 8.10). The patient

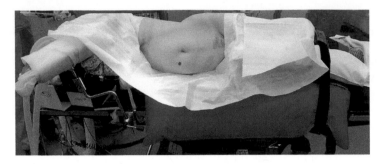

Photo 8.10 Right lateral position for splenic flexure mobilisation.

should be supported with his or her anterior abdominal wall level with the right edge of the operating table (11). The left arm is extended superiorly on a gutter board, so that the left elbow sits level with the nose. Place a back support in the lumbar curve and strap the legs to ensure safety and stability with slight leaning posteriorly. This position is required to allow uninhibited movement of the camera and instruments. Prepare the abdominal skin and drape as per local protocols. Once the splenic flexure mobilisation is complete, the position is then altered to as described above for medial to lateral dissection.

Place the first 10/12-mm port using an open technique into the left upper quadrant, mid-clavicular line, one hand's breadth below the costal margin. Alternatively a Visiport may be used for this first port insertion. Establish pneumoperitoneum with CO_2 and a pressure of 12 mm Hg. Under direct vision, place a further 10/12-mm port in the umbilicus, taking care to avoid the small bowel that has fallen there under gravity, and a 5-mm port in the left iliac fossa medial to the anterior superior iliac spine (Figure 8.3).

In this position, gravity is of assistance in providing retraction of the small bowel, stomach, and greater omentum. This presents the descending colon and splenic flexure, allowing mobilisation to be commenced without the need for a fourth port at this time.

Place a 10-mm 30° laparoscope through the umbilical port, a 5-mm atraumatic grasper through the left upper quadrant port, and the energy source for dissection through the left iliac fossa port. Divide the lateral attachments of the descending colon including the spleno-colic

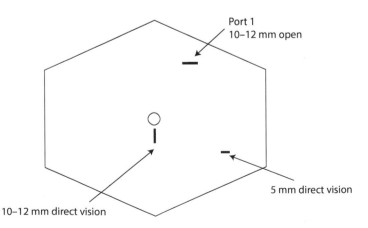

Figure 8.3 Ports for right lateral position for splenic flexure mobilisation.

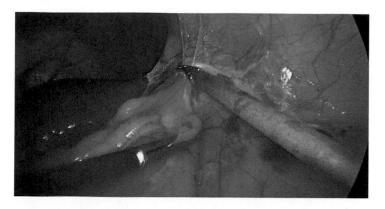

Photo 8.11 Mobilisation of the spleno-colic and phreno-colic ligaments.

and phreno-colic ligaments (Photo 8.11). Taking care not to erroneously mobilise the left kidney, dissect the descending mesocolon from Gerota fascia (Photo 8.12). This plane will be more anterior than initially expected. Continue in this plane, identifying the tail of the pancreas and, using mainly blunt dissection, separate this from the transverse mesocolon. This will present the inferior mesenteric vein (IMV) and open the lesser sac (Photo 8.13). Using sharp dissection, separate the greater omentum from the transverse colon, until the splenic flexure becomes a midline structure.

High division of the IMV at the inferior border of the pancreas at this stage can help improve the final length for anastomosis.

Minimal retraction with the left hand is required in this technique, reducing the risk to the marginal artery; however, one must be careful, especially in thin patients, to not damage the mesocolon and its vessels with the blunt dissecting instrument.

Upon completion of this step, the patient requires repositioning. Some advocate removal of the ports and dressing of the wounds (Frame et al. 2011), and others create a sealed unit around the ports while repositioning occurs (Photo 8.14). Place the patient in the Lloyd-Davies position as described in the medial to lateral section, and re-prepare the skin and re-drape. The vascular dissection is now completed as per the medial to lateral approach described previously.

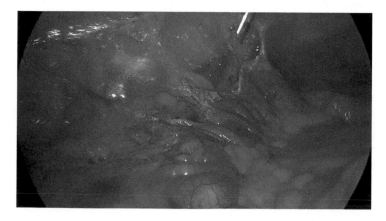

Photo 8.12 Lateral to medial Gerota fascia.

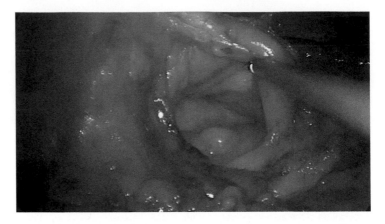

Photo 8.13 Lateral to medial opening lesser sac.

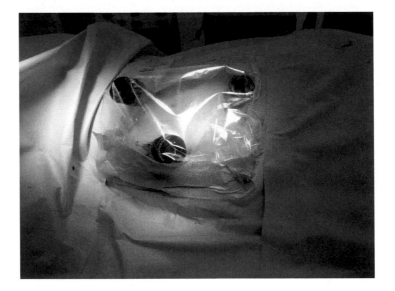

Photo 8.14 Sealed unit around the ports for repositioning.

KEY POINTS

- Clearly define your strategy at the start of the operation as this will aid with the setup and planning of the surgical technique adopted.
- Always mobilise the splenic flexure if there are any concerns regarding the tension of an anastomosis.
- During lateral to medial dissection, beware mobilising in too posterior a plane and potentially ending up behind the kidney.
- For sigmoid retraction by the assistant, consider placing the port higher for assistant comfort and ergonomics.

TAKE-HOME MESSAGE

Splenic flexure mobilisation is one of the most difficult steps to learn in laparoscopic colorectal surgery, but *never* omit it if you have concerns regarding the length of viable colon available for your tension-free anastomosis.

REFERENCES

1. Dobrowolski S, Haċ S, Kobiela J, Sledziński Z. Should we preserve the inferior mesenteric artery during sigmoid colectomy? *Neurogastroenterol Motil* 2009;21:1288–e123.
2. Masoni L, Mari FS, Favi F, Gasparrini M, Dall'Oglio A, Pindozzi F, Pancaldi A, Brescia A. Preservation of the inferior mesenteric artery via laparoscopic sigmoid colectomy performed for diverticular disease: Real benefit or technical challenge: A randomized controlled clinical trial. *Surg Endosc* 2013;27(1):199–206.
3. Fozard JBJ, Armitage NC, Schofield JB, Jones OM. ACPGBI position statement on elective resection for diverticulitis. *Colorectal Dis* 2011;13:(Suppl. 3), 1–11.
4. Dixon AR, Maxwell WA, Holmes JT. Carcinoma of the rectum: A 10-year experience. *Br J Surg* 1991;78:308–11.
5. Jamali FR, Soweid AM, Dismassi H, Bailey C, Leroy J, Marescaux J. Evaluating the degree of difficulty of laparoscopic colorectal surgery. *Arch Surg* 2008;143:762–8.
6. Kennedy R, Jenkins I, Finan PJ. Splenic flexure mobilization for anterior resection performed for sigmoid and rectal cancer: Controversial topics in surgery. *Ann R Coll Surg Engl* 2008;90:638–42.
7. Brennan DJ, Moynagh M, Brannigan AE, Gleeson F, Rowland M, O'Connell PR. Routine mobilization of the splenic flexure is not necessary during anterior resection for rectal cancer. *Dis Colon Rectum* 2007;50:302–7.
8. Katory M, Tang CL, Koh WL et al. A 6-year review of surgical morbidity and oncological outcome after high anterior resection for colorectal malignancy with and without splenic flexure mobilization. *Colorectal Dis* 2008;10:165–9.
9. Veldkamp R et al. Laparoscopic resection of colon cancer: Consensus of the European Association of Endoscopic Surgery (EAES). *Surg Endosc* 2004;18(8):1163–85.
10. Owens M, Barry M, Janjua AZ, Winter DC. A systematic review of laparoscopic port site hernias in gastrointestinal surgery. *The Surgeon* 2011;9(4):218–24.
11. Frame RJ, Wahed S, Mohiuddin MK, Katory M. Right lateral position for laparoscopic splenic flexure mobilization. *Colorectal Dis* 2011;13:e178–80.

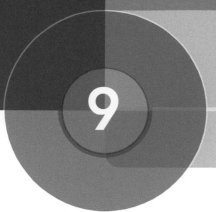

Laparoscopic sigmoid colectomy and high anterior resection

9

CHRIS MANN AND ANDREW S. MILLER

LEARNING OBJECTIVES

- Understand the indications and contraindications for sigmoid colectomy and high anterior resection.
- Understand the stepwise approach to setup, identifying anatomy and the procedure.
- Understand the principles of post-operative care in these patients.

BACKGROUND

The first laparoscopic colonic resection was reported in 1991 (1), and since then interest in the techniques involved have skyrocketed. Advancements in surgical techniques and technology have meant that now most colorectal operations are potentially amenable to the laparoscopic approach. Laparoscopic colonic resections have been found to be associated with reduced post-operative pain, faster return of bowel function, and a reduction in hospital stay. Although initially laparoscopic resections were performed for benign conditions, it has become an accepted technique for cancer resections with most recent studies demonstrating the short-term benefits to be maintained, along with equivalent oncological outcomes.

The indications for laparoscopic sigmoid colectomy and high anterior resection include colorectal carcinoma, endoscopically unresectable adenomatous polyps, sigmoid volvulus, inflammatory bowel disease, ischaemic colitis, and strictures and diverticular disease (including stricture and colovesical fistula). The only absolute contraindications to a laparoscopic approach are haemodynamic instability (e.g. if performed for diverticular bleeding or perforation), or cardiorespiratory disease that is severe enough to be compromised by pneumoperitoneum and the Trendelenburg position. Relative contraindications include morbid obesity, locally advanced tumours where a laparoscopic approach may threaten the oncological clearance, bowel obstruction, and extensive adhesions.

PREPARATION

Prior to surgery all patients should have a valid group and save, with two units of red cells available if pelvic dissection is anticipated. Bowel preparation is the choice of the surgeon. In our institution, all patients follow a low-residue diet for 72 hours prior to surgery and have a phosphate enema rectally on the day of surgery. Ideally, if the patient has undergone a colonoscopy/flexible sigmoidoscopy, the tumour or polyp should be tattooed in line with institutional guidelines. All patients are seen by a colorectal nurse specialist (CNS) preoperatively and sited for a stoma if appropriate. All patients are instructed in the Enhanced Recovery Protocol and receive preoperative carbohydrate drinks (e.g. Nutricia preOp) the evening before, and the morning of surgery, up to 2 hours pre-anaesthetic.

Patients must give consent to potential complications including bleeding, sepsis (wound, intra-abdominal, respiratory, urinary, wound), thromboembolic disease, cardiorespiratory complications, visceral injury (including bowel, spleen, and ureter), anastomotic leak, ileus, adhesions, hernia, and blood transfusion.

EXPOSURE

EQUIPMENT

Standard equipment should include a high-definition laparoscopic stack, a 30° 10-mm laparoscope, laparoscopic scissors, diathermy hook, atraumatic bowel grasping forceps, and suction/ irrigation. A laparoscopic clip applicator, laparoscopic stapler (bowel and vascular cartridges), and a range of endoluminal circular staplers should be available. The dissecting instrument is the surgeon's choice, however, dissection may be done with scissors, diathermy hook, or other energy device (e.g. Harmonic scalpel Ethicon, LigaSure, Covidien; Thunderbeat, Olympus). Other equipment that it is useful to have in theatre includes Endoloops, a laparoscopic paddle retractor, and a small wound edge protector for the extraction site (e.g. Alexis).

CORRECT THEATRE SETUP

The laparoscopic video stack is placed on the patient's left side caudally, with a slave video stack on the patient's right side (Figure 9.1). The entire abdomen is prepped and draped. We find it useful to use Steri-Strips to combine the camera lead, light lead, and gas tubing together to prevent entanglement. For the majority of the operation, both surgeon and assistant stand on the patient's right side, with the assistant standing on the operating surgeon's left.

APPROPRIATE PATIENT POSITIONING

In theatre, the patient is placed in the low Lloyd-Davies position, either on a beanbag or with shoulder and side supports to prevent movement during the operation as considerable tilting and head-down positioning of the operating table is used to facilitate surgery (Photo 9.1). The knees are flexed to prevent strain on the joints, and the legs positioned sufficiently low that the

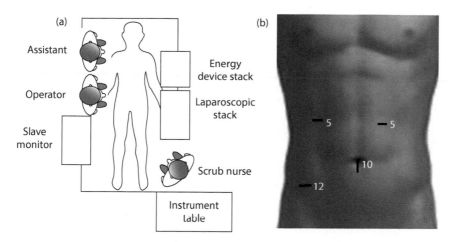

Figure 9.1 Equipment (a) and port (b) positioning.

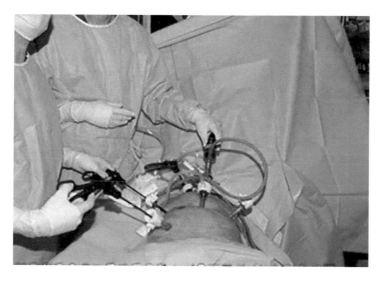

Photo 9.1 Patient in low Lloyd-Davies/beanbag position.

femurs are parallel with the floor and angulated so as to avoid common peroneal nerve palsy. It is important that the anus is at the edge of the table to allow insertion of the staple gun for anastomosis and that a digital rectal examination (DRE) is performed preoperatively to determine the size of the circular stapler device to be used. Both arms are wrapped, and the abdomen is shaved. A warming blanket is placed over the thorax of the patient. All patients should have a urethral catheter to decompress the bladder, prophylactic single-shot antibiotics, and deep vein thrombosis (DVT) prophylaxis (anti-thromboembolic stockings, low molecular weight heparin, and pneumatic calf compression). Nasogastric tubes are not routinely used.

SAFE ACCESS TECHNIQUE

Pneumoperitoneum is established with a standard open modified Hasson cut down infraumbilically to place a 10- to 12-mm port. This should be a vertical incision if a midline extraction site is to be used. High-flow (20 L/min) CO_2 at a pressure of 12 mm Hg is used for pneumoperitoneum. Other ports are inserted under direct vision. Port position is per surgeon preference; however, the positions we tend to use are shown in Figure 9.1. The 12-mm right iliac fossa port is inserted 2 cm above and medial to the anterior superior iliac spine. The 5 mm right sided port should be at least a hands-breadth above this and slightly more medial. All ports should be inserted perpendicular to the abdominal wall.

EXPOSURE OF THE OPERATING FIELD

An initial diagnostic laparoscopy is performed to assess for peritoneal disease, which may influence the decision to proceed. Following this the other ports are inserted under direct vision. The patient is tilted steeply head down (Trendelenburg) and right side down. The first step is to reflect the greater omentum over the transverse colon, dividing any adhesions required to do so. The small bowel is then stacked in the right upper quadrant to gain access to the pelvis and inferior mesenteric pedicle. If the stomach has been inflated during induction of anaesthesia, orogastric decompression may be required. Difficulty in keeping the small bowel out of the operating field may be aided by using an unfolded small swab gauze within the abdomen to keep the small bowel loops out of the pelvis. Occasionally an additional 5-mm port and grasper or even a paddle-retractor may be required. In the case of sudden loss of exposure, inadequate muscle relaxant or gas supply may be possible explanations.

In the case of malignancy, at this stage the tumour/tattoo is then located and an assessment is made to determine resectability.

VASCULAR DISSECTION

SAFE DISSECTION OF VASCULAR PEDICLE

The two major steps of dissection involve medial-to-lateral dissection to define and divide the inferior mesenteric artery pedicle, and lateral-to-medial mobilisation of the sigmoid/descending colon. Use an initial medial or lateral approach as operative findings dictate.

With the camera in the umbilical port, the assistant uses a grasper through the left-sided 5-mm port to lift the sigmoid colon up and caudally to tent the inferior mesenteric artery pedicle (Photo 9.2). The operating surgeon divides the peritoneum under and to the right of the pedicle at the level of the sacral promontory and continues this caudally, parallel with the sacrum into the posterior TME plane (Photo 9.3). This opens up a layer of adventitial tissue. Scoring the peritoneum allows air to enter into and open up the retroperitoneal space, directing further dissection – if this does not occur then the dissection must be altered either superiorly or inferiorly until the correct plane is found. In particular, in patients with greater adiposity, care must be taken not to enter a plane too deep with results in dissection under the ureter. Similarly, dissection too superiorly will enter the sigmoid mesocolon and cause bleeding.

The dissection then proceeds in a cranial direction towards the origin of the inferior mesenteric artery, with the operating surgeon using a grasper in his or her left hand to tent the pedicle superiorly. Care must be taken not to damage the sympathetic trunks that run along the aorta at the inferior mesenteric artery origin.

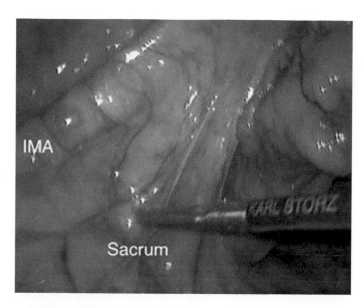

Photo 9.2 Lifting sigmoid to tent IMA pedicle.

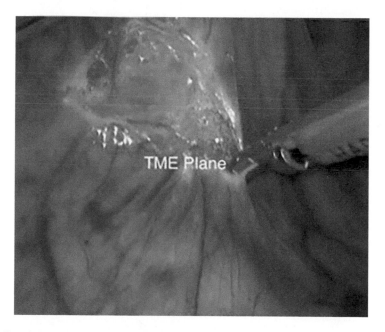

Photo 9.3 Opening up peritoneum under IMA pedicle.

IDENTIFICATION OF THE URETER

Using the left hand to retract the inferior mesenteric pedicle superiorly and the right hand to sweep downward, dissection continues under the pedicle on top of the fascia overlying the gonadals and left ureter until these structures are identified and swept inferiorly (Photos 9.4 and 9.5). Once beyond the ureter the dissection is extended in this plane to the left, up to

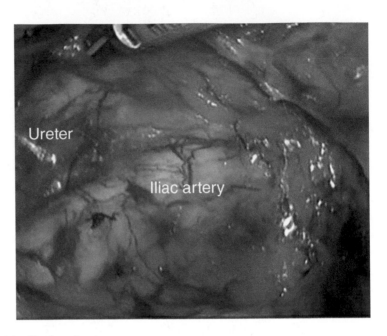

Photo 9.4 Identification of ureter.

the inferior mesenteric artery pedicle, and then continued behind the pedicle. Take care to avoid injury to the gonadal vein. The peritoneum over the inferior mesenteric pedicle is then divided and a window created to isolate the pedicle (Photo 9.6). The pedicle is then thinned down, being careful that the associated lymphatic tissue does not bleed. The vessel is either isolated and clipped using Hem-o-lok clips (Photo 9.7), or divided using a laparoscopic vascular

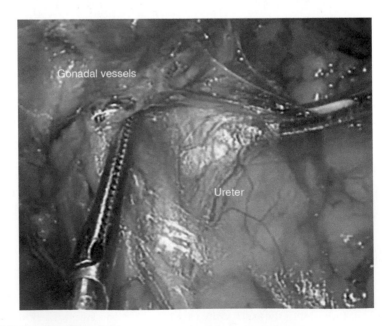

Photo 9.5 Ureter + gonadal vessels.

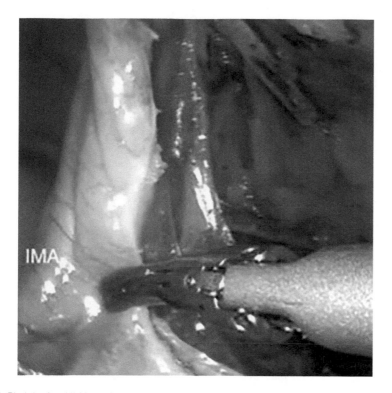

Photo 9.6 Skeletonised IMA pedicle.

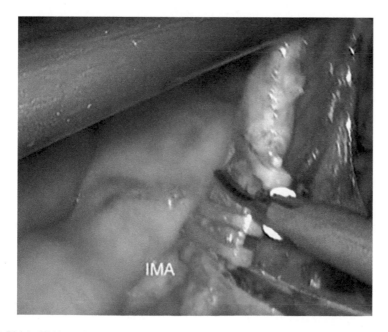

Photo 9.7 Divided IMA pedicle with clips.

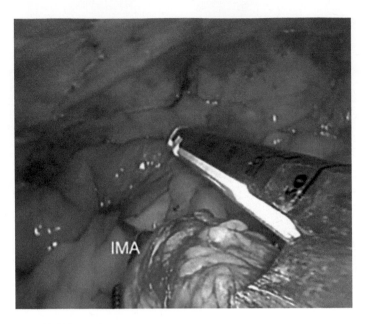

Photo 9.8 Divided IMA with stapler.

stapler (Photo 9.8), ensuring the left ureter is clear. When dividing using a stapler, it is useful to position a grasper on the pedicle to control any bleeding with pressure, followed by using an Endoloop or clip if necessary. For cancer operations, the inferior mesenteric artery is divided near its origin; for benign disease it can be divided more distally.

COMPLETION OF MEDIAL TO LATERAL DISSECTION

The assistant's grasper is then placed on the distal cut end of the inferior mesenteric artery pedicle and used to retract this superiorly. This allows dissection in the adventitial plane under the mesocolon (Photo 9.9), which can then be continued laterally and cranially under the descending colon and splenic flexure, separating the mesocolon from Gerota fascia – the majority of the dissection is done with gentle sweeping of the tissues, using the left hand to retract superiorly and the right to sweep downward. Any small vessels crossing this plane should be sealed as bleeding will obscure dissection. The dissection is continued to the lateral border of the descending colon. The inferior mesenteric vein is then isolated, clipped, and divided at the inferior border of the pancreas (Photo 9.10). Division of the inferior mesenteric vein is delayed until this stage as this allows the mesocolon to act as a barrier to prevent the small bowel entering the operating field. A swab is then left over the left ureter to allow identification from the lateral side.

LATERAL MOBILISATION

For mobilisation of the lateral attachments the assistant is then used to retract the sigmoid colon medially. This allows the lateral attachments of the sigmoid colon to be divided, and

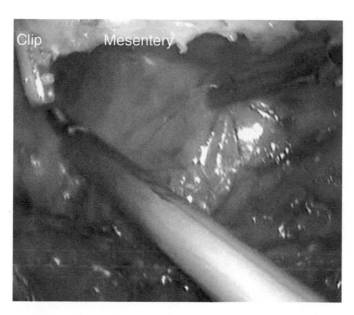

Photo 9.9 Dissection under descending colon.

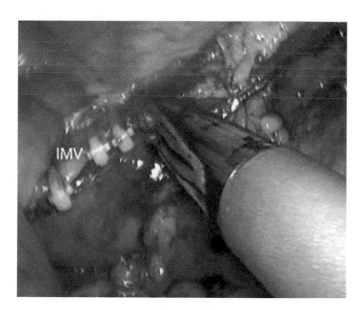

Photo 9.10 Dividing IMV.

the line of Toldt to be incised up to the splenic flexure, meeting up with the medial to lateral dissection (Photos 9.11 and 9.12). The swab positioned over the left ureter aids this and protects the ureter. The attachments to the spleen are divided, staying close to the splenic flexure.

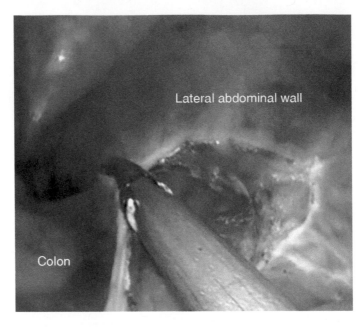

Photo 9.11 Division of lateral attachments of descending colon .

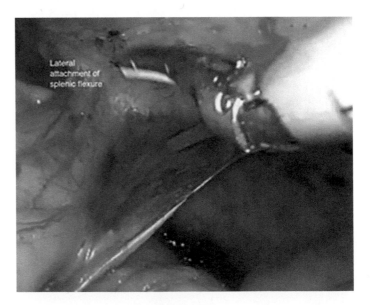

Photo 9.12 Division of lateral attachment of splenic flexure.

COMPLETION OF SPLENIC FLEXURE MOBILISATION

The patient is placed head up (reverse Trendelenburg), maintaining the right side down position. A further 5-mm port may be required to be placed in the epigastrium to do this. The assistant retracts the greater omentum attached to the distal transverse colon superiorly (Photo 9.13),

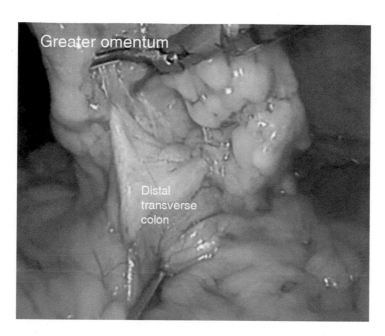

Photo 9.13 Greater omentum and distal transverse colon.

allowing the operator to detach this from the transverse mesocolon and to enter the lesser sac (Photo 9.14) – the differing appearance of omental and mesocolic fat aids dissection. This then allows the lateral dissection from below to be continued around the corner of the splenic flexure and to divide the mesentery of the distal transverse colon to fully mobilise the splenic flexure (Photo 9.15).

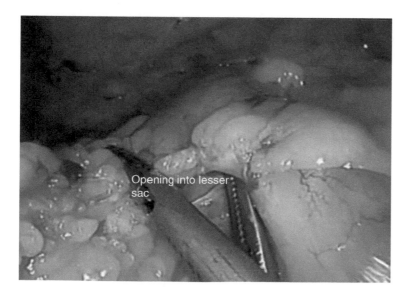

Photo 9.14 Opening into lesser sac.

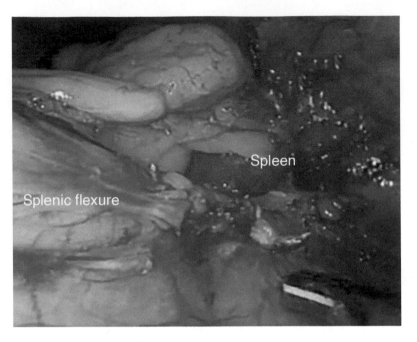

Photo 9.15 Splenic flexure fully mobilised.

DISSECTION INTO THE UPPER MESORECTUM

The patient is then returned to the Trendelenburg position, maintaining the right side down. The dissection is continued caudally in the loose areola tissue to enter the mesorectal plane between the mesorectum and the presacral fascia. The assistant retracts the rectum anteriorly and superiorly. This allows dissection in the posterior rectal plane as far as required. For diverticular disease, the mesorectum is then divided to the level of the bowel wall using an energy device at the level of the upper rectum. For cancer operations, the division of the mesorectum should leave an adequate distal margin. The rectum is then divided using an articulating linear endoscopic stapler (either 45 mm or 60 mm) with a bowel cartridge inserted through the right iliac fossa port (Photo 9.16). It is important that the stapler is placed at 90° to the bowel wall to avoid any areas of ischaemia. Occasionally more than one stapler firing is required, in which case care should be taken to avoid crossing of the staple lines. At this stage the dissection area should be assessed for haemostasis, and washout may be required. The mobility of the left colon is then reassessed confirming that it is sufficient for a tension-free anastomosis. A grasper from the right iliac fossa port is then placed on the specimen staple line ready for specimen extraction.

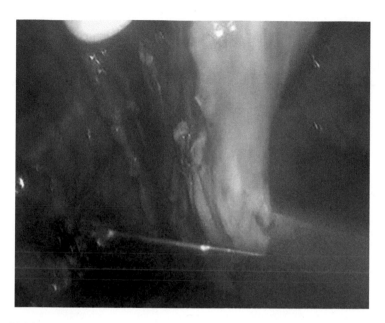

Photo 9.16 Division of upper rectum.

SPECIMEN EXTRACTION AND ANASTOMOSIS

SPECIMEN EXTRACTIONS

The site of extraction is surgeon preference – midline, left iliac fossa of Pfannenstiel. Our standard is a midline extraction site, enlarging the umbilical port wound to 3- to 4-cm muscle incision, depending on the size of the specimen. A wound protector/retractor (e.g. Alexis, Applied Medical) is routinely used (Photo 9.17). Delivery is assisted by the grasper placed on the specimen previously. It is important to not split the specimen, particularly in cancer cases, on delivery (Photo 9.18). The mesocolon is divided up to the bowel wall at an appropriate place to ensure adequacy of resection and blood supply (Photo 9.19). (Note that this can be performed laparoscopically to aid extraction.) Pulsatile flow within the marginal artery is assessed prior to ligating at the area of colonic transection. The colon is then sharply transected, allowing demonstration of an adequate blood supply. Our standard practice is to form an end-to-end circular stapler colorectal anastomosis rather than a side-to-end anastomosis. A 2–0 Prolene purse string suture is inserted in the cut end of the colon, before a circular stapler anvil (usually 29 mm) is inserted and the purse string tied (Photo 9.20). A loop is then tied in the purse string to facilitate manipulation inside the abdomen and to confirm stapler firing. The colon is then returned to the abdomen. At this point the extraction site can either be closed using a PDS suture, the wound extractor simply twisted, or a sterile glove can be used to seal the wound retractor (Alexis), which does have the added advantage of allowing a port to be inserted through a glove finger if required.

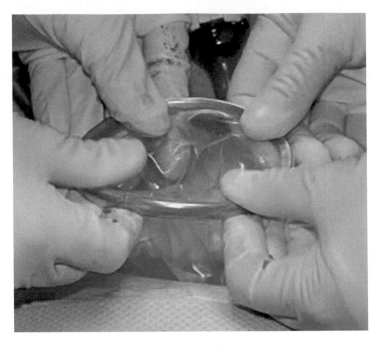

Photo 9.17 Wound edge protector for specimen extraction.

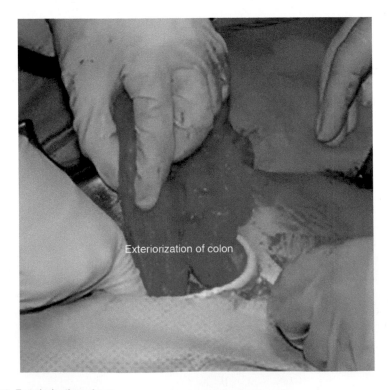

Exteriorization of colon

Photo 9.18 Exteriorisation of colon.

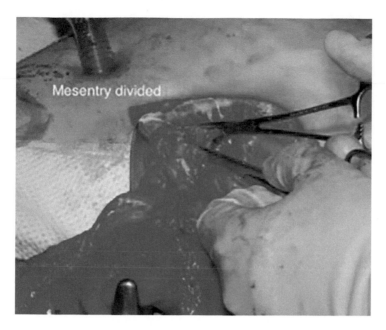

Photo 9.19 Division of colon mesentry.

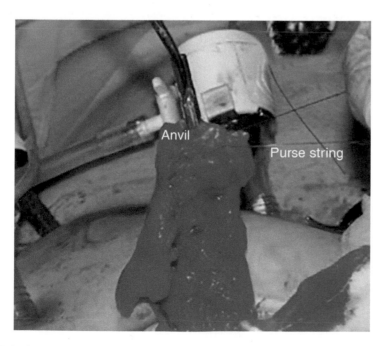

Photo 9.20 Anvil in proximal colon with purse string suture.

ANASTOMOSIS

Pneumoperitoneum is then re-established and the patient re-laparoscoped. Haemostasis is again checked. Correct orientation of the descending colon is then confirmed and torsion excluded as well as again ensuring that there is sufficient length for a tension-free anastomosis. The circular stapler is then inserted through the anus by an experienced assistant and manipulated under vision to the rectal staple line (Photo 9.21). We normally use a 29-mm curved CDH29 circular stapler. The spike is then fully deployed (Photos 9.22 and 9.23), ideally positioned just behind the rectal staple line. The anvil is then positioned on to the spike and fully engaged until a 'click' can be felt. Prior to closing the gun and firing, it is important to again recheck descending colon orientation, as well as to ensure that no errant small bowel or pelvic side wall has been caught. The anvil is slowly closed under operating surgeon command until fully closed, when it is fired (Photo 9.24). It is important to partially unwind the staple gun prior to removal. The two donuts are checked for completeness. Air inflation into the rectum using a rigid sigmoidoscope with intra-abdominal saline irrigation, while occluding the colon proximal to the anastomosis, is used to look for bubbles, indicative of an anastomotic defect. In these cases, the anastomosis can be laparoscopically oversewn prior to repeating the leak test. A drain is not routinely used, but if used is introduced via an existing port site.

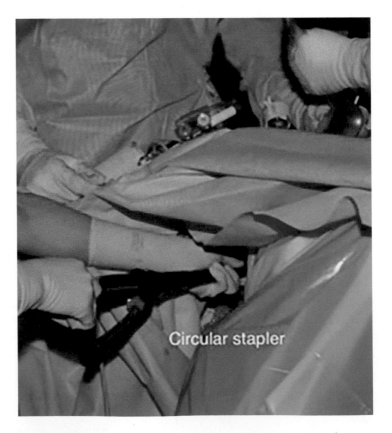

Photo 9.21 Circular stapling gun.

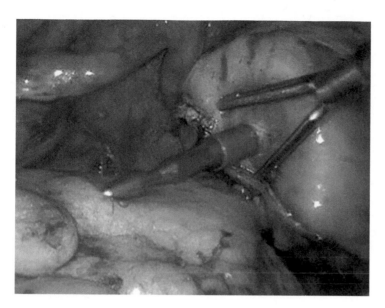

Photo 9.22 Spike deployed.

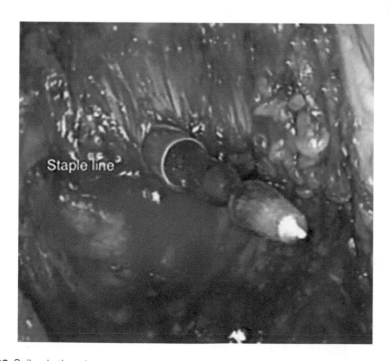

Photo 9.23 Spike deployed.

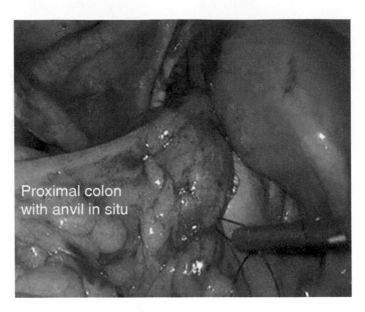

Proximal colon
with anvil in situ

Photo 9.24 Anvil/spike clicked in place for anastomosis.

CLOSURE

The remaining ports are then watched to check for bleeding, and attempts are made to ensure all gas is expelled from the abdomen. The 12-mm laparoscopic ports are closed with 0-Ethibond (Ethicon) on a J-needle. Then 3–0 Vicryl Rapide (Ethicon) and glue are used for the skin. An ultrasound-guided transversus abdominis plane block is usually inserted at the end of the operation.

LOOP ILEOSTOMY

It is unusual to need to defunction a laparoscopic sigmoid colectomy or high anterior resection. Defunctioning is performed with a loop ileostomy to reduce the potential clinical consequences of an anastomotic leak. It should be considered if the patient factors indicate a higher-than-normal risk of anastomotic leak – immunosuppression, steroid treatment, vascular disease, and in cases where laparoscopic suturing is needed to reinforce the anastomosis. If a loop ileostomy is formed, the orientation should be checked at relaparoscopy to ensure no rotation has occurred and that the appropriate end is spouted.

KEY POINTS

- Set up operating room and patient.
- Identify the anatomy.
- Follow a stepwise approach.

OVERALL PERFORMANCE

Post-operatively, patients follow the Enhanced Recovery After Surgery protocol. They all receive regular antiemetics, simple analgesia including non-steroidal anti-inflammatory drugs, low-dose opiate patient-controlled analgesia, and thromboprophylaxis (this continues for 28 days post-operatively for cancer cases), as well as receiving post-operative nutrition drinks. They would be expected to be tolerating oral intake and eating the evening of the surgery, and to sit out of bed. At day 1, patients will be expected to have full oral intake, be walking, and have the urethral catheter removed.

Our criteria for discharge are tolerating fluids and light diet, mobilising, adequate analgesia, patient happy to go home, and stoma competency (if appropriate). All patients should have contact details of a clinical nurse specialist or discharging ward to contact if any concerns. Patients are seen early (within 2 weeks) in our follow-up clinics.

TAKE-HOME MESSAGE

- Using an ordered stepwise approach enhances surgical progression and hence patient safety.

REFERENCE

1. Jacobs M, Verdeja JC, Goldstein HS. Minimally invasive colon resection (laparoscopic colectomy). *Surg Laparosc Endosc* 1991;1:144–50.

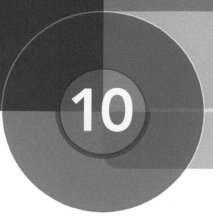

Laparoscopic total mesorectal excision for rectal cancer

10

MANFRED ODERMATT, NUNO FIGUEIREDO,
AND AMJAD PARVAIZ

LEARNING OBJECTIVES

- Understand that laparoscopic total mesorectal excision (TME) is a challenging technique, with increased difficulty due to the male pelvis, bulky tumours, bony confines of anatomy, preoperative chemoradiation, and so on.
- Recognise solutions for challenges encountered during TME by understanding the concept of standardisation of the operative technique, which is applicable to all patients undergoing laparoscopic TME surgery.
- Become familar with the concept of the modular approach, as the operation is divided into simple steps for task completion and teaching and training. This system of teaching provides a valuable tool for better feedback to trainees with a focus on each of the steps.
- Be aware of specific intra-operative difficulties that can be encountered during the surgery, and understand suggested solutions.

BACKGROUND AND INTRODUCTION

Minimally invasive colorectal surgery has become the standard of care for many conditions in the last decade (1,2). However, laparoscopic rectal cancer surgery took a long time to be widely accepted. Like all new developments, it went through three distinct phases characteristic for any fundamental change, described by Schopenhauer: First, it was ridiculed: 'rectal cancer surgery could never be done properly through keyhole surgery'; second, it was violently opposed and all its supporters were considered outlaws; and last, it was accepted as being self-evident and 'how could it ever be done otherwise…'.

Three major factors contributed to this change in paradigm: advances in video-imaging technology, improvement of surgical tools, and growing clinical evidence of better outcomes.

In 2002, Lacy et al. published a seminal trial for minimally invasive colon cancer surgery, showing that the laparoscopic approaches had better short-term outcomes (3). On both sides of the Atlantic, the multicentre non-inferiority Clinical Outcomes of Surgical Therapy (COST) (4) and Colon Carcinoma Laparoscopic or Open Resection (COLOR) (5) trials followed, demonstrating that the laparoscopic approach had similar recurrence rates compared to open colon surgery. With earlier recovery of bowel function, less need of analgesics, shorter lengths of stay, and similar morbidity and mortality, these studies allowed laparoscopic colon resections to become an acceptable alternative to open surgery.

The Medical Research Council (MRC) Conventional versus Laparoscopic-Assisted Surgery in Colorectal Cancer (CLASICC) trial (6) was the first large study to also include rectal cancer patients. However, lack of surgical proficiency and the high rates of conversion could have accounted for a set of confusing data on short-term outcomes after laparoscopic-assisted anterior resection for rectal cancer, delaying its acceptance. In the long-term analysis (7), the higher positivity of circumferential resection margins observed in the laparoscopic anterior resection group has not resulted in higher local recurrence rates, demonstrating that altogether the laparoscopic approach to rectal cancer is feasible and oncologically acceptable.

From our Korean colleagues came the first robust evidence supporting laparoscopic resection for low rectal cancer. The Comparison of Open versus Laparoscopic Surgery for Mid and Low Rectal Cancer after Neoadjuvant Chemoradiotherapy (COREAN) trial was a non-inferiority, randomised controlled trial, for patients with cT3N0-2 mid or low rectal cancer without distant metastasis after preoperative chemo-radiotherapy, done between 2006 and 2009 including three centres in Korea. In 2010, the short-term outcomes and surrogate oncological markers were published (8). For the laparoscopic group the rates of positive radial margin or incomplete total mesorectal excision were low (2.9% and 4.7%, respectively), median lymph node yield was 17, and conversion to open surgery and peri-operative complications were low (1.2% and 21.2%, respectively). The follow-up paper published in 2014 confirmed these excellent results (9). In 340 patients submitted to either laparoscopic or open surgery, the 3-year disease-free survival was similar (79.2% and 72.5%, respectively) and mortality rates did not differ (12% and 15%, respectively). There were 14 patients in the laparoscopic surgery group and 19 in the open surgery group who died of rectal cancer.

In the West, the oncological safety of laparoscopic rectal cancer surgery was finally confirmed by the long-term results of the COLOR II trial published in 2015 (10). COLOR II demanded not only a quality assessment of the specimen by the pathologist but also of the participating surgeons' level of technical proficiency as a prerequisite for being accepted as a participating centre. This study showed that in minimally invasive rectal surgery the rates of loco-regional recurrence, disease-free survival, and overall survival were similar to those of open surgery.

To be accepted as a surgeon contributing data to the COST, CLASICC, or COLOR trials, at least 20 laparoscopic colorectal cases were required. However, the CLASICC trial authors suggested that 20 cases were not sufficient as conversion rates fell from 38% in year 1 to 16% in year 6 (7).

Laparoscopic TME is more demanding than colonic cancer resection because of the technical constraints raised by operating in the narrow and deep pelvis. A good technique combined with autonomic nerve preservation are prerequisites for functional and oncological safety (11,12).

This raises the key issue of teaching and training, and the need for a standardised surgical curriculum for the laparoscopic rectal surgeon, as a higher number of minimum cases than previously required might be necessary to minimise learning curve effects (13,14). Supervised training has been shown to shorten the proficiency gain curve in all levels of surgical proficiency, without compromising patient safety.

In our view, the best way of overcoming the learning curve and 'flattening' the proficiency curve is the modular approach (15) when teaching laparoscopic TME (16).

PREOPERATIVE INVESTIGATION

After rectal carcinoma has been diagnosed by biopsy, staging is undertaken by a computed tomography (CT) scan of the chest, abdomen, and pelvis. Magnetic resonance imaging of the pelvis is routinely performed to assess the relationship of the tumour to the mesorectal fascia and the sphincter.

In the case of low rectal carcinoma and/or suspicious T1 versus T2 lesions, we often employ endo-anal ultrasonography to better visualise the exact tumour location and its relationship to the sphincter complex.

Once the staging is complete, each case is discussed in the multidisciplinary tumour board meeting. Preoperative radiotherapy is restricted to patients with mrT4 lesions, mrT3 with threatened/involved mesorectal fascia, or N2/extramesorectal involved lymph nodes.

PATIENT PREPARATION

- Operative risk is assessed by an anaesthetist in an outpatient setting.
- Mechanical bowel preparation is advised for all patients undergoing mid- or low-rectal cancer resection with low anastomosis defunctioned by an ileostomy. We prescribe two sachets of Picolax (sodium picosulfate) the day before surgery.
- A modified enhanced recovery programme as popularised by Henrik Kehlet is applied in all patients, however, with exception of a more selective use of an epidural catheter for post-operative pain control.
- All patients are marked preoperatively for loop ileostomy in case of anastomosis or end colostomy in case of abdominoperineal resection by the stoma nurse.
- Informed consent is signed by the patient.

EXPOSURE

POSITIONING AND SETUP

- The patient is brought to a modified Lloyd-Davies position on an operating table that allows maximal head down and side tilting during surgery (Figure 10.1).
- To avoid the patient slipping during the head down position, a vacuum beanbag is used.
- We avoid any additional support devices. Shoulder supports can result in brachial plexus injury, particularly in patients with high body mass index (BMI).
- Sequential compression devices are placed on the lower extremities.
- A prophylactic single-shot antibiotic is administered before the start of the operation.
- Digital rectal examination in the relaxed patient is essential to assess tumour height in relation to the sphincter and mobility.

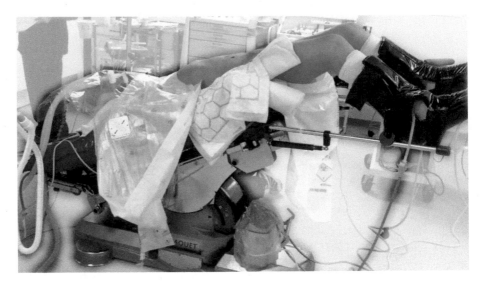

Figure 10.1 Patient positioning.

- The operating surgeon and next to him the assistant holding the camera stand to the right-hand side of the patient. Another assistant is required to stand on the left-hand side of the patient in order to provide traction and countertraction during the operation (Figure 10.2).
- Monitors are placed on both sides and on the lower left side of the patient so that all surgeons have appropriate views during the different steps of the operation.

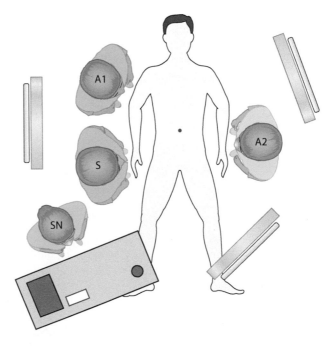

Figure 10.2 Set up.

EQUIPMENT

- High-definition camera and monitor system
- 30° 10-mm laparoscope
- Atraumatic bowel graspers
- Monopolar hook electrocautery and additionally a harmonic scalpel (Harmonic) or bipolar energy device (LigaSure)
- Wound protection self-retractor (Alexis)
- Articulating endoscopic linear stapler for division of the rectum

SAFE ACCESS TECHNIQUE

For access and pneumoperitoneum a modified Hasson technique at the umbilicus is used. The umbilical port is a 10- to 12-mm trocar and is used for the 10 -mm 30° camera. The following ports are placed under vision after pre-peritoneal injection of a local anaesthetic (Figure 10.3). A 5-mm port is inserted on the left side at the level of the umbilicus and the outer border of the rectus muscle. A second 5-mm port is placed on the right side at just above the level of the umbilicus and the lateral border of the rectus muscle. A third 5-mm port is placed in the mid-clavicular line below the costal margin. This port is helpful to retract the rectum out of the pelvis during the total mesorectal excision. Then the patient is brought in a head down position to make the small bowel leave the pelvis by gravity. This leads to a safe placement of a 12-mm port around 2.5 cm medial to the anterior superior iliac spine. All ports are inserted perpendicularly to the skin, which results in less fatigue for the surgeon during a lengthy operation.

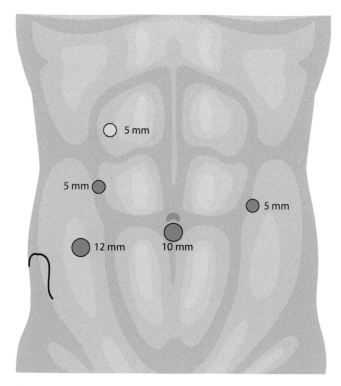

Figure 10.3 Port placement.

EXPOSURE OF THE OPERATING FIELD

Optimal exposure at any stage of the procedure is essential for accurate and safe laparoscopic surgery. For the mobilisation of the left colon, good exposure is achieved by having the patient in a steep head down and right tilt position. This will hold the small bowel out of the pelvis and to the upper right abdomen. The omentum with the attached transverse colon is brought cranially and placed under the left liver lobe. If the stomach is distended, deflation by a naso- or orogastric tube is necessary. The tube will be removed after the operation. In case of a short mesentery of the small bowel or in case of patients with higher BMI we routinely place a small swab at the edge of the small bowel convolute in order to prevent bowel loops from gliding into the operating field by peristalsis. To expose the course of the inferior mesenteric artery (IMA)/superior rectal artery, the mesentery of the sigmoid colon is lifted up at the level of the pelvic brim by the assistant standing on the left side of the patient. Sustained traction is applied. The operating surgeon looks from the medial to the sigmoid mesentery.

VASCULAR DISSECTION

SAFE DISSECTION OF THE VASCULAR PEDICLE

The dissection is started by using a monopolar cautery hook inserted through the 12-mm working port. With an additional grasper the mesentery is additionally brought under tension. The power setting of the electrocautery is on 25 Watts for both coagulation and cutting. In our experience, this setting allows for minimal charring of the tissues leading to precise dissection. First, the peritoneum is scored at the level of the pelvic brim in a caudocranial fashion (parallel and below to the IMA/superior rectal artery) in the direction of the duodeno-jejunal junction (Figure 10.4 and Photo 10.1). When opening the peritoneum with the cautery hook, air enters the retroperitoneal space. This air is like a roadmap for further dissection. If no air spreads, the entry point is too low or too high and the dissection plane has to be changed. Dissection is performed at the upper border of the air bubbles in order not to enter the plane leading below the ureter and the gonadal vessels. Once the peritoneum is incised alongside and below the IMA/superior rectal artery, the vessel is supported by a grasper. The loose fatty tissue is divided until a shiny surface appears which indicates that the right embryologic plane for further dissection has been found. As long as the IMA has not been divided yet, the dissection stays close to the vascular pedicle until its origin at the aorta is clearly identified. When pursuing the plane to the root of the IMA, care must be taken not to damage the sympathetic roots that run parallel at that point. By using gentle traction and countertraction and teasing off the adjacent fatty tissue of the vessel the clean surface of the IMA can be exposed. Once the appropriate planes have been identified in the beginning, further dissection from medial to lateral is achieved by using mainly blunt dissection on top of a thin layer of fascia overlying both left ureter and gonadal vessels (Figure 10.5). If the ureter appears to be uncovered, dissection is a layer too deep. Once the left ureter has been safely identified, the IMA is ligated and divided near its origin. This is carried out by making a blunt window around the IMA proximal to the ascending left colic artery. We divide the IMA between Hem-o-Lock clips (Photo 10.2 and Figure 10.6). Important at this stage is to avoid prolonged thermal dissection at the root of the IMA as this may result in injury to the main trunk of the autonomic nerves that run at this level near to the vessel. For the same reason, the IMA is divided leaving a stump of 0.5–1 cm length.

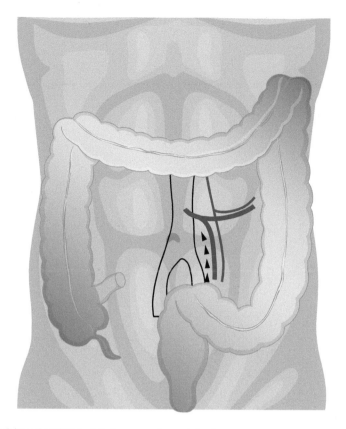

Figure 10.4 Incision of peritoneum below superior rectal artery.

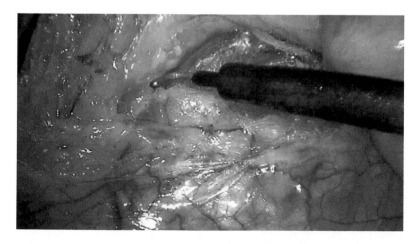

Photo 10.1 Scoring of the peritoneum below the superior rectal artery.

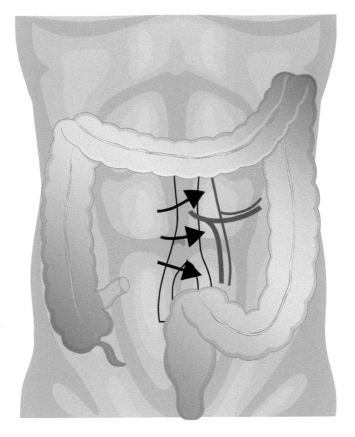

Figure 10.5 Medial to lateral mobilisation.

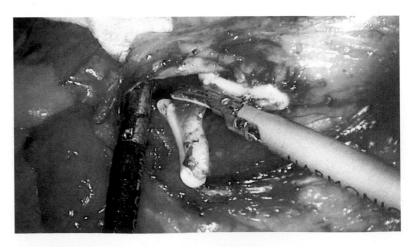

Photo 10.2 Division of inferior mesenteric artery.

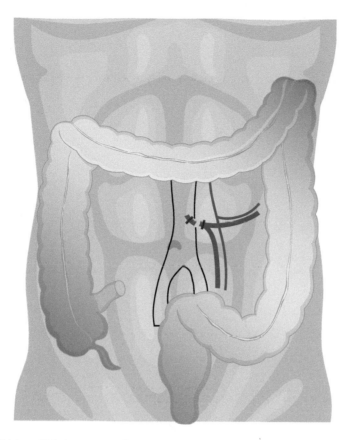

Figure 10.6 Division of inferior mesenteric artery.

DISSECTION OF THE MESENTERY AND DIVISION OF INFERIOR MESENTERIC VEIN

Once the inferior mesenteric artery has been divided, the focus turns on the inferior mesenteric vein. However, we attempt to delay the division of the vein as long as possible during medial to lateral mobilisation (Photo 10.3). By supporting the inferior mesenteric vein by a grasper, a curtain is created preventing the small bowel from gliding into the operating field from above. Furthermore, the vein may help in defining the correct plane in difficult cases. By scoring the peritoneum medial to the inferior mesenteric vein and lifting the vein up, the right dissection plane can be found promptly. During medial to lateral dissection small and easily bleeding vessels are often encountered between the two layers of Gerota and mesocolic fascia that should be pre-emptively sealed as they result in staining of the correct plane making their identification difficult. Once the dissection has reached the lateral border of the descending colon and proximal sigmoid, attention is focused on the pancreas. The border of the pancreas is identified, and a thin covering layer is incised in order to enter the plane on top of the pancreas where a swab is placed which will facilitate splenic flexure mobilisation at a later stage. This swab will serve as a protection and reference point of the pancreas when completing the dissection coming from the lesser sac. When the medial to lateral dissection has been completed, the inferior mesenteric vein is clipped and divided just below the border of the pancreas (Figure 10.7 and Photo 10.4).

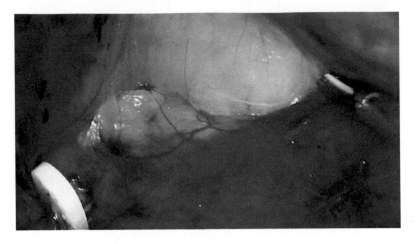

Photo 10.3 Medial to lateral dissection.

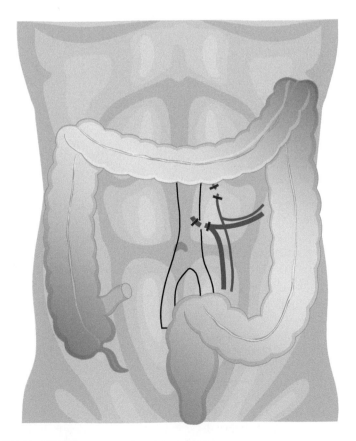

Figure 10.7 Division of inferior mesenteric vein.

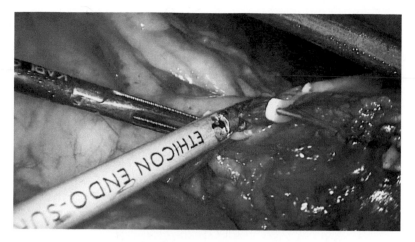

Photo 10.4 Division of inferior mesenteric vein.

MOBILISATION

LATERAL MOBILISATION

After completion of the mobilisation from medial there should be only a thin peritoneal layer left between Toldt's line and the left colon, which is divided by the monopolar hook. Dissection begins from the sigmoid colon and advances towards the spleen (Figure 10.8 and Photo 10.5). The attachments to the spleen have to be divided while staying close to the turn of the splenic flexure. Any traction on the spleen, which can result in considerable bleeding, has to be avoided.

MOBILISATION OF THE LEFT-SIDED TRANSVERSE COLON

To completely free the splenic flexure, the left-sided mesentery of the transverse colon has to be divided above the pancreas (Figure 10.9). This can be achieved from inframesocolic or from the lesser sac. We normally choose the second option. To enter the lesser sac either the gastrocolic ligament has to be divided or the greater omentum has to be detached from the transverse colon. Then, the cranial layer of the mesentery of the transverse colon is divided over the previously placed swab, which protects the pancreas (Photo 10.6). The splenic flexure should now be completely freed from any attachments.

LAPAROSCOPIC TOTAL MESORECTAL EXCISION

STEP 1: POSTERIOR DISSECTION

If the medial to lateral mobilisation of the colon has been in the right embryologic plane so far, the mesorectal plane is found by continuing the dissection caudally (Figure 10.10). To expose the area of interest, the rectum is elevated and retracted anteriorly by the assistant. The dissection proceeds close to the dorsal aspect of the superior rectal artery. Following the natural angle of the superior rectal artery leads automatically to the correct embryological plane. Only monopolar hook dissection is performed in order to always accurately visualise the separation of the correct cobweb planes. At this, the cautery is used in small and short tissue contacts that

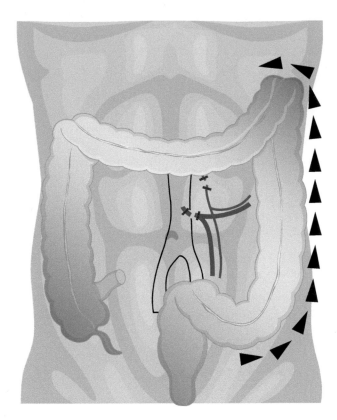

Figure 10.8 Lateral dissection line.

we call the 'paint-brush technique'. Charring of the tissue indicates that there is not enough traction and countertraction. During mesorectal excision in particular, dissection takes place on 'the yellow side of the white' cobwebs. When continuing the dissection posteriorly, it is crucial to stay between the hypogastric nerves. The posterior dissection is carried out down to the top of the Waldeyer fascia which divides the retrorectal space in an upper and a lower compartment (Photo 10.7).

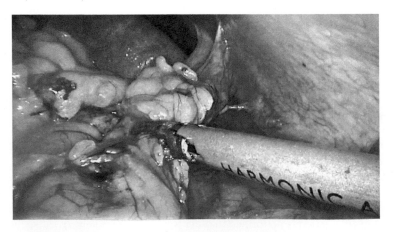

Photo 10.5 Lateral mobilisation towards the spleen.

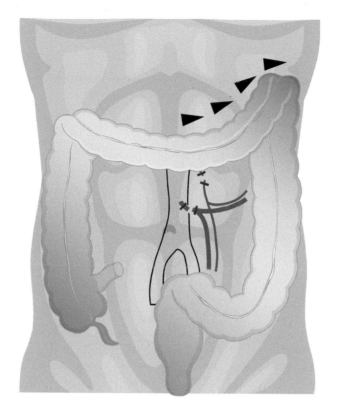

Figure 10.9 Entering the lesser sac.

STEP 2: HIGH RIGHT LATERAL DISSECTION

The rectum is retracted cephalad and towards the left (Figure 10.11 and Photo 10.8). The right pararectal peritoneum is scored (Photo 10.9). The operating surgeon applies traction on the rectum and the assistant countertraction on the sidewall. The right pararectal attachments are divided in a posterior-anterior direction. Care must be taken not to injure the right hypogastric

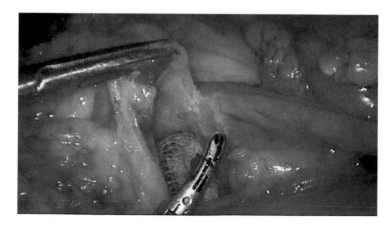

Photo 10.6 Division over pancreas swab.

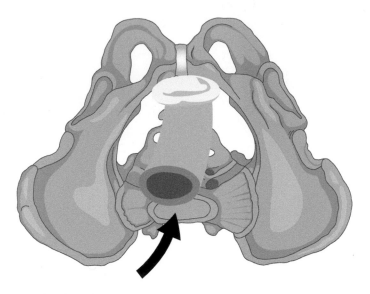

Figure 10.10 Posterior dissection.

nerve posterolaterally as it comes close to the specimen, and its normal course can be distorted due to traction on the specimen. Therefore, traction should be moderate and dissection should allow the hypogastric nerve to separate from the specimen without being injured.

STEP 3: ANTERIOR DISSECTION

The anterior dissection (Figure 10.12) requires special preparation to have optimal exposure. In order to achieve better exposure, the fundus of the uterus in female patients and the bladder's peritoneal fold in male patients is elevated to the abdominal front wall using a transabdominal suture (Photos 10.10 and 10.11). Slightly below the fold the peritoneum is scored by diathermy. Then the free peritoneal edge of the specimen is grasped by the operator's left hand and dorsal traction is applied. Meanwhile, countertraction on the anterior pelvic wall is provided by a small pledget held by the atraumatic grasper of the assistant standing on the patient's left

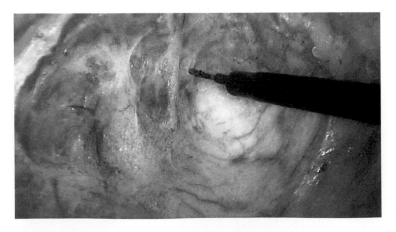

Photo 10.7 Dorsal dissection.

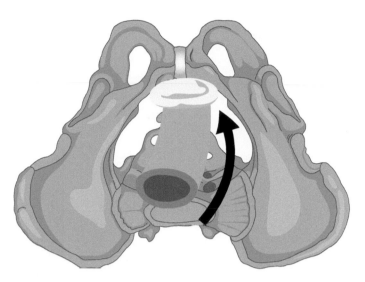

Figure 10.11 Right lateral dissection.

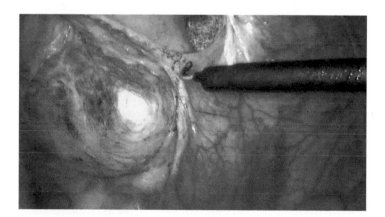

Photo 10.8 Right peritoneal fold.

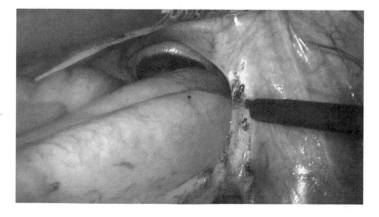

Photo 10.9 Right anterolateral peritoneal fold.

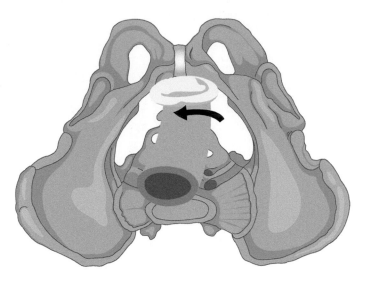

Figure 10.12 Anterior dissection.

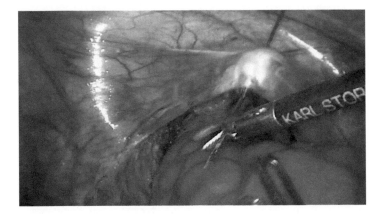

Photo 10.10 Hitch-up of anterior peritoneal fold overlying the bladder.

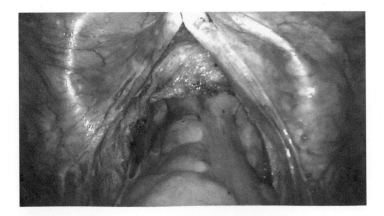

Photo 10.11 Hitch-up of bladder.

side. Anterior dissection continues as far down as sufficient traction and countertraction can be maintained.

STEP 4: HIGH LEFT LATERAL DISSECTION

Dissection continues on the left pararectal side (Figure 10.13). The rectum is retracted anteriorly and to the right. The remaining peritoneal layer that holds the specimen in place is scored and the pararectal attachments divided (Photo 10.12). Care must be taken not to dissect too wide as this may result in injury of the left ureter or the left hypogastric nerve.

STEP 5A: ANTERIOR DISSECTION IN MALES

The rectum is retracted out of the pelvis and dorsally. Countertraction on the anterior pelvic wall is applied by the assistant. In anteriorly located tumours, the plane between the Denonvilliers facia and the seminal vessels is dissected (Photo 10.13). This dissection has to be precise in order not to risk bleeding or injury of the seminal vesicles or the prostate. However, there is no need to use special energy devices other than the monopolar hook, as this tool is more precise. In posterior tumours, the dissection can also be performed dorsally to the Denonvilliers fascia as long as the mesorectal fascia stays intact.

STEP 5B: ANTERIOR DISSECTION IN FEMALES

The hitched up uterus helps to visualise the anterior pelvis. Traction and countertraction are applied in analogy to male patients. The mesorectal fascia is dissected off the posterior vaginal wall where perforation has to be avoided.

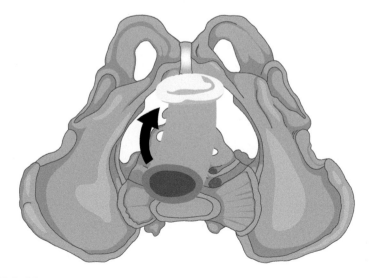

Figure 10.13 Left lateral dissection.

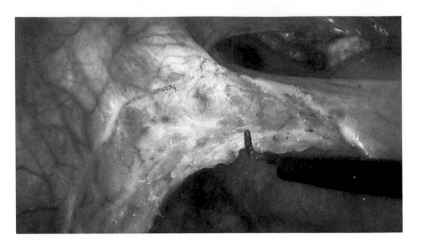

Photo 10.12 Left lateral dissection.

STEP 6: DEEP RIGHT AND LEFT POSTEROLATERAL DISSECTION, EXPOSURE OF ERIGENT PILLARS

Dissection continues anteriorly and posteriorly to the sidewall attachments so that these two areas eventually can be joined up (Photos 10.14 and 10.15). At this, the sidewall attachments are dissected in a posterior to anterior direction rather than from the top. Anterolateral and on the level of the coccyx, branches of the lower hypogastric plexus have to be preserved. Further dissection continues towards the pelvic floor.

STEP 7: COMPLETION OF DISSECTION

The rectal tube is fully mobilised circumferentially (Photo 10.16) down to the pelvic floor where dissection is accomplished by using the harmonic scalpel or other energy device as traction and countertraction are difficult to achieve. Especially the dense fibers of the ano-coccygeal raphe have to be divided to facilitate subsequent stapling (Photo 10.17).

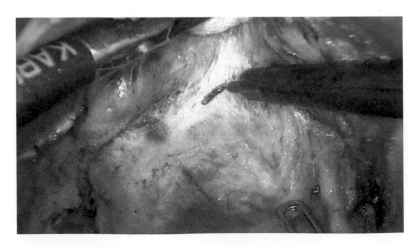

Photo 10.13 Anterior dissection in males.

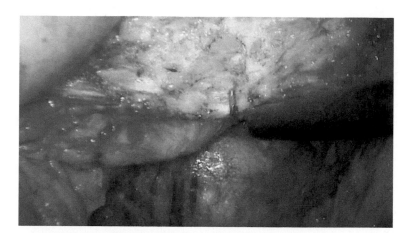

Photo 10.14 Deep right lateral dissection.

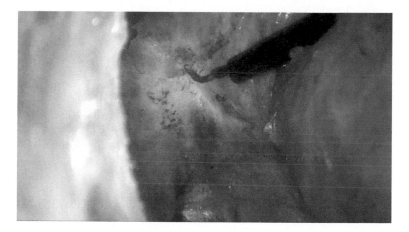

Photo 10.15 Deep left lateral dissection.

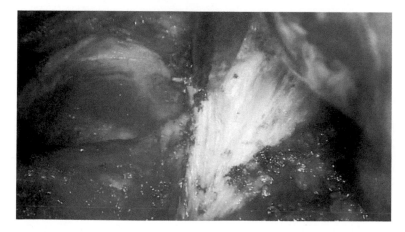

Photo 10.16 Deep anterior dissection.

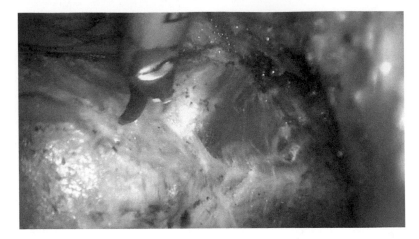

Photo 10.17 Posterior raphe.

STEP 8: RECTAL WASHOUT

The rectum is washed out and irrigated with aqueous Betadine.

STEP 9: STAPLING

An articulating endoscopic linear stapler is used to divide the rectum. In dependence of the thickness of the bowel wall, a purple or green cartridge is chosen. We prefer a cartridge length of 45 mm as it is easier to manipulate in the narrow pelvis. Most of the time, two firings are necessary. The rectum is retracted out of the pelvis and posteriorly. The stapler is inserted from the right lateral side encompassing the rectum. Then the stapler is maximally articulated and rotated counterclockwise into a vertical position (Photo 10.18). This allows for an anteroposterior staple line flush on the level of the pelvic floor (Photo 10.19). If more firings are necessary, the staple lines should meet exactly and not cross each other.

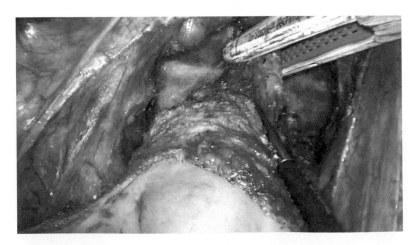

Photo 10.18 Insertion of stapler vertically.

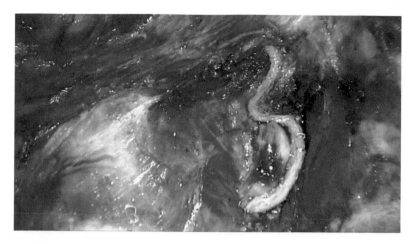

Photo 10.19 Stapler line.

ANASTOMOSIS

SAFE EXTRACTION OF THE SPECIMEN

The mobility and length of the left colon is assessed. A tension-free anastomosis is crucial. A grasper is placed at the distal end of the specimen. To extract the specimen, the umbilical port site incision is enlarged to about 5 cm. We use a self-retractor plastic wound protector (Alexis) to facilitate exteriorisation of the specimen. The specimen with the adjacent mesentery and corresponding vascular pedicle is resected. Before dividing the marginal artery at the level of the trans-section, its pulsatile blood flow is assessed.

ANASTOMOSIS

In our hands, we perform an end-to-end rather than a side-to-end circular stapler anastomosis. The stapler anvil is attached to the descending colon end using a purse-string suture. Then, the exteriorised bowel is put back into the abdominal cavity. To seal the extraction site, we pull a surgical glove over the self-retractor wound protector and use one of the glove fingers for camera port insertion. After having established the pneumoperitoneum, the descending colon is aligned anatomically and any torsion excluded. The bowel end with the anvil is brought into the pelvis to reassure that a tension-free anastomosis is possible. The stapler gun is inserted transanally by an experienced assistant. We normally use a 29-mm curved ultraluminal stapler (CDH29A). The spike has to be brought out centrally and just beside the staple line (Photo 10.20). In case of more than one staple line, the spike ideally perforates so that the meeting point of the two staple lines is incorporated into the anastomosis. The anvil is then docked to the rod (Photo 10.21). Before fully closing the stapler, the alignment and torsion of the mobilised colon are checked once again. Small bowel positioned under the descending colon should be retracted medially. Then, the stapler is fully closed and fired. The integrity of the two doughnuts is checked. A flexible sigmoidoscopy is performed to assess the integrity of the anastomosis. The pelvis is irrigated, and leaks are excluded by insufflating the colon with air (Photo 10.22). A transabdominal drain through the left 5-mm port site is placed next to the anastomosis.

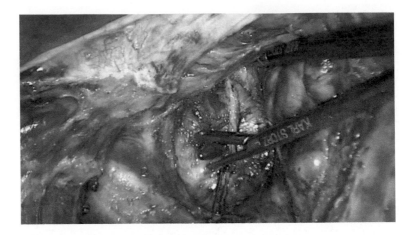

Photo 10.20 Insertion of circular stapler transanally.

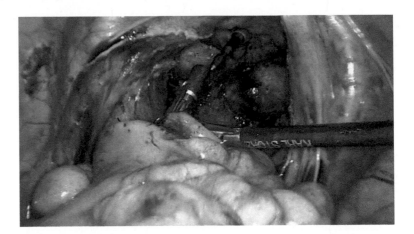

Photo 10.21 Docking anvil.

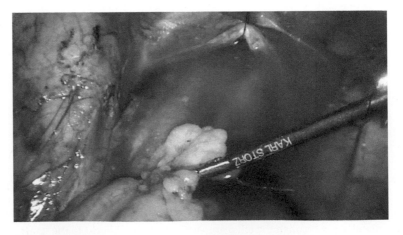

Photo 10.22 Bubble test.

LOOP ILEOSTOMY

We routinely perform a loop ileostomy after a total mesorectal excision with primary anastomosis unless an abdominoperineal resection is intended. A mobile ileal loop in proximity to the caecum is brought up to the abdominal wall for creation of an ileostomy in a standard fashion.

CONCLUSIONS

Laparoscopic rectal resection remains a challenging and technically demanding procedure. Following the principles of a standardised approach, some of these difficulties can be overcome. It is particularly useful to have this model while teaching and training this technique. Clinical evidence suggests that laparoscopic rectal cancer surgery is at par with open surgery for the oncological outcomes with the added benefit of better short-term outcomes associated with minimal access surgery. With advancement in both tools and technical skills of surgeons, it should become the gold standard of care for patients with rectal cancer.

KEY POINTS (COMMON INTRA-OPERATIVE DIFFICULTIES)

- *Lack of exposure.* Distended, hypermobile, or fluid-filled bowel loops can be difficult to handle. Incomplete mechanical bowel preparation before surgery due to delayed beginning may be one reason. Inadvertent gastric insufflation by the anaesthetist or insufficient muscle relaxation are further reasons for limited intra-peritoneal space.
- *Difficulty identifying IMA.* In patients with lipomatous mesocolon/retroperitoneal fat, identification of the reference points like the iliac artery may be made difficult. There is a risk of dissecting into the mesosigmoid, causing bleeding, or too deep behind the ureter. When in doubt, it is mostly possible to enter the correct plane at the level of the duodenojejunal junction by dissecting beneath the inferior mesenteric vein.
- *Intra-operative bleeding.* Intra-operative bleeding can vary from minor to a life-threatening incident. In laparoscopic TME, bleeding can occur during several steps:
  - When approaching the root of the IMA, surrounding lymphatic tissue may bleed when sealed insufficiently.
  - In medial to lateral mobilisation, small vessels running in between the two planes may bleed and stain the correct plane. Therefore, all these vessels have to be sealed meticulously.
  - When dissecting the IMV or identifying the border of the pancreas, forceful retraction of the mesocolon may cause injury to the IMV. Applying the Hem-o-lock clips without division of the vein before extensive dissection under the mesocolic curtain may simplify management in case of bleeding.
  - Separating the recto-prostatic (Denonvilliers) or recto-vaginal fascia may cause bleeding due to rich blood supply at these areas. Slow and meticulous dissection is obligatory.
  - If the bleeding source is not identifiable and controlled promptly, direct pressure by a swab and patience are always a good idea as in open surgery and will often stop the bleeding completely. Sometimes an extra port allows prolonged direct compression by an assistant, while the surgeon can continue the procedure around the bleeding site. On this way, bleeding control may become easier at a later stage. Uncontrollable

and haemodynamically relevant bleeders necessitate prompt conversion to an open procedure without any delay.

- *Splenic flexure mobilisation.* When mobilising the left colon, the take-down of the splenic flexure is often one of the most difficult steps. Adhesions of the greater omentum are common and bothersome. It is often prudent to take down these adhesions first in order not to get confused. The different appearances of omental and mesocolic fat are helpful to guide dissection.
- *Difficulty with posterior vaginal wall/previous hysterectomy.* Laparoscopic preparation in scarred tissue is difficult even for the expert laparoscopic surgeon. Insertion of a swab forceps into the vagina may help to delineate the course of dissection. Fortunately, iatrogenic holes in the vaginal back wall are repaired by simple suture and normally heal without any problems. Adhesions of colon to the bladder are less forgiving. Thermal dissection may lead to bladder wall necrosis and delayed bladder perforation days after surgery.
- *Tumour location/inking.* Early cancers or precancerous lesions not amenable to endoscopic resection or lesions where adequate endoscopic resection are questionable (>sm2) need preoperative tattooing by the endoscopist. If a flexible sigmoidoscope is available, clearly visible lesions are localised by endoscopy.
- *Difficulty with stapler.* In the narrow deep pelvis, stapling of the rectum at the level of the pelvic floor by one firing is often impossible. Rather than using a 60-mm cartridge, a 45-mm cartridge offers the advantage of better manoeuvrability and allows stapling at the lowest possible point. For this advantage, we deliberately take into account two firings.

TAKE-HOME MESSAGE

- Laparoscopic rectal cancer surgery remains the next frontier for the colorectal surgeons. Standardisation of technique, operative work-up, and perioperative care remain the key issues in predicting better short- and long-term oncological results. In order to get excellent oncological outcomes, the concept of precision surgery with particular attention to anatomy of the 'Holy Plane' remain the key steps to success.

REFERENCES

1. Laparoscopic surgery for colorectal cancer—NICE technology appraisal guidance [TA105]. August 2006; http://www.nice.org.uk/guidance/ta105
2. Hemandas AK, Abdelrahman T, Flashman KG, Skull AJ, Senapati A, O'Leary DP, Parvaiz A. Laparoscopic colorectal surgery produces better outcomes for high risk cancer patients compared to open surgery. *Ann Surg* 2010 Jul;252(1):84–9.
3. Lacy AM, García-Valdecasas JC, Delgado S, Castells A, Taurá P, Piqué JM, Visa J. Laparoscopy-assisted colectomy versus open colectomy for treatment of non-metastatic colon cancer: A randomised trial. *Lancet* 2002 Jun 29;359(9325):2224–9.
4. Clinical Outcomes of Surgical Therapy Study Group. A comparison of laparoscopically assisted and open colectomy for colon cancer. *N Engl J Med*. 2004 May 13;350(20):2050–9.

5. Veldkamp R, Kuhry E, Hop WC, Jeekel J, Kazemier G, Bonjer HJ et al. COlon cancer Laparoscopic or Open Resection Study Group (COLOR). Laparoscopic surgery versus open surgery for colon cancer: Short-term outcomes of a randomised trial. *Lancet Oncol* 2005 Jul;6(7):477–84.

6. Guillou PJ, Quirke P, Thorpe H, Walker J, Jayne DG, Smith AM, Heath RM, Brown JM; MRC CLASICC trial group. Short-term endpoints of conventional versus laparoscopic-assisted surgery in patients with colorectal cancer (MRC CLASICC trial): Multicentre, randomised controlled trial. *Lancet* 2005 May 14–20;365(9472):1718–26.

7. Jayne DG, Guillou PJ, Thorpe H, Quirke P, Copeland J, Smith AM, Heath RM, Brown JM; UK MRC CLASICC Trial Group. Randomized trial of laparoscopic-assisted resection of colorectal carcinoma: 3-year results of the UK MRC CLASICC Trial Group. *J Clin Oncol* 2007 Jul 20;25(21):3061–8.

8. Kang SB, Park JW, Jeong SY, Nam BH, Choi HS, Kim DW et al. Open versus laparoscopic surgery for mid or low rectal cancer after neoadjuvant chemoradiotherapy (COREAN trial): Short-term outcomes of an open-label randomised controlled trial. *Lancet Oncol* 2010 Jul;11(7):637–45.

9. Jeong SY, Park JW, Nam BH, Kim S, Kang SB, Lim SB et al. Open versus laparoscopic surgery for mid-rectal or low-rectal cancer after neoadjuvant chemoradiotherapy (COREAN trial): Survival outcomes of an open-label, non-inferiority, randomised controlled trial. *Lancet Oncol* 2014 Jun;15(7):767–74.

10. Bonjer HJ, Deijen CL, Abis GA, Cuesta MA, van der Pas MH, de Lange-de Klerk ES et al.; COLOR II Study Group. A randomized trial of laparoscopic versus open surgery for rectal cancer. *N Engl J Med* 2015 Apr 2;372(14):1324–32.

11. Chand M, Bhoday J, Brown G, Moran B, Parvaiz A. Laparoscopic surgery for rectal cancer. *J R Soc Med* 2012 Oct;105(10):429–35.

12. McGlone ER, Khan OA, Conti J, Iqbal Z, Parvaiz A. Functional outcomes following laparoscopic and open rectal resection for cancer. *Int J Surg* 2012;10(6):305–9.

13. Mackenzie H, Miskovic D, Ni M, Parvaiz A, Acheson AG, Jenkins JT, Griffith J, Coleman MG, Hanna GB. Clinical and educational proficiency gain of supervised laparoscopic colorectal surgical trainees. *Surg Endosc* 2013 Aug;27(8):2704–11.

14. Miskovic D, Ni M, Wyles SM, Kennedy RH, Francis NK, Parvaiz A et al. National training programme in laparoscopic colorectal surgery in England. Is competency assessment at the specialist level achievable? A study for the national training programme in laparoscopic colorectal surgery in England. *Ann Surg* 2013 Mar;257(3):476–82.

15. Hemandas A, Flashman KG, Farrow J, O'Leary DP, Parvaiz A. Modular training in laparoscopic colorectal surgery maximizes training opportunities without clinical compromise. *World J Surg* 2011 Feb;35(2):409–14.

16. Miskovic D, Foster J, Agha A, Delaney CP, Francis N, Hasegawa H et al. Standardization of laparoscopic total mesorectal excision for rectal cancer: A structured international expert consensus. *Ann Surg* 2015 Apr;261(4):716–22.

PART 3

CLOSURE

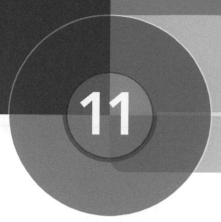

Enhanced recovery and post-operative care

11

PAUL HENDRY AND ALAN HORGAN

LEARNING OBJECTIVES

- Outline the principles of an enhanced recovery programme.
- Understand the evidence base supporting each of the individual components.

INTRODUCTION

The Enhanced Recovery After Surgery (ERAS) pathway combines a series of measures that reduce the perioperative stress response following surgery, thereby minimising post-operative organ dysfunction and promoting faster recovery (1).

This model of care covers the entire perioperative period applying evidence-based practice where available. It targets the main obstacles to recovery; pain, gastrointestinal dysfunction, and immobility. In reducing these consequences of surgery it has become possible to improve early post-operative function, reduce post-operative complications, and shorten inpatient hospital stay. This has been demonstrated in both case series from dedicated centres and by randomised controlled trials (2–5). The ongoing problem facing ERAS is that the data quality from the many studies is often low. Despite overwhelming enthusiasm and seemingly unquestionable results, there is a scarcity of true randomised controlled trials. This has resulted in the Cochrane database falling short of recommending ERAS as the standard of care (6).

ERAS AND THE LAPAROSCOPE

Although the potentially beneficial role of laparoscopic surgery within an ERAS protocol was initially challenged (7), its value has become clear with up to a 2.5-day reduction in length of stay and reduced number of readmissions from >20% to <5% (8). This, however, was a small study and the open surgery group was a historical cohort. Recent evidence from randomised controlled trials (RCTs) has confirmed this 2-day reduction in length of stay. Moreover, regression analysis confirms laparoscopy as the only predictive factor to reduce both length of stay and post-operative morbidity in segmental colectomy for colon cancer (9,10). The improved short-term outcomes confirmed in meta-analysis have to be balanced with longer operative time (11).

Benefits of laparoscopic surgery are less clear in the longer term with similar fatigue scores at 1 month after surgery irrespective of an open or laparoscopic approach (12). However, patients undergoing laparoscopic surgery are more likely to report full functional recovery within 12 months of surgery (90% in laparoscopic versus 58% of undergoing open resection), and they are more likely to have resumed activities such as driving or personal hobbies within that year (13).

Where an incision is required either for specimen extraction or conversion to open procedure, then a smaller, lower abdominal incision is less painful and results in less respiratory compromise (14). Transverse incisions may also reduce pain, but the evidence is less clear (15,16).

The laparoscope complements the enhanced recovery ethos. Following laparoscopic surgery it may be easier to promote early mobilisation and diet while open surgery still toils under the memory of traditional practice, with extended fasting and protracted bedrest. Laparoscopy improves patient outcome in relation to post-operative complications, pain, and length of stay (17–19) with comparable oncological outcomes (20). As we approach the horizon of single port access and robotic surgery, their role in colorectal surgery is still being debated, although interestingly, a clear benefit has not been demonstrated thus far.

PREADMISSION, EDUCATION, AND COUNSELLING

All ERAS protocols highlight the importance of preoperative patient education. Appropriately detailed preoperative information should be the standard in any surgical unit. Preoperative counselling has itself been demonstrated to ameliorate preoperative anxiety leading to improved post-operative pain control and reduced length of stay (21,22). Written and oral ERAS guidance emphasising the potential achievements of early recovery have been shown to promote overall protocol compliance and indeed early post-operative recovery (23,24). The role of a dedicated ERAS nurse in the preoperative counselling process improves patient satisfaction; however, it has not been shown to improve other outcomes (25). Within laparoscopic surgery, interventions aimed at improving patients' relaxation prior to surgery have been shown to improve post-operative fatigue levels (26).

PREOPERATIVE OPTIMISATION

It is generally accepted that preassessment and appropriate medical optimisation are important in maintaining standards and improving outcomes. However, often the necessity for surgery precludes any prolonged preoperative interventions. Abstinence from tobacco and alcohol prior to surgery, even in the relatively short term, has been shown to improve outcomes. Pre-habilitation exercise programmes have not been as successful (27–29).

MECHANICAL BOWEL PREPARATION

It has long been established that mechanical bowel preparation (MBP) has a deleterious effect on patients. It prolongs fasting, is distressing for the patient, places patients at risk of fluid and electrolyte imbalance, and is associated with post-operative colonic ileus. This has been well known to anaesthetists, often resulting in a requirement for large volumes of intra-operative intravenous fluids. A Cochrane Review has not demonstrated any difference in post-operative anastomotic leak rate wound infection, or mortality between those receiving MBP and those receiving nothing or a simple enema. It has been recommended that oral mechanical bowel preparation should therefore be omitted (30).

Although much of this evidence is in open surgery, one paper has already demonstrated its safety in laparoscopic surgery (31). MBP may facilitate finding smaller tumours in laparoscopic surgery; however, appropriate endoscopic tattooing should negate this issue. It may be appropriate that patients requiring defunctioning loop ileostomy should receive preoperative MBP as some surgeons feel that an enema alone is not sufficient in these patients.

FASTING/CARBOHYDRATE LOADING

Historically, patients undergoing colorectal surgery are subjected to prolonged periods of fasting before and after surgery. However, fasting from midnight does not confer any additional advantage over patients allowed clear fluids up to 2 hours before surgery. It does not reduce gastric content nor does it reduce gastric pH (32). Most anaesthetists now safely recommend clear fluids up to 2 hours before theatre (33). This is more acceptable for patients, reducing both thirst and anxiety (34).

A preoperative clear carbohydrate-based drink can be safely administered prior to this 2-hour window (35,36) and permits patients to undergo surgery in a metabolically fed state. These carbohydrate drinks have been shown to reduce post-operative insulin resistance (37), minimise protein and nitrogen losses, and preserve lean body mass and muscle strength (38). Overall patients report less thirst and anxiety (34), recover faster, and have a 1-day shorter length of stay when undergoing open abdominal surgery (39,40). They are also suitable for well-controlled diabetic patients (41). Within laparoscopic (cholecystectomy) surgery, preoperative carbohydrate (CHO) loading has been shown to reduce post-operative nausea, vomiting, and pain (42).

PRE-MEDICATION

Pre-anaesthetic sedatives may be associated with a reduced time to mobilisation and return of diet, and clearly long-acting sedatives should be avoided (43). The combination of appropriate patient education and preoperative carbohydrate loading along with avoidance of mechanical bowel preparation can help reduce preoperative patient anxiety and therefore the requirement for a preoperative sedative (34).

DEEP VEIN THROMBOSIS PROPHYLAXIS

Due to the nature of their pathology (cancer) and the mechanism of surgery (pelvic), colorectal patients undergoing surgery without thromboprophylaxis have up to 30% risk of DVT and 1% risk of fatal pulmonary embolism (PE) (44). Therefore, these patients should receive low molecular weight heparin, ideally beginning the night before surgery, combined with graduated compression stockings (45). Although there is evidence that this should continue up to a month after open surgery (46), it is disputed in laparoscopic surgery as these patients recover faster and will therefore have improved post-operative mobility (47).

ANTIMICROBIAL AND SKIN PREP

A single shot of antibiotics should be administered prior to the start of the procedure. The type of antibiotic should be decided by local protocol. In prolonged cases (more than 4 hours) or if there is major blood loss (>1500 mL) a further dose should be considered. There is no role for routine administration of prolonged courses of antibiotics (48,49).

NASOGASTRIC INTUBATION

There is no role for routine nasogastric intubation in elective colorectal surgery. In select cases, relief of gastric dilatation may aid surgery but their prolonged use results in a delay to oral intake and increases the risk of respiratory complications (50). Nasogastric tubes are associated with a delayed recovery of gastrointestinal function supported by meta-analysis in open surgery (50). There is no difference in wound infection or anastomotic leak rate. In laparoscopic surgery, compared to open surgery, the requirement for nasogastric decompression appears even less (51).

PERIOPERATIVE NORMOTHERMIA

Intra-operative hypothermia is associated with increased incidence of wound infection (52), cardiac complications (53), and bleeding (54). Intra-operative warming and maintenance of normothermia during major abdominal surgery have been demonstrated to reduce blood loss and reduce both septic (55,56) and cardiac complications (57).

Despite the fact that laparoscopic procedures may reduce exposure of the peritoneal cavity, these procedures are often longer; therefore, intra-operative warming devices should be employed as per open surgery.

STANDARD ANAESTHETIC

The complexities of anaesthesia may be beyond this chapter; however, there are desirable features of any ERAS anaesthetic. Use of short-acting induction agents and muscle relaxants combined with, when appropriate, neuromuscular blockade allow faster recovery from anaesthesia without a hangover and therefore earlier mobilisation and enteral feeding. The benefits of epidural anaesthetic in open surgery are not seen in laparoscopic surgery, where spinal anaesthetic or patient-controlled analgesia (PCA) is associated with shorter length of stay (58).

PERIOPERATIVE FLUID MANAGEMENT

Correct fluid balance plays a significant role in positive patient outcomes. The dangers of hypo-perfusion due to intravascular depletion are well established in emergency surgery. Much routine fluid management was extrapolated from this resulting in large volumes of intra-operative fluid administration. However, the effect of such dramatic volumes of water, sodium, and chloride have been shown to be deleterious in routine elective cases and can result in intestinal edema and prolonged ileus (59,60).

Aided by the reduction in fasting period, CHO/fluid loading, and omission of oral MBP a more restrictive intravenous fluid regimen has emerged as part of the ERAS protocol. Goal-directed fluid regimens through devices such as the esophageal Doppler are promoted as a method of reducing intra-operative splanchnic hypoperfusion through targeted fluid boluses. When compared with traditional fluid regimen their use demonstrates clear benefits in length of stay and recovery of gastrointestinal function (61); however, more recent papers highlight the lack of difference between outcomes for groups following a restrictive fluid regimen and goal-directed regimen (62–64). Clearly the type of fluid is also significant with appropriate balance of sodium and chloride being as important as the fluid load (65).

Fluid requirements in laparoscopic resections are potentially different to open surgery; there is less bowel handling, no open abdominal cavity, and no epidural anaesthesia. However, the head down position and pneumoperitoneum may adversely affect cardiac output requiring appropriate consideration (66).

Although there is no universally agreed point at which intravenous fluid therapy should discontinue, the return to oral intake and discontinuation of IV fluids should be undertaken at the earliest point after surgery. There is clear evidence that excessive volumes of fluids, sodium, and chloride are associated with prolonged gastrointestinal dysfunction and other measured side effects (59). It would appear that the best way to avoid such issues is early discontinuation of intravenous therapy and resumption of oral fluids (65).

INTRA-ABDOMINAL DRAINS

Traditionally drains were used as an early warning of anastomotic leakage or to drain post-operative collections; however, they are not effective for the former nor sufficient in the latter. Drains are associated with pain and discomfort and act as an impediment to mobilisation. Meta-analysis has confirmed that routine drainage of the abdominal cavity does not confer any advantage (67). There is no role for the routine use of surgical drains (67,68), even in TME. If pelvic drainage is employed irrigation-suction drains should be avoided (69).

URINARY CATHETERS

Short-term use of urethral catheters allows monitoring of fluid balance. Minimising duration of catheterisation reduces the risk of urinary tract infection and its impediment to mobilisation. Within laparoscopic surgery, early removal (day 1) is feasible, but there is an associated 20% risk of urinary retention. Predictors of retention are prolonged operation time and increased intravenous fluid volume in the intra-operative and early post-operative periods (70).

POST-OPERATIVE ANALGESIA

Duration of pain following laparoscopic surgery is shorter than for open procedures. As soon as patients tolerate oral food and therefore oral analgesia, they may be eligible for discharge (71). Although pain from port sites may be significantly less, there is usually an extraction site and about 10% of laparoscopic resections will require conversion (72). Small transverse incisions low in the abdomen should be employed where possible (14).

Within open surgery, epidural anaesthesia blocks sympathetic activity attenuating the post-operative stress response. This mainstay of open surgery is, however, associated with a longer length of hospital stay and slower return of bowel function when compared with spinal analgesia and opioid PCA in laparoscopic surgery (73). Overall the length of hospital stay reported in all participants of this study was low with even the 'slower' epidural group having a median length of stay of 3.7 days. Use of an epidural, especially a mid-thoracic epidural in patients undergoing laparoscopic colonic resection, results in an earlier passage of flatus, stool, and tolerance of diet when compared with parenteral opioid analgesia. There was also better pain relief in the first 2 post-operative days (though no difference in readiness for discharge or actual length of stay) (74). Low thoracic epidural had a similar benefit in requirement of analgesia in the first 2 days post-surgery (period of epidural); however, there was no benefit demonstrated from a gastrointestinal point of view, measured by time to first passage of stool. A single-shot injection of intrathecal morphine has been demonstrated to be as effective in relation to postoperative nausea and return of gastrointestinal function (oral diet) but with the addition of faster recovery of mobility and discharge from hospital in patients undergoing laparoscopic colorectal resection (75).

Traditionally the benefit of epidural anaesthesia has been in relation to early return of gastrointestinal function. Within laparoscopic surgery the duration of requirement for strong analgesia is much shorter, and with early recovery of gastrointestinal function oral analgesia requirements may be addressed by oral medication within 24 hours of surgery (71).

Transversus abdominis plane (TAP) blocks have become increasingly popular serving the role of covering the extraction site and in several case series have been shown to have a potential role in reducing length of hospital stay as part of an ERAS protocol (76,77). In comparison to epidural anaesthesia, continuous infusion to provide posterior TAP analgesia was non-inferior to epidural analgesia with a higher success rate for placement. There are no randomised controlled trials comparing TAP blocks with intrathecal spinal analgesia.

During the post-operative recovery period a combination of paracetamol and NSAIDs can be utilised as an opioid-sparing strategy. Although recent case series have suggested potential increase in anastomotic leaks associated with the use of NSAIDs (78), this has not been borne out in meta-analysis (79). NSAIDs have long been a useful adjunct to post-operative analgesia, and results of case series do not yet justify the discontinuation of established practices of administering NSAIDs in this setting. There is still considerable uncertainty in this area and with regard to the effects of inhibiting the COX subtypes.

PERIOPERATIVE NUTRITIONAL CARE/ILEUS

Reduction of post-operative gastrointestinal dysfunction is felt to be the key to reducing overall recovery time. Return of gastrointestinal function allows parenteral therapy to discontinue, diet to restart, and patient comfort to improve. No single element has been demonstrated to eradicate post-operative ileus; however, laparoscopic surgery results in a faster return of gastrointestinal function and resumption of diet (19).

In open surgery, routine post-operative laxatives such as oral magnesium hydroxide have been demonstrated to reduce time to first passage to stool but with no difference in oral intake or length of hospital stay (80). Use of chewing gum reduced duration of ileus (81), as does Alvimopan (opioid antagonist) in open colorectal resection (82).

Traditionally post-operative diet has been reintroduced cautiously; ERAS programmes have demonstrated that diet can safely be reintroduced immediately following surgery, even in the presence of an anastomosis. In the absence of colonic function small bowel activity will be present (83). Therefore, tolerance of oral diet may itself be a more objective evaluation of gut function.

There is no benefit to maintain patients nil by mouth following colorectal surgery, and indeed there may be a detrimental effect on mortality. Early feeding is not associated with any major complications including anastomotic leak but can be associated with increased bloating, nausea, and vomiting (84,85). Early feeding should therefore be included within a programme of care that promotes recovery of gastrointestinal function.

Post-operative nausea and vomiting (PONV) affects a significant percentage of patients undergoing major abdominal surgery (86) with females, non-smokers, and those who suffer motion sickness at greatest risk. Laparoscopy, avoidance of opiates, and minimised volumes of intravenous sodium and water are all of benefit in reducing PONV. Preoperative scoring of patients and prophylactic administration of antiemetics or simply administering prophylactic antiemetics to all patients undergoing major abdominal surgery due to the low risks and low costs associated with the drugs may improve PONV.

The mainstay of perioperative nutrition in ERAS is oral diet, which can be supplemented with oral nutritional supplements to increase caloric intake (87). These can also in part maintain nitrogen equilibrium (88). In significantly malnourished patients and if started over 10 days preoperatively, supplementary nutrition can improve post-operative infectious complications and anastomotic leak rate (89). Results related to the role of immunonutrition are heterogeneous but do suggest a potential role in reducing complications and length of hospital stay.

EARLY MOBILISATION

Even short periods of immobility are detrimental to recovery, with a negative effect on respiratory function, risk of DVT, and loss of muscle mass and strength. This requires regular reinforcement and education of patients and the overcoming of obstacles such as patient bed-side entertainment systems (90). Successful mobilisation on day 1 is a predictor of reduced length of stay (91).

SUMMARY

Many elements of the ERAS protocol have been extrapolated from other areas of research, and this results in general weakness in evidence for many components of the protocol. Similarly the shift towards laparoscopy means that again the evidence for perioperative care components is extrapolated from open surgery. Although the benefit of laparoscopic surgery within an ERAS programme was initially unclear, recent papers have demonstrated that there is a significant improvement in length of stay recovery of gastrointestinal function, complications, and abdominal wall hernias. These results are more reproducible outside the major ERAS centres where strict compliance with all ERAS elements is difficult. Moreover, in regression analysis the greatest predictor of improved outcome is indeed laparoscopic surgery. It is easier to follow other elements of protocol when combined with laparoscopy, and if you could only have one element of the ERAS protocol it would surely be the laparoscope. The feasibility of a 23-hour stay following laparoscopic major colorectal resection within and ERAS protocol has already been demonstrated (71).

KEY POINTS

- Patient education and managing expectations are paramount to a successful patient centered ERAS program of care.
- All ERAS interventions are building blocks to achieve early mobilization and return to oral intake.
- Early discharge from hospital is consequence of an early overall recovery but should not be considered the sole aim of ERAS.

TAKE-HOME MESSAGES

A properly executed enhanced recovery programme will enhance the patient's perioperative experience.

Most of the elements of the Enhanced Recovery After Surgery programme are evidence based.

Some of the traditional ways to treat patients in the perioperative period are not only unhelpful but can be harmful.

REFERENCES

1. Lassen K, Soop M, Nygren J, Cox PBW, Hendry PO, Spies C et al. Consensus review of optimal perioperative care in colorectal surgery: Enhanced Recovery After Surgery (ERAS) group recommendations. *Arch Surg* 2009;144(10):961–9.
2. Basse L, Hjort Jakobsen D, Billesbølle P, Werner M, Kehlet H. A clinical pathway to accelerate recovery after colonic resection. *Ann Surg* 2000 Jul;232(1):51–7.
3. Varadhan KK, Neal KR, Dejong CHC, Fearon KCH, Ljungqvist O, Lobo DN. The Enhanced Recovery After Surgery (ERAS) pathway for patients undergoing major elective open colorectal surgery: A meta-analysis of randomized controlled trials. *Clin Nutr* 2010 Aug 1;29(4):434–40.
4. Wind J, Polle SW, Fung Kon Jin PHP, Dejong CHC, Meyenfeldt von MF, Ubbink DT et al. Systematic review of enhanced recovery programmes in colonic surgery. *Br J Surg* 2006;93(7):800–9.
5. Serclová Z, Dytrych P, Marvan J, Nová K, Hankeová Z, Ryska O et al. Fast-track in open intestinal surgery: Prospective randomized study (Clinical Trials Gov Identifier no. NCT00123456). *Clin Nutr* 2009 28(6):618–24.
6. Spanjersberg WR, Reurings J, Keus F, van Laarhoven CJ. Fast track surgery versus conventional recovery strategies for colorectal surgery. In W.R. Spanjersberg (Ed.) *Cochrane Database of Systematic Reviews*. Wiley, Chichester, UK, 2011. Issue 2. Art. No.: CD007635.
7. Basse L, Jakobsen DH, Bardram L, Billesbølle P, Lund C, Mogensen T et al. Functional recovery after open versus laparoscopic colonic resection. *Ann Surg* 2005 Mar;241(3):416–23.

8. King PM, Blazeby JM, Ewings P, Franks PJ, Longman RJ, Kendrick AH et al. Randomized clinical trial comparing laparoscopic and open surgery for colorectal cancer within an enhanced recovery programme. *Br J Surg* 2006;93(3):300–8.

9. Vlug MS, Wind J, Hollmann MW, Ubbink DT, Cense HA, Engel AF et al. Laparoscopy in combination with fast track multimodal management is the best perioperative strategy in patients undergoing colonic surgery: A randomized clinical trial (LAFA-study). *Ann Surg* 2011 Dec;254(6):868–75.

10. Zhuang C-L, Huang D-D, Chen F-F, Zhou C-J, Zheng B-S, Chen B-C et al. Laparoscopic versus open colorectal surgery within enhanced recovery after surgery programs: A systematic review and meta-analysis of randomized controlled trials. *Surg Endosc* 2015;29(8):2091–100.

11. Reza MM, Blasco JA, Andradas E, Cantero R, Mayol J. Systematic review of laparoscopic versus open surgery for colorectal cancer. *Br J Surg* 2006 Aug;93(8):921–8.

12. Kennedy RH, Francis EA, Wharton R, Blazeby JM, Quirke P, West NP et al. Multicenter randomized controlled trial of conventional versus laparoscopic surgery for colorectal cancer within an enhanced recovery programme: EnROL. *J Clin Oncol* 2014 Jun 10;32(17):1804–11.

13. King PM, Blazeby JM, Ewings P, Kennedy RH. Detailed evaluation of functional recovery following laparoscopic or open surgery for colorectal cancer within an enhanced recovery programme. *Int J Colorectal Dis* 2008 May 9;23(8):795–800.

14. O'Dwyer PJ, McGregor JR, McDermott EW, Murphy JJ, O'Higgins NJ. Patient recovery following cholecystectomy through a 6 cm or 15 cm transverse subcostal incision: A prospective randomized clinical trial. *Postgrad Med J* 1992 Oct;68(804):817–9.

15. Brown SR, Goodfellow PB. Transverse verses midline incisions for abdominal surgery. *Cochrane Database of Systematic Reviews* 2010, Issue 4. Art. No.: CD005199.

16. Seiler CM, Deckert A, Diener MK, Knaebel H-P, Weigand MA, Victor N et al. Midline versus transverse incision in major abdominal surgery: A randomized, double-blind equivalence trial (POVATI: ISRCTN60734227). *Ann Surg* 2009 Jun;249(6):913–20.

17. Abraham NS, Young JM, Solomon MJ. Meta-analysis of short-term outcomes after laparoscopic resection for colorectal cancer. *Br J Surg* 2004 Sep 20;91(9):1111–24.

18. Kennedy GD, Heise C, Rajamanickam V, Harms B, Foley EF. Laparoscopy decreases postoperative complication rates after abdominal colectomy: Results from the national surgical quality improvement program. *Ann Surg* 2009 Apr;249(4):596–601.

19. Tjandra JJ, Chan MKY. Systematic review on the short-term outcome of laparoscopic resection for colon and rectosigmoid cancer. *Colorectal Dis* 2006 Jun;8(5):375–88.

20. Green BL, Marshall HC, Collinson F, Quirke P, Guillou P, Jayne DG et al. Long-term follow-up of the Medical Research Council CLASICC trial of conventional versus laparoscopically assisted resection in colorectal cancer. *Br J Surg* 2013 Jan;100(1):75–82.

21. Kiecolt-Glaser JK, Page GG, Marucha PT, MacCallum RC, Glaser R. Psychological influences on surgical recovery. Perspectives from psychoneuroimmunology. *Am Psychol* 1998 Nov;53(11):1209–18.

22. Egbert LD, Battit GE, Welch CE, Bartlett MK. Reduction of postoperative pain by encouragement and instruction of patients. A study of doctor-patient rapport. *N Engl J Med* 1964 Apr 16;270(16):825–7.

23. Halaszynski TM, Juda R, Silverman DG. Optimizing postoperative outcomes with efficient preoperative assessment and management. *Crit Care Med* 2004 Apr;32(Supplement):S76–S86.

24. Disbrow EA, Bennett HL, Owings JT. Effect of preoperative suggestion on postoperative gastrointestinal motility. *West J Med* 1993 May;158(5):488–92.

25. Forster AJ, Clark HD, Menard A, Dupuis N, Chernish R, Chandok N et al. Effect of a nurse team coordinator on outcomes for hospitalized medicine patients. *Am J Med* 2005 Oct;118(10):1148–53.

26. Kahokehr A, Broadbent E, Wheeler BRL, Sammour T, Hill AG. The effect of perioperative psychological intervention on fatigue after laparoscopic cholecystectomy: A randomized controlled trial. *Surg Endosc* 2012 Jun;26(6):1730–6.

27. Tonnesen H, Rosenberg J, Nielsen HJ, Rasmussen V, Hauge C, Pedersen IK et al. Effect of preoperative abstinence on poor postoperative outcome in alcohol misusers: Randomised controlled trial. *BMJ* 1999 May 15;318(7194):1311–6.

28. Lindström D, Sadr Azodi O, Wladis A, Tønnesen H, Linder S, Nåsell H et al. Effects of a perioperative smoking cessation intervention on postoperative complications: A randomized trial. *Ann Surg* 2008 Nov;248(5):739–45.

29. Lindström D, Sadr Azodi O, Bellocco R, Wladis A, Linder S, Adami J. The effect of tobacco consumption and body mass index on complications and hospital stay after inguinal hernia surgery. *Hernia* 2007 Apr;11(2):117–23.

30. Güenaga KF, Matos D, Wille-Jørgensen P. Mechanical bowel preparation for elective colorectal surgery. *Cochrane Database of Systematic Reviews* 2011, Issue 9. Art. No.: CD001544. DOI: 10.1002/14651858.CD001544.pub4.

31. Zmora O, Lebedyev A, Hoffman A, Khaikin M, Munz Y, Shabtai M et al. Laparoscopic colectomy without mechanical bowel preparation. *Int J Colorectal Dis* 2006 Oct;21(7):683–7.

32. Brady M, Kinn S, Stuart P. Preoperative fasting for adults to prevent perioperative complications. *Cochrane Database of Systematic Reviews* 2003, Issue 4. Art. No.: CD004423.

33. Søreide E, Ljungqvist O. Modern preoperative fasting guidelines: A summary of the present recommendations and remaining questions. *Best Pract Res Clin Anaesthesiol* 2006 Sep;20(3):483–91.

34. Hausel J, Nygren J, Lagerkranser M, Hellström PM, Hammarqvist F, Almström C et al. A carbohydrate-rich drink reduces preoperative discomfort in elective surgery patients. *Anesth Analg* 2001 Nov;93(5):1344–50.

35. Nygren J, Thorell A, Jacobsson H, Larsson S, Schnell PO, Hylén L et al. Preoperative gastric emptying. Effects of anxiety and oral carbohydrate administration. *Ann Surg* 1995 Dec;222(6):728–34.

36. Lobo DN, Hendry PO, Rodrigues G, Marciani L, Totman JJ, Wright JW et al. Gastric emptying of three liquid oral preoperative metabolic preconditioning regimens measured by magnetic resonance imaging in healthy adult volunteers: A randomised double-blind, crossover study. *Clin Nutr* 2009 Dec 1;28(6):636–41. Available at http://eutils.ncbi.nlm.nih.gov/entrez/eutils/elink.fcgi?dbfrom=pubmed&id=19500889&retmode=ref&cmd=prlinks

37. Soop M, Nygren J, Thorell A, Weidenhielm L, Lundberg M, Hammarqvist F et al. Preoperative oral carbohydrate treatment attenuates endogenous glucose release 3 days after surgery. *Clin Nutr* 2004 Aug;23(4):733–41.

38. Yuill KA, Richardson RA, Davidson HIM, Garden OJ, Parks RW. The administration of an oral carbohydrate-containing fluid prior to major elective upper-gastrointestinal surgery preserves skeletal muscle mass postoperatively—A randomised clinical trial. *Clin Nutr* 2005 Feb;24(1):32–7.

39. Noblett SE, Watson DS, Huong H, Davison B, Hainsworth PJ, Horgan AF. Pre-operative oral carbohydrate loading in colorectal surgery: A randomized controlled trial. *Colorectal Dis* 2006 Sep;8(7):563–9.

40. Svanfeldt M, Thorell A, Hausel J, Soop M, Rooyackers O, Nygren J et al. Randomized clinical trial of the effect of preoperative oral carbohydrate treatment on postoperative whole-body protein and glucose kinetics. *Br J Surg* 2007;94(11):1342–50.

41. Gustafsson UO, Nygren J, Thorell A, Soop M, Hellström PM, Ljungqvist O et al. Pre-operative carbohydrate loading may be used in type 2 diabetes patients. *Acta Anaesthesiol Scand* 2008 Mar 7;52(7):946–51.

42. Singh BN, Dahiya D, Bagaria D, Saini V, Kaman L, Kaje V et al. Effects of preoperative carbohydrates drinks on immediate postoperative outcome after day care laparoscopic cholecystectomy. *Surg Endosc* 2015;29(11):3267–72.

43. Walker KJ, Smith AF. Premedication for anxiety in adult day surgery. *Cochrane Database of Systematic Reviews* 2009, Issue 7. Art. No.: CD002192.

44. Fleming FJ, Kim MJ, Salloum RM, Young KC, Monson JR. How much do we need to worry about venous thromboembolism after hospital discharge? A study of colorectal surgery patients using the National Surgical Quality Improvement Program database. *Dis Colon Rectum* 2010 Oct;53(10):1355–60.

45. Rasmussen MS, Jørgensen LN, Wille-Jørgensen P. Prolonged thromboprophylaxis with low molecular weight heparin for abdominal or pelvic surgery. In M.S. Rasmussen MS (Ed.) *Cochrane Database of Systematic Reviews* 2009, Issue 1. Art. No.: CD004318.

46. Huo MH, Muntz J. Extended thromboprophylaxis with low-molecular-weight heparins after hospital discharge in high-risk surgical and medical patients: A review. *Clin Ther* 2009 Jun;31(6):1129–41.

47. Verheijen PM, Stevenson ARL, Stitz RW, Clark DA, Clark AJ, Lumley JW. Prolonged use of thromboprophylaxis may not be necessary in laparoscopic colorectal surgery. *Int J Colorectal Dis* 2011 Jun;26(6):755–9.

48. Nelson RL, Glenny AM, Song F. Antimicrobial prophylaxis for colorectal surgery. In RL Nelson (Ed.) *Cochrane Database of Systematic Reviews* 2009, Issue 1. Art. No.: CD001181.

49. Steinberg JP, Braun BI, Hellinger WC, Kusek L, Bozikis MR, Bush AJ et al. Timing of antimicrobial prophylaxis and the risk of surgical site infections: Results from the Trial to Reduce Antimicrobial Prophylaxis Errors. *Ann Surg* 2009 Jul;250(1):10–6.

50. Verma R, Nelson RL. Prophylactic nasogastric decompression after abdominal surgery. *Cochrane Database of Systematic Reviews* 2007, Issue 3. Art. No.: CD004929. DOI: 10.1002/14651858.CD004929.pub3.

51. Shussman N, Brown MR, Johnson MC, Da Silva G, Wexner SD, Weiss EG. Does nasogastric tube decompression get used less often with laparoscopic and hand-assisted compared with open colectomy? *Surg Endosc* 2013 Dec;27(12):4564–8.

52. Kurz A, Sessler DI, Lenhardt R. Perioperative normothermia to reduce the incidence of surgical-wound infection and shorten hospitalization. Study of Wound Infection and Temperature Group. *N Engl J Med* 1996 May 9;334(19):1209–15.

53. Frank SM, Fleisher LA, Breslow MJ, Higgins MS, Olson KF, Kelly S et al. Perioperative maintenance of normothermia reduces the incidence of morbid cardiac events. A randomized clinical trial. *JAMA* 1997 Apr 9;277(14):1127–34.

54. Schmied H, Kurz A, Sessler DI, Kozek S, Reiter A. Mild hypothermia increases blood loss and transfusion requirements during total hip arthroplasty. *Lancet* 1996 Feb 3;347(8997):289–92.

55. Melling AC, Ali B, Scott EM, Leaper DJ. Effects of preoperative warming on the incidence of wound infection after clean surgery: A randomised controlled trial. *Lancet* 2001 Sep 15;358(9285):876–80.

56. Wong PF, Kumar S, Bohra A, Whetter D, Leaper DJ. Randomized clinical trial of perioperative systemic warming in major elective abdominal surgery. *Br J Surg* 2007;94(4):421–6.

57. Elmore JR, Franklin DP, Youkey JR, Oren JW, Frey CM. Normothermia is protective during infrarenal aortic surgery. *J Vasc Surg* 1998 Dec;28(6):984–92, discussion 992–4.

58. Levy BF, Scott MJP, Fawcett WJ, Day A, Rockall TA. Optimizing patient outcomes in laparoscopic surgery. *Colorectal Dis* 2011 Nov;13 Suppl 7(s7):8–11.

59. Lobo DN. Fluid overload and surgical outcome. *Ann Surg* 2009 Feb;249(2):186–8.

60. Brandstrup B, Tønnesen H, Beier-Holgersen R, Hjortsø E, Ørding H, Lindorff-Larsen K et al. Effects of intravenous fluid restriction on postoperative complications: Comparison of two perioperative fluid regimens. *Ann Surg* 2003 Nov;238(5):641–8.

61. Noblett SE, Snowden CP, Shenton BK, Horgan AF. Randomized clinical trial assessing the effect of Doppler-optimized fluid management on outcome after elective colorectal resection. *Br J Surg* 2006;93(9):1069–76.

62. Srinivasa S, Taylor MHG, Singh PP, Yu T-C, Soop M, Hill AG. Randomized clinical trial of goal-directed fluid therapy within an enhanced recovery protocol for elective colectomy. *Br J Surg* 2013 Jan;100(1):66–74.

63. Brandstrup B, Svendsen PE, Rasmussen M, Belhage B, Rodt SÅ, Hansen B et al. Which goal for fluid therapy during colorectal surgery is followed by the best outcome: Near-maximal stroke volume or zero fluid balance? *Br J Anaesth* 2012 Aug;109(2):191–9.

64. Challand C, Struthers R, Sneyd JR, Erasmus PD, Mellor N, Hosie KB, Minto G. Randomized controlled trial of intraoperative goal-directed fluid therapy in aerobically fit and unfit patients having major colorectal surgery. *Br J Anaesth* 2012;108(1):53–62.

65. Powell-Tuck J, Gosling P, Lobo DN, Allison SP. British consensus guidelines on intravenous fluid therapy for adult surgical patients. GIFTASUP. 2008. Ref Type: Report; 2011.

66. Levy BF, Fawcett WJ, Scott MJP, Rockall TA. Intra-operative oxygen delivery in infusion volume-optimized patients undergoing laparoscopic colorectal surgery within an enhanced recovery programme: The effect of different analgesic modalities. *Colorectal Dis* 2012 Jul;14(7):887–92.

67. Karliczek A, Jesus EC, Matos D, Castro AA, Atallah AN, Wiggers T. Drainage or non-drainage in elective colorectal anastomosis: A systematic review and meta-analysis. *Colorectal Dis* 2006 May;8(4):259–65.

68. Jesus EC, Karliczek A, Matos D, Castro AA, Atallah AN. Prophylactic anastomotic drainage for colorectal surgery. *Cochrane Database of Systematic Reviews* 2004, Issue 4. Art. No.: CD002100.

69. Yeh CY, Changchien CR, Wang J-Y, Chen J-S, Chen HH, Chiang J-M et al. Pelvic drainage and other risk factors for leakage after elective anterior resection in rectal cancer patients: A prospective study of 978 patients. *Ann Surg* 2005 Jan;241(1):9–13.

70. Kin C, Rhoads KF, Jalali M, Shelton AA, Welton ML. Predictors of postoperative urinary retention after colorectal surgery. *Dis Colon Rectum* 2013 Jun;56(6):738–46.

71. Levy BF, Scott MJP, Fawcett WJ, Rockall TA. 23-hour-stay laparoscopic colectomy. *Dis Colon Rectum* 2009 Jul;52(7):1239–43.

72. Buchanan GN, Malik A, Parvaiz A, Sheffield JP, Kennedy RH. Laparoscopic resection for colorectal cancer. *Br J Surg* 2008 Jul;95(7):893–902.

73. Levy BF, Scott MJ, Fawcett W, Fry C, Rockall TA. Randomized clinical trial of epidural, spinal or patient-controlled analgesia for patients undergoing laparoscopic colorectal surgery. *Br J Surg* 2011 May 17;98(8):1068–78.

74. Taqi A, Hong X, Mistraletti G, Stein B, Charlebois P, Carli F. Thoracic epidural analgesia facilitates the restoration of bowel function and dietary intake in patients undergoing laparoscopic colon resection using a traditional, nonaccelerated, perioperative care program. *Surg Endosc* 2007 Feb;21(2):247–52.

75. Virlos I, Clements D, Beynon J, Ratnalikar V, Khot U. Short-term outcomes with intrathecal versus epidural analgesia in laparoscopic colorectal surgery. *Br J Surg* 2010 Sep;97(9):1401–6.

76. Conaghan P, Maxwell-Armstrong C, Bedforth N, Gornall C, Baxendale B, Hong L-L et al. Efficacy of transversus abdominis plane blocks in laparoscopic colorectal resections. *Surg Endosc* 2010 Oct;24(10):2480–4.

77. Favuzza J, Brady K, Delaney CP. Transversus abdominis plane blocks and enhanced recovery pathways: Making the 23-h hospital stay a realistic goal after laparoscopic colorectal surgery. *Surg Endosc* 2013 Jul;27(7):2481–6.

78. Gorissen KJ, Benning D, Berghmans T, Snoeijs MG, Sosef MN, Hulsewe KWE et al. Risk of anastomotic leakage with non-steroidal anti-inflammatory drugs in colorectal surgery. *Br J Surg* 2012 May;99(5):721–7.

79. Burton TP, Mittal A, Soop M. Nonsteroidal anti-inflammatory drugs and anastomotic dehiscence in bowel surgery: Systematic review and meta-analysis of randomized, controlled trials. *Dis Colon Rectum* 2013 Jan;56(1):126–34.

80. Hendry PO, van Dam RM, Bukkems SF, McKeown DW, Parks RW, Preston T et al.; Enhanced Recovery After Surgery (ERAS) Group. Randomized clinical trial of laxatives and oral nutritional supplements within an enhanced recovery after surgery protocol following liver resection. *Br J Surg* 2010 Aug;97(8):1198–206.

81. Parnaby CN, MacDonald AJ, Jenkins JT. Sham feed or sham? A meta-analysis of randomized clinical trials assessing the effect of gum chewing on gut function after elective colorectal surgery. *Int J Colorectal Dis* 2009 May;24(5):585–92.

82. Delaney CP, Wolff BG, Viscusi ER, Senagore AJ, Fort JG, Du W et al. Alvimopan, for postoperative ileus following bowel resection: A pooled analysis of phase III studies. *Ann Surg* 2007 Mar;245(3):355–63.

83. Catchpole BN. Review article. *Aust N Z J Surg* 1989 Mar;59(3):199–208.

84. Andersen HK, Lewis SJ, Thomas S. Early enteral nutrition within 24 h of colorectal surgery versus later commencement of feeding for postoperative complications. *Cochrane Database of Systematic Reviews* 2006, Issue 4. Art. No.: CD004080.

85. Lewis SJ, Andersen HK, Thomas S. Early enteral nutrition within 24 h of intestinal surgery versus later commencement of feeding: A systematic review and meta-analysis. *J Gastrointest Surg* 2009 Mar;13(3):569–75.

86. Chatterjee S, Rudra A, Sengupta S. Current concepts in the management of postoperative nausea and vomiting. *Anesthesiol Res Pract* 2011;2011(10):748031–10.

87. Smedley F, Bowling T, James M, Stokes E, Goodger C, O'Connor O et al. Randomized clinical trial of the effects of preoperative and postoperative oral nutritional supplements on clinical course and cost of care. *Br J Surg* 2004 Jul 27;91(8):983–90.

88. Soop M, Carlson GL, Hopkinson J, Clarke S, Thorell A, Nygren J et al. Randomized clinical trial of the effects of immediate enteral nutrition on metabolic responses to major colorectal surgery in an enhanced recovery protocol. *Br J Surg* 2004 Sep 20;91(9):1138–45.

89. Waitzberg DL, Saito H, Plank LD, Jamieson GG, Jagannath P, Hwang T-L et al. Postsurgical infections are reduced with specialized nutrition support. *World J Surg* 2006 Aug;30(8):1592–604.

90. Papaspyros S, Uppal S, Khan SA, Paul S, O'Regan DJ. Analysis of bedside entertainment services' effect on post cardiac surgery physical activity: A prospective, randomised clinical trial. *Eur J Cardiothorac Surg* 2008 Nov;34(5):1022–6.
91. Smart NJ, White P, Allison AS, Ockrim JB, Kennedy RH, Francis NK. Deviation and failure of enhanced recovery after surgery following laparoscopic colorectal surgery: Early prediction model. *Colorectal Dis* 2012 Oct;14(10):e727–34.

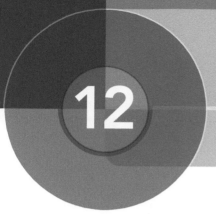

12

Complications of laparoscopic colorectal surgery

S NADIA GILANI AND TOM CECIL

LEARNING OBJECTIVES

- Increase awareness and improve management of the complications of laparoscopic colorectal surgery.

INTRODUCTION

Laparoscopic colorectal surgery when performed by adequately experienced and skilled surgeons reduces length of stay, enhances recovery, and results in better cosmesis following bowel resection. The National Institute for Health and Care Excellence (NICE) in 2006 recommended that every patient suitable for laparoscopic colorectal cancer resection should be offered the option of laparoscopic surgery (1). This led to the formation of the Lapco National training programme that has contributed to a dramatic increase in the numbers of laparoscopic colorectal resections in the United Kingdom. However, limitations inherent to laparoscopic surgery, such as loss of depth perception, reduced tactile feedback, and reduced range of motion have created a necessity for new training modalities as minimally invasive surgery requires skills that are not routinely used during open surgery. It has been well documented that inexperienced surgeons on their learning curve have a higher risk of both laparoscopic-specific and colorectal-specific complications (2). Mentorship training programmes can reduce the number of cases and complications required to achieve competency in laparoscopic surgery, but complications can still occur in the most skilled and experienced hands. In this chapter we hope that increasing awareness of the potential complications of laparoscopic colorectal surgery will allow avoidance of many of these pitfalls and better management should they occur.

TUMOUR LOCALISATION

Identifying the location and extent of colonic disease is the primary step in planning the treatment strategy. Precise localisation of tumours is a critical aspect of the minimally invasive approach to colorectal surgery. Loss of tactile sensation and inability to palpate colonic tumours in laparoscopic surgery makes identification of colorectal pathology more difficult than in open surgery (3). Furthermore, the setup of equipment and the positioning of the patient generally focus on one side of the abdomen. Some investigators have reported removing the wrong segment of the colon during laparoscopic colorectal surgery (4). In a survey involving members of the American Society of Colon and Rectal Surgeons, 6.5% of the respondents reported resection of a wrong segment in at least one case, which required conversion to a standard laparotomy for a correct operation (5). This is almost certainly an underreported complication, and the authors have personally had two cases in over 1000 cases where a tumour was left behind due to dual pathology (see Case report 1).

Although colonoscopy is accurate for localisation of tumours in the rectum and caecum, it is inaccurate in other areas (6). The error rate of preoperative colonoscopy in locating tumours is as high as 12%, whereas the incidence of synchronous lesions in patients with colorectal

CASE REPORT 1: Missed tumour

Colonoscopy revealed a stenosing splenic flexure tumour in a 71-year-old male, and a computed tomography (CT) scan identified a T3 transverse colon cancer (Photo 12.1); the man was treated with a laparoscopic right hemicolectomy. He presented 6 months later with abdominal distension. A CT scan confirmed an obstructing sigmoid cancer (Photo 12.2) that, with hindsight, was missed at the time of initial diagnosis and at surgery and was the stenosing cancer seen at initial colonoscopy with a separate synchronous transverse colon tumour (Photo 12.3).

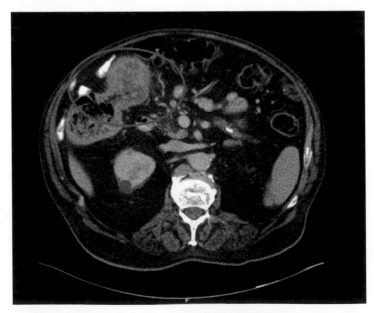

Photo 12.1 Tumour at proximal transverse colon thought to be tumour seen at colonoscopy.

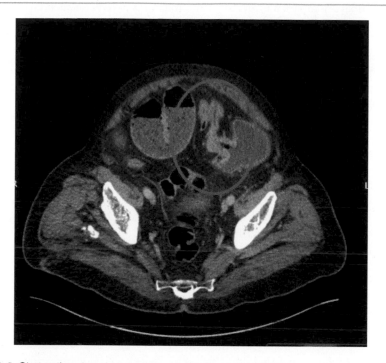

Photo 12.2 Obstructing sigmoid tumour presenting 6 months later.

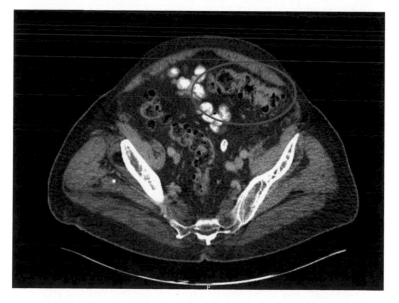

Photo 12.3 Sigmoid tumour was visible on original scan, with hindsight note the long loopy sigmoid that led the endoscopist to believe he was at the splenic flexure.

cancer varies from 2% to 11% for carcinoma and from 27% to 60% for adenoma (7). The risk of synchronous lesions may make preoperative colonoscopy even less reliable, especially if there is an obstructive lesion.

Vignati et al. reported a 14% error rate for preoperative endoscopic localisation that led to difficulty with intra-operative localisation in 4.8% of the cases, which was mainly due to non-palpable lesions (8). Therefore, even though colonoscopy can accurately localise lesions, its success is heavily dependent on the experience of the endoscopist.

An effective localisation method preoperatively is essential for preventing this problem. Ideally the surgeon who is going to perform the surgery should meet the patient in the outpatient setting and correlate all the preoperative information. The entire colon and rectum should be evaluated, usually with colonoscopy. If the colonoscopy is incomplete or there is any doubt, a barium enema or computed tomography colonography should be performed (9). A staging CT of chest, abdomen, and pelvis should be performed and the tumour location correlated with the endoscopic assessment. Colonic tattooing can precisely localise small or flat colonic malignancies or previously snared malignant polyps that are not visible on CT scan (10). The tattoo persists for a long time, which enables the subsequent surgical operation to be suitably scheduled (Photo 12.4).

The use of preoperative tattooing for localising colorectal lesions in both conventional and laparoscopic approaches has been reported to be effective in more than 90% of cases (11). Accurate tattooing helps the surgeon identify an appropriate margin of tissue for resection, avoiding additional manipulation of tumour intra-operatively. Multiple, carefully placed, intramural injections should be made circumferentially in the colonic wall close to the lesion to maximise the surgeon's ability to localise the lesion (12). It is important that the operator clearly documents the relationship of the tattoo to the lesion. There are various tinting methods, but two-step ink injection, which includes injecting saline before reported as less than 1% (13). There have been episodic reports of perforation, colon abscess, or inflammatory pseudo-tumour with necrosis of the perivisceral fat. Transmural injections can result in diffuse intra-abdominal staining and may predispose to adhesion formation (14).

Surgeons should be prepared to use colonoscopy intra-operatively if the tumour is not localised preoperatively, or the preoperative marking cannot be reliably identified during surgery. However, an intra-operative colonoscopy performed during laparoscopic surgery carries an increased risk of conversion due to bowel distention and the potential for post-operative

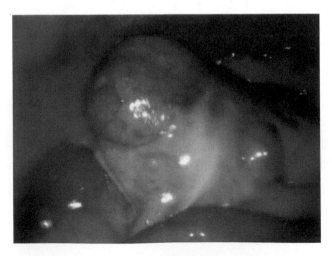

Photo 12.4 Colonic tattoo in caecum seen at laparoscopy.

complications such as prolonged bowel distension and increased morbidity (15). When intra-operative colonoscopy is utilised, carbon dioxide insufflation may be preferable as its rapid absorption lessens the risk of a persistently distended colon interfering with surgery (16).

BLEEDING

Bleeding presents a set of challenges to the laparoscopic colorectal surgeon that with proper thought preparation and an effective strategy to a large part can be prevented or managed safely. Meticulous attention to haemostasis allows the surgeon to maintain a good view and stay in the correct planes. Major vascular injury generally occurs due to a combination of poor views, difficult or distorted anatomy, or technical failure when sealing major vessels.

MINOR BLEEDING

Accumulation of small volumes of blood leads to absorption of light staining of planes resulting in a poor view and impaired appreciation of the anatomy. Careful use of diathermy or energy devices to take down adhesions and open planes followed by blunt dissection in the correct plane needs to be accompanied by careful haemostasis of minor bleeding. Small tonsil swabs that easily fit down a 10-mm port can help to dry planes and provide gentle retraction (Photo 12.5).

The use of suction to aspirate blood rather than irrigation that spreads and dilutes blood helps maintain good vision. Particular care needs to be taken in handling the omentum, small bowel and colonic mesentery, and splenic adhesions, avoiding tearing, and if bleeding occurs controlling with careful diathermy or sealing, or if persistent packing with swabs in addition to the pressure of the pneumoperitoneum. Maintenance of good haemostasis allows a good view of planes but also avoids the risk of post-operative haemorrhage from small vessels that may bleed without the intra-operative pneumoperitoneum.

A preventable common minor vascular injury is to the inferior epigastric vessels. These injuries can be easily prevented as they occur during placement of secondary trocars, which should be placed under direct vision and with prior transillumination of the abdominal wall. Careful laparoscopic inspection of the port sites at the end of the procedure when trocars are removed can identify bleeding that can be controlled by use of an EndoClose if necessary (Photo 12.6).

MAJOR BLEEDING

Vascular injury is a major cause of death from laparoscopy, with reported mortality rate of 15% (17). The incidence of bleeding can vary from 0.5% (Barcelona Trial) to 4.8% (CLASICC Trial) (18).

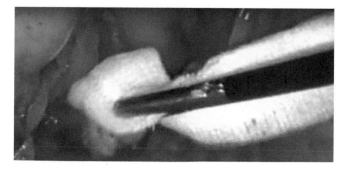

Photo 12.5 Use of tonsil swab for haemostasis.

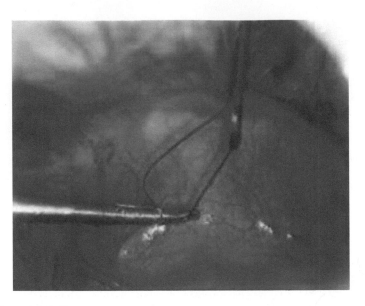

Photo 12.6 Use of EndoClose.

Due to the tamponade effect of pneumoperitoneum on major blood vessels, bleeding may not be apparent until after the laparoscopic procedure has been concluded. Thin people are at higher risk of vascular injury as the distance between the anterior abdominal wall and the retroperitoneal structures can be as little as 2 cm (19). The right common iliac artery is particularly prone to injury as it takes off directly below the umbilicus. Vascular injuries occur mainly in patients undergoing oncologic resections and those with difficult anatomic exposure, owing to previous operation, recurrent tumour, or radiation therapy. Injuries to the main vascular structures like the aorta, inferior vena cava, and the iliac vessels may need immediate conversion and surgical repair. Most of the injuries can be repaired by primary suture. Few injuries need interposition grafts, patch venoplasty, or venous ligation. Abandoning the use of blind Veres needles in favour of an open Hassan technique (20) reduces the risk of direct injury to major vessels.

During right-sided dissection the superior mesenteric artery can be mistaken for the ileocolic artery. A submesenteric tunnel beneath the mesentery of the right colon can be created to clarify the vascular anatomy when in doubt. Retracting on the caecum will usually identify and demonstrate the ileocolic trunk. Injury to the superior mesenteric trunk can devascularise the small bowel and requires immediate reconstruction by a vascular surgeon.

Careful identification of the aorta, iliacs, and inferior mesenteric artery (IMA) are important in left-sided resection. It is possible especially with the patient tilted to the right to dissect under the left iliac vessel, mistaking it for the IMA (see Case report 2).

CASE REPORT 2: Bleeding

A 52-year-old female recently discharged after laparoscopic surgery for sigmoid cancer by a locum surgeon in a neighboring hospital presented as an emergency with a cold left foot. Her CT scan revealed transection of left iliac (Photo 12.7) confirmed on CT arteriogram (Photo 12.8), and left hydronephrosis and hydroureter (Photo 12.9). She underwent vascular reconstruction and ureteric reconstruction.

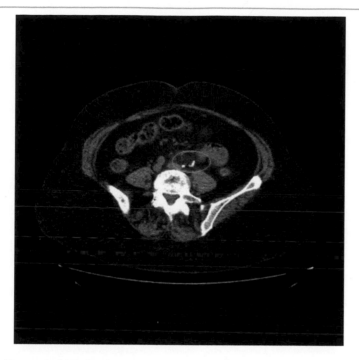

Photo 12.7 Transaction with staples across left iliac artery.

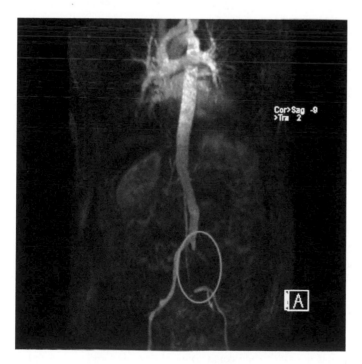

Photo 12.8 Arteriogram confirming transection of left external iliac.

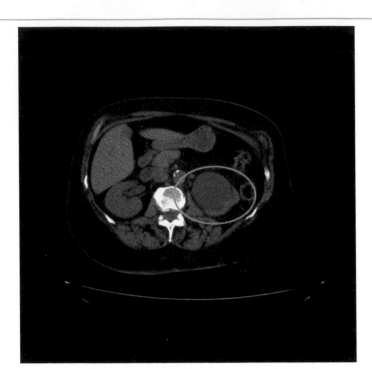

Photo 12.9 Left hydronephrosis on CT due to transection of left ureter with the artery.

During left-sided resections, especially when performing a high tie ligation to obtain maximum bowel length, care must be taken to preserve the left branch of the middle colic artery. Dissection on the anterior surface of the pancreas and opening the transmesenteric window into the lesser sac is carried out to prevent devascularisation of the entire left colon by damage to the marginal artery. The splenic vein on the posterior part of the pancreas can be damaged while expanding the submesenteric tunnel cranially during medial to lateral mobilisation of the left colon. If the submesenteric plane is opened correctly, the gonadal vessels will remain in their retroperitoneal position.

STRATEGY FOR PREVENTION AND TREATMENT

It is necessary to have a range of equipment available in order to deal with bleeding. Rapid access to diathermy, energy devices, EndoLoop, laparoscopic clips, laparoscopic suturing, and laparoscopic vascular staplers as well as swabs, suction, and additional ports are all necessary. Using the correct devices to divide or seal a major vessel is important. Large vessels need a vascular stapler if larger than the available clips or if too big to seal with energy devices. Calcified atherosclerotic vessels may not seal with energy devices, and if there is doubt an EndoLoops or clip can be simply applied to secure a vascular pedicle following division.

Maintenance of haemostasis, good views, and the correct planes and anatomy are crucial to avoiding injury or catastrophic incorrect division of major vessels. If there is doubt and the origin of the vessel is not clear, then conversion is warranted and the surgeon should avoid the temptation to use a 'blind' vascular stapler.

If dealing with major bleeding, the surgeon should stay calm and start with control of the bleeding using an adequate suction system without irrigation. The open principles of distal and proximal control of bleeding are equally applicable to laparoscopic surgery, and additional ports may be required for this. Once controlled and adequately visualised the bleeding can often be stopped with clips, an EndoLoop, or sutures. Venous bleeding even when substantial can often be controlled and stopped with adequate pressure and/or the use of haemostatic agents such as TachoSil. If the bleeding cannot be controlled or there is doubt over the anatomy, there should be no hesitation in conversion to open surgery and pressure should be applied while this happens.

ANASTOMOTIC LEAKAGE

Anastomotic leakage is a serious and potentially life-threatening but recognised complication of colorectal surgery (Photo 12.10).

Literature review suggests various incidence rates of anastomotic leak in laparoscopic colorectal surgery, ranging between 2.5% and 12%, and account for almost one third of the mortality post-colorectal surgery (21,22). It is more common following left-sided anastomosis than right-sided ileocolic anastomosis, with anastomosis located within the rectum being over seven times more likely to leak than an ileocolic (right colon) anastomosis and almost four times more likely to leak than a colo-colic anastomosis (left colon) (23). For pelvic procedures, the leak rate also depends on the height of anastomosis. Lopez-Kostner et al. in 1998 showed that anastomotic leak was 8.4% in below 10-cm anastomosis when compared with 0.14% leak rate in above 15 cm (24). Rullier et al. found that the risk of leakage was six times higher for anastomoses situated less than 5 cm from the anal verge than for those situated above 5 cm (25).

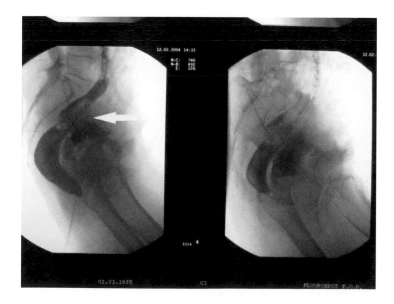

Photo 12.10 A contrast radiograph showing an anastomotic leak.

Recent studies have suggested that anastomotic leak rate after surgery for colorectal cancer compromises not only the immediate prognosis but in addition may be associated with worse long-term survival and/or increased rate of local recurrence after a potentially curative resection (26).

Extensive information is available on the risk factors for anastomotic leakage which apply equally to laparoscopic or open surgery and include male gender, smoking, obesity, alcohol abuse, preoperative radiotherapy, preoperative steroid and non-steroidal anti-inflammatory drugs use, longer duration of operation, preoperative transfusion, contamination of operative field, and timing during duty hours (27).

RIGHT-SIDED ANASTOMOSIS

Most right-sided ileocolic anastomoses are performed extracorporeally, either stapled or hand sewn. This requires adequate mobilisation of both the terminal ileum and transverse colon with division of the right colic or right colic branch of the middle colic. Failure to adequately mobilise the colon can lead to damage of the mesentery and its blood supply and technical difficulty in performing the anastomosis if the bowel cannot be adequately delivered out of the abdomen. Care needs to be taken to ensure there is no twist on the mesentery, and it is worth spending time prior to the specimen extraction to orientate and align the mobilised colon at the end of laparoscopic mobilisation. Right-sided colonic mobilisation with a medial to lateral approach can be challenging and tiring to surgeons on their learning curves, and it is important to concentrate for the anastomosis. Teamwork on the learning curve and recognition of surgeon fatigue are important in reducing anastomotic complications.

LEFT-SIDED ANASTOMOSIS

Laparoscopic left-sided anastomoses are most often stapled intra-corporeally. Once again adequate colonic mobilisation is key to allow exteriorisation of the specimen and placement of the anvil into a well-vascularised bowel, avoiding traction injuries to the mesentery and marginal artery blood supply. To achieve this it may be necessary to fully mobilise the splenic flexure and then ensure a tension-free anastomosis. It is the author's practice to do this first if it is likely to be necessary. It is also important to adequately mobilise the rectal stump and divide the mesocolon or mesorectum to allow the gun to adequately reach a well-vascularised but free staple line.

Rectal anastomosis poses several challenges for the laparoscopic surgeon (28). Morino et al. reported a leak rate of 17% in 100 rectal cancers below 12 cm but as high as 25% in those who were not defunctioned (29). Leroy et al. reported a leak rate of 20% in 98 rectal cancers below 15 cm (17/83 anterior resections) (30). Both studies concluded that all laparoscopic rectal cancers should be defunctioned. The current laparoscopic stapling devices angulate to a maximum of 65° making horizontal division of the rectum difficult from the side. This is often overcome by stapling in a vertical direction, which may impact on blood supply to the rectal stump. The staples are deployed at the same time as the in-built knife divides the rectum, and this often results in several firings with the potential to create steps and dog-ears in the transverse staple line. If this is not excised by the circular stapler, the integrity of the anastomosis may be compromised. Division of the rectum without tactile sensation can also make it difficult to locate the tumour and also be sure that an adequate length of mesorectum is being removed. Opinion is divided regarding the requirement for a rectal washout. In our unit it is the policy to staple below the tumour, wash out the rectum below the closed staple line, and then divide through the washed rectum. This is probably of greater importance in dealing with very low tumours with a close distal margin. This triple stapling technique is possible but challenging laparoscopically.

Anecdotally there is a feeling among laparoscopic colorectal surgeons that the problems with anastomotic technique alluded to above do impact on rectal anastomotic leakage. The consequences of leakage are important both in terms of immediate morbidity and mortality and in terms of long-term functional outcome with 50% of patients with a clinical leak ending up with a permanent stoma in our unit. An alternative for low anastomosis reported by some surgeons is the use of open staplers through a slightly wider Pfannenstiel incision than that required for extraction of the specimen. This combines some of the potential advantages of a laparoscopic approach such as laparoscopic splenic flexure mobilisation with a reduced risk of splenic trauma, good views, reduced blood loss, and a reduced incision with better cosmesis and earlier recovery, and also allows the use of horizontal staplers, rectal washout, and easy formation of a defunctioning ileostomy if necessary (31). In our experience this can work well but requires adequate laparoscopic mobilisation of the rectum of the pelvic floor for easy use of a small Pfannenstiel for triple stapling.

LAPAROSCOPIC MANAGEMENT OF ANASTOMOTIC LEAKS

The laparoscopic surgeon should have a low threshold to suspect an anastomotic leak if there is any deviation from the expected path of recovery following laparoscopic surgery. Due to the associated significant morbidity, it is imperative to identify the problem as early as possible, and a CT scan is most commonly used to obtain an objective test of anastomotic integrity. Leaks needing surgical treatment can be managed with re-laparoscopy and washout with defunctioning and drainage and/or resection of the anastomosis. A study by Wind et al. showed evidence that laparoscopic re-intervention may be beneficial for patients with anastomotic leakage following laparoscopic colorectal surgery (32). The study showed that the morbidity rate, hospital stay, intensive care unit admission, and incisional hernia rate were reduced in the laparoscopic when compared with the open re-intervention group. However, the decision must be made early to improve patient outcome.

WOUND COMPLICATIONS

SUPERFICIAL WOUND INFECTION

Superficial wound infections are one of the common complications of colorectal surgery. The combination of contamination, major surgery, and debilitated patients is associated with a high risk of wound infection. The incidence is significantly lowered with the frequent use of plastic wound protectors during specimen retrieval after laparoscopic resection. Superficial wound infections can be recognised by cellulitis, induration, tenderness, and purulent discharge from the wound. They are mostly managed by opening the wound and draining the pus with daily dressings to allow healing by secondary intention.

PORT SITE/INCISIONAL HERNIA

Port site hernias are associated with significant morbidity (34). The incidence of port site hernia is reported between 0.65% and 2.8% (33). It has a proportional rise with the increase in size of the port site incision and trocar. They can present early in the post-operative period or late during follow-up.

CASE REPORT 3: Port site hernia

A 64-year-old woman developed prolonged ileus post-laparoscopic colorectal procedure. A CT scan confirmed a port site hernia and a return to theatre was necessary to repair the defect (Photo 12.11). The hernia was not clinically evident even assessing after the CT.

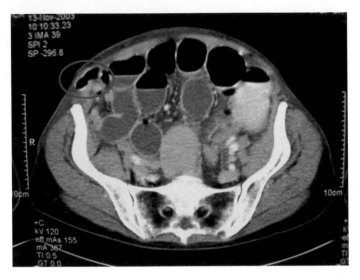

Photo 12.11 CT demonstrating 10-mm port site hernia that was not palpable clinically despite the patient being thin.

The clinical course of port site hernia depends on the extent and nature of herniated content. Symptoms of early trocar site hernia consist of a painful lump at the trocar site or persistent or intermittent ileus when a CT scan is helpful in diagnosis (34). Management includes surgical exploration of the port site with laparoscopy or laparotomy depending on the extent and nature of herniated content. It is recommended that the fascial layer of all trocar sites greater than 5 mm must be closed (35). In obese patients, devices such as the EndoClose can facilitate. Awareness of the need to close the fascia in all ports over 5 mm can eliminate this complication, which significantly increases morbidity and prolong hospital stay (see Case report 3).

PORT SITE METASTASIS

The exact incidence of port site metastases following laparoscopic colorectal surgery for cancer is unknown but is believed to be as low as 0.85% (36). The rate of port site complications following laparoscopic surgery is about 21 per 100,000 cases. Although port site metastases are now reported less frequently, this unfortunate consequence of laparoscopic colorectal surgery for cancer can still occur if precautions to prevent it from happening are not taken. Reports have shown most port site metastases are associated with advanced tumours involving the serosal layer and diffuse peritoneal carcinomatosis (37). This may suggest that it is related to the advanced nature of the tumour rather than to the laparoscopic technique. Other factors and mechanisms that may contribute to the occurrence of port site metastases have also been suggested. These include the technical skills of the surgeon, tumour manipulation during laparoscopy, hematological spread, and the adherence of tumour cells to the surface of the instruments or ports with subsequent implantation in the trocar sites (38). The type of trocars (reusable or disposable, traumatic or non-traumatic), pneumoperitoneum, and the rate of CO_2 gas insufflation may also play a role in tumour dissemination (39).

Meticulous surgical technique during entry and exit at all the port sites, minimal tumour handling, extraction of the specimen through an abdominal incision wide enough to allow easy passage of the specimen, isolation of the specimen within a bag before its extraction, wound protection during tumour extraction, and the desufflation of pneumoperitoneum before trocar extraction have resulted in a decrease in port site metastases.

CONVERSION

No agreed-on definition of conversion exists, and debate remains as to the impact of conversion on outcomes and if it should be considered a complication. The authors' definition of conversion is 'an incision made in order to progress intra-abdominal dissection', often an extended Pfannenstiel or targeted incision, if there is lack of progress. Conversion rates under 10% have been reported for elective laparoscopic colectomy for cancer (40), while others have reported higher conversion rates up to 25% when benign, malignant, elective, and emergency colorectal resections are included (41). Predictors of conversion include body mass index (BMI), ASA grade, type of resection, and surgeon seniority. Buchanan et al. identified rectal cancer resections to have an increased conversion rate over colonic resections, but this decreased with experience (42). Tekkis et al. have reported an almost twofold conversion rate for left-sided resection than for right-sided resection: 15.3% versus 8.1% (43).

Conversions did not significantly increase morbidity or prolong hospital stay in 3526 resections (44). In contrast in the Conventional versus Laparoscopic-Assisted Surgery in Colorectal Cancer (CLASICC) trial, conversion was associated with a poor outcome and high mortality of 10% (18).

Others have proposed the concept of laparoscopy followed by 'adaption' to the most appropriate operation be it open, a hybrid combination of laparoscopy with targeted incision, or a totally laparoscopic procedure.

Early conversion especially when progress is not being made is recommended to minimise errors due to tiredness or technical difficulties and should not be perceived as a complication. In contrast there is little doubt that late conversion is associated with increased morbidity, mortality, operating time, and hospital stay and should be considered a complication (45).

When in doubt, either help is required from a more experienced laparoscopic surgeon or a decision should be made to convert early. In situations where technical difficulties arise requiring late conversion, help from a senior colleague who is neither tired nor 'emotionally involved' is recommended.

IATROGENIC INJURIES

There are limited data regarding iatrogenic injuries in laparoscopic colorectal surgery. The main risks are vessel injury, damage to the spleen, and bowel and ureteric injuries.

INJURY TO BOWEL

Iatrogenic perforation of the bowel can occur either during small bowel manipulation or adhesiolysis by inadvertent diathermy injury or direct trauma during the operation. The incidence is reported as <0.01% (46). The risk of thermal injury is increased with conventional monopolar diathermy and has several shortcomings in laparoscopic surgery including difficulty with haemostasis and excessive smoke production, making the use of additional tools like sutures or clips necessary. The bipolar vessel sealers are popular devices as they shorten dissection time and are cost effective. Damage to the small bowel can also occur by direct trauma from instrumentation of the bowel out of the field of view or by pulling the small bowel back into the trocars during manipulation. In laparoscopic cases bowel injuries should be sutured immediately with primary repair or resection with anastomosis considered, as it might be difficult to localise later. During laparoscopy the pneumoperitoneum may prevent enteric contents leaking from the small bowel, and injuries can easily be missed. Care must be taken as delayed presentation of bowel injuries carries a high mortality.

SPLENIC INJURY

The incidence of iatrogenic splenic injury is underestimated as it is often not documented. The incidence is reported as 0.006% (47). Splenic injury results in increased blood loss, longer hospital stay, and higher mortality and infection rates and is therefore considered a poor prognostic factor (47). Splenic injury can be reduced by achieving good exposure, avoiding undue traction, and careful division of splenic ligaments and adhesions. If the spleen is injured preservation is desirable and often feasible with careful diathermy, packing, and use of newer haemostatic agents such as TachoSil, which can be used down a laparoscopic port. In the authors' experience splenic injury is less common with laparoscopic mobilisation than the open approach due to better views and the reduced likelihood of tearing off adhesions.

URETERIC INJURY

It is estimated that ureter damage occurs in 1% of the laparoscopic colorectal resections (48). Failure to recognise the ureter secondary to severity of disease process, inadequate dissection techniques, or inability to identify anatomical relations can result in ureteric injury. As a rule of thumb no structure should be divided in the pelvis or near the pelvic brim without identification of the ureter along its entire course. Identification of the ureter can be accomplished by recognising the iliac artery as the ureter will always cross it and ureteric vermiculation will help differentiate it from gonadal vessels (see Case report 4).

Ureteric stents or illumination can also be planned preoperatively to help in identification in difficult cases. Ureteric injuries have a very low morbidity rate if promptly identified and repaired. Post-operatively, ureteric injury can be diagnosed by measuring creatinine levels in drain fluid, ultrasound of the kidneys, or CT or intravenous urogram.

CASE REPORT 4: Ureteric injury

A patient discharged day 5 after laparoscopic anterior resection presented unwell with peritonitis day 8. A CT revealed free fluid and a pelvic collection around the anastomosis (Photo 12.12).

A laparotomy revealed widespread purulent fluid with no obvious anastomotic dehiscence, and the abdomen was washed out, a stoma fashioned, and a large drain left in the pelvis. The drainage fluid changed from pus to urine, and an intravenous urogram was organised that showed a ureteric injury (Photo 12.13) that was successfully stented. The patient made a full recovery.

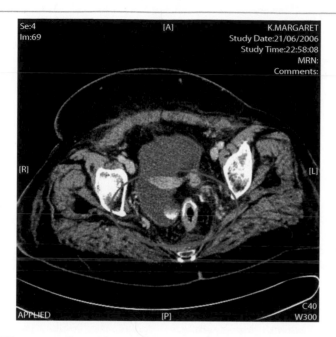

Photo 12.12 CT scan revealing pelvic collection next to the anastomosis in a patient with peritonitis.

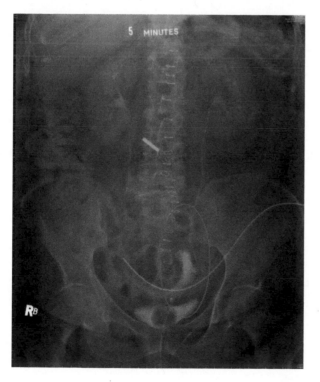

Photo 12.13 An intravenous urogram revealing a delayed left ureteric injury almost certainly due to inadvertent thermal injury.

SUMMARY

We hope that by discussing and sharing our experience of complications we will have given you insight into the many potential pitfalls of laparoscopic colorectal surgery and will help you to avoid some of these errors but also importantly to be aware and recognise when they do occur. It has always been our policy to involve senior colleagues in helping to manage our complications: a 'phone-a-friend approach', and we hope that with awareness and this approach, you can manage your patients as safely as possible and achieve the best outcomes for them.

KEY POINTS

- Preoperative localisation of the tumour is paramount.
- The right equipment and preparation are key for haemostasis and vascular control.
- Concentrate for the anastomosis and defunction if at all worried.
- Close all the fascia for all ports greater than 5 mm and use a wound protector.
- Convert if struggling or in doubt and never hesitate to ask for a second opinion.

TAKE-HOME MESSAGE

Laparoscopy is a tool not a religion.

REFERENCES

1. Green CJ et al. The influence of NICE guidance on the uptake of laparoscopic surgery for colorectal cancer. *J Public Health* 2009;31(4):541–5.
2. Miskovic D et al. Learning curve and case selection in laparoscopic colorectal surgery: Systematic review and international multicenter analysis of 4852 cases. *Dis Colon Rectum* 2012;55(12):1300–10.
3. Cho YB et al. Tumor localization for laparoscopic colorectal surgery. *World J Surg* 2007;31(7):1491–5.
4. Wexner SD et al. Laparoscopic colorectal surgery—Are we being honest with our patients? *Dis Colon Rectum* 1995;38(7):723–7.
5. Louis MA et al. Correlation between preoperative endoscopic and intraoperative findings in localizing colorectal lesions. *World J Surg* 2010;34(7):1587–91.
6. Piscatelli N, Hyman N, Osler T. Localizing colorectal cancer by colonoscopy. *Arch Surg* 2005;140(10):932–5.
7. Vaziri K, Choxi SC, Orkin BA. Accuracy of colonoscopic localization. *Surg Endosc* 2010;24(10):2502–5.
8. Vignati P, Welch JP, Cohen JL. Endoscopic localization of colon cancers. *Surg Endosc* 1994;8(9):1085–7.
9. Brady AP, Stevenson GW, Stevenson I. Colorectal cancer overlooked at barium enema examination and colonoscopy: A continuing perceptual problem. *Radiology* 1994;192(2):373–8.
10. Johnson CD et al. Accuracy of CT colonography for detection of large adenomas and cancers. *N Engl J Med* 2008;359(12):1207–17.

11. Arteaga-Gonzalez I et al. The use of preoperative endoscopic tattooing in laparoscopic colorectal cancer surgery for endoscopically advanced tumors: A prospective comparative clinical study. *World J Surg* 2006;30(4):605–11.

12. Yeung JM, Maxwell-Armstrong C, Acheson AG. Colonic tattooing in laparoscopic surgery—Making the mark? *Colorectal Dis* 2009;11(5):527–30.

13. Park JW et al. The usefulness of preoperative colonoscopic tattooing using a saline test injection method with prepackaged sterile India ink for localization in laparoscopic colorectal surgery. *Surg Endosc* 2008;22(2):501–5.

14. Feingold DL et al. Safety and reliability of tattooing colorectal neoplasms prior to laparoscopic resection. *J Gastrointest Surg* 2004;8(5):543–6.

15. Brullet E et al. Intraoperative colonoscopy in patients with colorectal cancer. *Br J Surg* 1992;79(12):1376–8.

16. Souma Y et al. The role of intraoperative carbon dioxide insufflating upper gastrointestinal endoscopy during laparoscopic surgery. *Surg Endosc* 2009;23(10):2279–85.

17. Krishnakumar S, Tambe P. Entry complications in laparoscopic surgery. *J Gynecol Endosc Surg* 2009;1(1):4–11.

18. Reza MM et al. Systematic review of laparoscopic versus open surgery for colorectal cancer. *Br J Surg* 2006;93(8):921–8.

19. Philips PA, Amaral JF. Abdominal access complications in laparoscopic surgery. *J Am Coll Surg* 2001;192(4):525–36.

20. McKernan JB, Champion JK. Access techniques: Veress needle—Initial blind trocar insertion versus open laparoscopy with the Hasson trocar. *Endosc Surg Allied Technol* 1995;3(1):35–8.

21. Schlachta CM et al. Could laparoscopic colon and rectal surgery become the standard of care? A review and experience with 750 procedures. *Can J Surg* 2003;46(6):432–40.

22. Vignali A et al. Factors associated with the occurrence of leaks in stapled rectal anastomoses: A review of 1014 patients. *J Am Coll Surg* 1997;185(2):105–13.

23. Goriainov V, Miles AJ. Anastomotic leak rate and outcome for laparoscopic intra-corporeal stapled anastomosis. *J Minim Access Surg* 2010;6(1):6–10.

24. Lopez-Kostner F et al. Total mesorectal excision is not necessary for cancers of the upper rectum. *Surgery* 1998;124(4):612–7; discussion 617–8.

25. Rullier E et al. Risk factors for anastomotic leakage after resection of rectal cancer. *Br J Surg* 1998;85(3):355–8.

26. Law WL et al. Anastomotic leakage is associated with poor long-term outcome in patients after curative colorectal resection for malignancy. *J Gastrointest Surg* 2007;11(1):8–15.

27. Konishi T et al. Risk factors for anastomotic leakage after surgery for colorectal cancer: Results of prospective surveillance. *J Am Coll Surg* 2006;202(3):439–44.

28. Cecil TD, Taffinder N, Gudgeon AM. A personal view on laparoscopic rectal cancer surgery. *Colorectal Dis* 2006;8(Suppl 3):30–2.

29. Morino M et al. Laparoscopic total mesorectal excision: A consecutive series of 100 patients. *Ann Surg* 2003;237(3):335–42.

30. Leroy J et al. Laparoscopic total mesorectal excision (TME) for rectal cancer surgery: Long-term outcomes. *Surg Endosc* 2004;18(2):281–9.

31. Cartmell MT et al. A defunctioning stoma significantly prolongs the length of stay in laparoscopic colorectal resection. *Surg Endosc* 2008;22(12):2643–7.

32. Wind J et al. Laparoscopic reintervention for anastomotic leakage after primary laparoscopic colorectal surgery. *Br J Surg* 2007;94(12):1562–6.

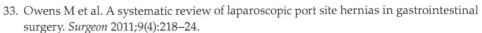

33. Owens M et al. A systematic review of laparoscopic port site hernias in gastrointestinal surgery. *Surgeon* 2011;9(4):218–24.
34. Bevan KE et al. Respect for the laparoscopic port site: Lessons in diagnosis, management, and prevention of port-site hernias following laparoscopic colorectal surgery. *J Laparoendosc Adv Surg Tech A* 2010;20(5):451–4.
35. Yamamoto M, Minikel L, Zaritsky E. Laparoscopic 5-mm trocar site herniation and literature review. *JSLS* 2011;15(1):122–6.
36. Cook TA, Dehn TC. Port-site metastases in patients undergoing laparoscopy for gastrointestinal malignancy. *Br J Surg* 1996;83(10):1419–20.
37. Whelan RL, Lee SW. Review of investigations regarding the etiology of port site tumor recurrence. *J Laparoendosc Adv Surg Tech A* 1999;9(1):1–16.
38. Tseng LN et al. Port-site metastases. Impact of local tissue trauma and gas leakage. *Surg Endosc* 1998;12(12):1377–80.
39. Balli JE et al. How to prevent port-site metastases in laparoscopic colorectal surgery. *Surg Endosc* 2000;14(11):1034–6.
40. King PM et al. Randomized clinical trial comparing laparoscopic and open surgery for colorectal cancer within an enhanced recovery programme. *Br J Surg* 2006;93(3):300–8.
41. Newman CM et al. The majority of colorectal resections require an open approach, even in units with a special interest in laparoscopic surgery. *Colorectal Dis* 2012;14(1):29–34; discussion 42–3.
42. Buchanan GN et al. Laparoscopic resection for colorectal cancer. *Br J Surg* 2008;95(7):893–902.
43. Tekkis PP, Senagore AJ, Delaney CP. Conversion rates in laparoscopic colorectal surgery: A predictive model with, 1253 patients. *Surg Endosc* 2005;19(1):47–54.
44. Jones OM, Lindsey I, Cunningham C. Laparoscopic colorectal surgery. *BMJ* 2011;343:d8029.
45. Tan PY et al. Laparoscopically assisted colectomy: A study of risk factors and predictors of open conversion. *Surg Endosc* 2008;22(7):1708–14.
46. Levy BS, Soderstrom RM, Dail DH. Bowel injuries during laparoscopy. Gross anatomy and histology. *J Reprod Med* 1985;30(3):168–72.
47. Malek MM et al. Comparison of iatrogenic splenectomy during open and laparoscopic colon resection. *Surgical Laparosc Endosc Percutan Tech* 2007;17(5):385–7.
48. Nam YS, Wexner SD. Clinical value of prophylactic ureteral stent indwelling during laparoscopic colorectal surgery. *J Korean Med Sci* 2002;17(5):633–5.

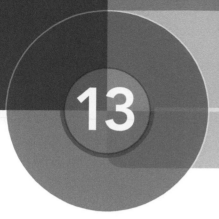

13

Laparoscopic surgery for inflammatory bowel disease (IBD)

JAMES HOLLINGSHEAD, TAN ARULAMPALAM, AND SHARMILA GUPTA

LEARNING OBJECTIVES

- Understand the role of laparoscopic surgery in inflammatory bowel disease.
- Appreciate the range of available surgical options, and the factors that influence the choice of operation.
- Understand the technical differences between colorectal resections for colitis and for colorectal cancer.
- Appreciate the available approaches to laparoscopic resection for Crohn's disease.
- Appreciate the place of laparoscopic surgery within the wider context of the multidisciplinary management of IBD.

INTRODUCTION

Many of the laparoscopic operations carried out on those with inflammatory bowel disease (IBD) are similar to those carried out for cancer described elsewhere in this book. The patient cohort however is very different. While they are frequently younger with a better underlying physiological reserve, they may also be significantly malnourished as a result of their IBD, immunosuppressed from their treatment, or acutely unwell with a substantial systemic inflammatory response. A multidisciplinary team (MDT) approach should be taken, and where possible management of these patients should be discussed at an MDT meeting involving gastroenterologists, surgeons with a specialist interest in IBD, radiology, specialist IBD nurses, and a member of the nutrition team. Although this is not covered in detail in this operative book, it is vital to achieving good outcomes.

Laparoscopic surgery in IBD has potential advantages over open surgery in terms of faster recovery and improved cosmesis (1,2). The cosmetic advantage can be particularly important in a group of younger patients coming to terms with the diagnosis of a chronic illness. Additionally many patients with inflammatory bowel disease will need multiple abdominal operations over their lifetime, and the reduced adhesion formation with each laparoscopic procedure is a major benefit for the next operation.

Standard enhanced recovery programmes are often used post-operatively in those undergoing laparoscopic (and open) surgery for IBD, but there is little evidence in this setting and, especially in Crohn's disease, they may need to be modified to take account of specific circumstances (3). Where there has been significant preoperative bowel distension or extensive inflammation there will be an increased risk of post-operative ileus. Where gastric distension or significant ileus develops post-operatively, it is important that this is recognised and that intravenous fluids and nasogastric drainage are established. Where ileus is prolonged, or a patient develops complications, then early consideration should be given to parenteral nutrition, especially as these patients will frequently have been malnourished preoperatively.

COLITIS

EMERGENCY SURGERY

PREOPERATIVE MANAGEMENT

Patients with acute severe colitis who require emergency surgery will usually have had initial medical treatment under a gastroenterology team. Where medical management fails to improve the patient's condition, the patient will need surgery. The planning of a colectomy takes time, and patients can take time to agree to an operation. It is therefore important that the surgical team and stoma nurse specialist are involved at an early stage in all patients who may require emergency colectomy (4).

The physiological condition of a patient, who is not responding to medical treatment of his or her colitis, will usually deteriorate over time. The earlier that surgery can be carried out, the better the condition of the patient, and therefore the outcomes. This needs to be balanced against the risk of carrying out a colectomy on a patient who would have recovered if only medical treatment had been given additional time to take effect. The ultimate outcome of delay is perforation with peritonitis. This currently accounts for around 5% of emergency colectomies in the United Kingdom, but most patients should be having surgery well before this stage in order to be in a reasonable condition at the time of their surgery (5). Of those admitted to hospital with acute colitis who recover with medical management alone, one in three will have elective or emergency colectomy in the future, usually within the next 2 years.

The decision of when to operate is multidisciplinary. Historically any patient who was not responding to intravenous steroids within 3 days would have surgery planned within the next few days. A stool frequency of more than eight per day on the third day of IV steroids was 85% predictive of colectomy on that admission (6).

Availability of additional medical therapies has complicated this decision-making process. A calcineurin inhibitor (Tacrolimus or Cyclosporin) or infliximab will result in a response in 70%–80% of patients who have not responded to steroids alone, but of those who respond one third will subsequently have a colectomy within the next year, and the lifetime colectomy risk is 60%–88% (7,8). Consideration of treatment with one of these agents is reasonable despite the additional delay before surgery. Cyclosporin is cheaper, and has the theoretical advantage of a half-life of only a few hours, and can therefore be fully excreted before surgery begins, and infliximab is associated with a small increased risk of septic perioperative complications. Whichever is used it is important that they are introduced early so that a rapid assessment of effect may be carried out, and that where surgery is required it is not delayed for too long. Provided this is the case colectomy outcomes in those who have had failed rescue therapy are similar to those who proceed to colectomy after treatment with IV steroids alone (9). Use of multiple sequential rescue therapies is not recommended by current guidelines due to the risk of delayed surgery with associated increased morbidity (4).

Where acute colitis does not respond to medical treatment, surgery will be required. This group of patients is acutely unwell, immunosuppressed, and often poorly nourished. Pelvic surgery and panproctocolectomy is to be avoided. The operation of choice is therefore a subtotal colectomy with end ileostomy, and where possible this should be carried out laparoscopically.

THEATRE SETUP

The surgeon will require access to both left and right sides during surgery. Both arms therefore need wrapping by the patient's sides. As a minimum, a second screen is required in addition to the main laparoscopic stack so that the operative side can change without needing to move the main stack. While access to the perineum is not usually required, having the ability for the surgeon or an assistant to stand between the patient's legs may be helpful for access to the transverse colon or splenic flexure. The intra-abdominal space is often limited if there is any ileus associated with the acute colitis, and a nasogastric tube in addition to the urinary catheter may be useful.

The required ports will be a combination of those needed for a left- and a right-sided operation: three lateral ports on each side. With a 5-mm camera these can all be 5-mm diameter apart from the right iliac fossa port, which should be 12 mm to allow use of a stapler. Additional 5-mm ports carry minimal morbidity and should be inserted where they make dissection easier. An additional port at the umbilicus is often useful for transverse colon and splenic flexure dissection. Many surgeons prefer to use a 10-mm camera that will therefore require 10-mm port placement.

COLONIC MOBILISATION

There is no need to carry out high mesenteric division in an acute colitis. A medial to lateral dissection as carried out for a cancer resection therefore mobilises much more mesentery than is necessary. With a lateral to medial dissection the mesenteric division can take place flush with the bowel with much less mobilisation.

Surgeon's preference varies as to the order of mobilisation. The transverse colon is often the area that surgeons are least familiar with from cancer resections, and the anatomy of the middle colic vessels may be variable. Some prefer to start with the transverse colon dissection, while others prefer to start with the right or left side and work sequentially. The resection carried out is the same regardless of the order.

The right colon is best mobilised laterally to medially. The small bowel should be swept into the pelvis and left iliac fossa, and some lateral tilt and a small amount of head-up may be helpful here. The colon should be gently retracted towards the midline and the white line of the lateral peritoneal reflection divided. Care is needed when retracting friable inflamed colon – if there is doubt as to whether this can be done safely it is better to convert than to cause an intraoperative perforation and widespread contamination. The retrocolic plane is now developed with a combination of sharp dissection and blunt dissection under direct vision. It is easy to enter the plane behind the perinephric fat by mistake. As the dissection continues medially the lateral part of the duodenum will be seen and should be swept posteriorly, taking care to allow an energy device to cool before touching the duodenum. The mesentery is then divided close to the bowel, using either an energy device or clips.

If the lateral to medial plane becomes difficult to follow, then the dissection can switch instead to a medial to lateral one as described in Chapter 6. Alternatively, the same plane can be entered from below the mesentery of the terminal ileum, or from the hepatic flexure after mobilising the transverse colon.

The transverse colon needs both mesentery and omentum dissecting in order to mobilise it. The omentum may either be dissected off the colon and left *in situ*, or removed with the specimen. With open surgery the omentum was usually removed to reduce the risk of subsequent adhesions, and while this is less of a concern with a laparoscopic approach, most surgeons will still remove it.

Initially the omentum is positioned above the transverse colon in the upper abdomen. Two graspers, one held by the assistant and one in the non-operating hand of the surgeon, are used to lift separate points on the transverse colon towards the anterior abdominal wall in order that the transverse mesocolon is stretched directly upward from the retroperitoneum. Slow dissection through the mesentery close to the colon should allow the lesser sack to be entered, with branches of the middle colic vessels identified and secured with either an energy device or clips.

The transverse colonic mobilisation is completed by bringing the patient to a head-up position with the omentum folded down towards the pelvis. Traction on the transverse colon towards the pelvis places the gastrocolic omentum under tension, and allows this to be divided, joining on to the left- and right-sided dissections at the colonic flexures.

The left colonic mobilisation is carried out lateral to medial in a similar fashion to the right. The mesenteric division should take place close to the bowel with preservation of the inferior mesenteric artery, as this will provide better blood supply to the long rectal/sigmoid stump. Future proctectomy will also be made easier as this can start by dividing the inferior mesenteric artery (IMA), and proceed by following it down behind the mesorectum.

The distal division should be in the distal sigmoid colon, not at the rectosigmoid junction or upper rectum. The small additional amount of colonic mucosa left *in situ* does not significantly alter any morbidity from proctitis, and makes subsequent proctectomy easier. It also gives the option of bringing the stapled end to the anterior abdominal wall as a mucous fistula.

SPECIMEN RETRIEVAL/STOMA FORMATION

Either the distal or the proximal end of the specimen should be divided in order to retrieve the specimen. If the bowel is severely inflamed, or the patient's physiological condition is poor, then a mucous fistula should be considered. This is most easily achieved by dividing the terminal ileum laparoscopically, leaving a grasper each on the TI and on the caecum, and then extracting the specimen caecum first through a Pfannenstiel incision. The distal division is then made extracorporally at a suitable point for creating the mucous fistula in or underneath the Pfannenstiel.

If there is no intention to make a mucous fistula then the distal division can be made laparoscopically and the specimen retrieved sigmoid first via the ileostomy site. A per-anal Foley catheter left in the rectal stump may be useful to help relieve buildup of pressure in the rectal stump where there is some inflammation and no mucous fistula is created.

ELECTIVE SURGERY

PREOPERATIVE MANAGEMENT

Elective surgery for colitis may be indicated for quality of life in chronically poorly controlled disease or in steroid-dependent disease to avoid serious side effects of medication.

Long-standing colitis is associated with an increased malignancy risk, and these patients should be on surveillance programmes. Cancer will be found in the resection specimens of 19% of patients undergoing colectomy for low-grade dysplasia (10). With high-grade dysplasia 40%–50% will have a synchronous cancer (10,11), and where there is a dysplasia-associated lesion or mass (DALM) the risk approaches 60% (12). More than one third of patients with a colitis-associated colorectal cancer will have dysplasia elsewhere in the colon, and 15% will have a synchronous cancer (11). Colectomy is therefore currently recommended in all patients with operable cancer, DALM, or dysplasia, except where the dysplasia is confined to a polyp that can be resected endoscopically (4).

The safest option in the short term is a subtotal colectomy with end ileostomy as carried out in the emergency setting. This is the best option where a patient is on systemic steroids, is unwell or poorly nourished, or has significant comorbidities precluding a more major procedure. If this is the only procedure carried out, then rectal surveillance for dysplasia is important as in the long term 10%–15% will develop cancer in the rectal stump (13).

Given the cancer risk, poor compliance with surveillance, and symptoms from inflammation in the residual rectum, most patients benefit from proctectomy. If they are fit then this can be carried out as a proctocolectomy in one sitting, but otherwise a completion proctectomy should be considered after recovery from the initial subtotal colectomy.

Where a patient wishes to avoid a permanent ileostomy following colectomy, there are two potential options, although some patients will not be suitable for either. An ileoanal pouch may be carried out at the time of proctectomy. In women there is a threefold increase in infertility after open pouch surgery (14), although this risk may be lower after laparoscopic surgery (15). If there is relative rectal sparing an ileorectal anastomosis has the advantage of avoiding this risk, and of the small risk of erectile and/or ejaculatory dysfunction due to autonomic pelvic nerve damage in men.

LAPAROSCOPIC SUBTOTAL COLECTOMY

This operation is carried out in a similar fashion electively as it is in the emergency situation above. There is not normally any need for a mucous fistula, but the rectal/sigmoid stump should still be left long and the IMA preserved as this makes finding the correct plane for any future proctectomy much easier.

When colectomy is carried out because of dysplasia or malignancy, it should be performed as the cancer operations described elsewhere in this book. The vessels should be divided close to their origin to allow mesenteric lymph node resection, and this is usually easiest done with a medial to lateral dissection. Dysplasia in colitis is a multifocal phenomenon: dysplasia in one area is often associated with undetected early malignancy elsewhere in the colon, and synchronous cancers are common. The mesentery should therefore be divided high throughout the colon, and not just at the point of concern.

ILEORECTAL ANASTOMOSIS

An ileorectal anastomosis allows resection of the colon without either a stoma or any pelvic dissection, and was the main operation for ulcerative colitis prior to the development of the ileoanal pouch.

The main indication now is in patients who have colitis with rectal sparing, and where a pouch is either not possible due to Crohn's disease, or because the patient wishes to avoid the fertility risk from pelvic surgery. Long-term results in selected patients with ulcerative colitis

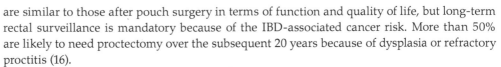
are similar to those after pouch surgery in terms of function and quality of life, but long-term rectal surveillance is mandatory because of the IBD-associated cancer risk. More than 50% are likely to need proctectomy over the subsequent 20 years because of dysplasia or refractory proctitis (16).

No special laparoscopic technique is needed: a subtotal colectomy is carried out as above, and then a stapled end-to-end ileorectal anastomosis carried out with a transanal staple gun.

PROCTECTOMY

A proctectomy may be carried out either as part of a proctocolectomy, as a subsequent procedure in someone with ulcerative colitis who has previously had a subtotal colectomy, or as the only procedure in a patient with severe perianal Crohn's or Crohn's proctitis. Only 50% of women who have had a proctectomy (with or without pouch formation) will conceive within 1 year of trying, and this must be discussed with the patient where appropriate as part of the consent process.

Port positions should be as for an anterior resection; although in a completion proctectomy the right iliac fossa port may be 5 mm instead of 12 mm as there is no need for any laparoscopic stapler. This port needs to be placed medially enough that the instrument placed through it can reach the distal pelvis, and for pouch surgery a more medial port gives better access for cross-stapling the rectum just above the dentate line.

In the absence of malignancy a close rectal dissection has some advantages over a total mesenteric excision. The dissection is further from pelvic autonomic nerves, reducing the risk of damage to these. The residual mesorectum may help to reduce symptomatic small bowel adhesions deep into the pelvis.

Where there is malignancy, or rectal dysplasia which is associated with a risk of occult malignancy, a formal total mesorectal excision should be performed (see Chapter 10). This is carried out identically to an anterior resection for cancer in other circumstances and will not be re-described here.

For a close rectal dissection the posterior plane between the rectum and mesorectum is followed first. If there has been previous surgery the rectal stump will first need dissecting free from any adhesions; otherwise the plane is simply continued from the close mesenteric plane followed on the colon. The harmonic scalpel may be used to divide the mesorectum directly on the rectal muscle and should be sufficient to seal any vessels that cross this plane. Once the plane has been followed as far as possible posteriorly, it may be followed around to either side. An assistant should provide longitudinal traction of the rectum up and out of the pelvis.

Anteriorly the peritoneum should be divided posterior to the peritoneal reflection instead of anteriorly as would be done in a cancer operation. This keeps the plane of dissection posterior to Denonvilliers fascia, which in turn protects the neurovascular bundle on the back of the prostate in the male. The assistant's grasper may now be more usefully employed in an A-frame inserted initially under the divided edge of peritoneum, and as the dissection deepens behind the vagina or prostate, and used to provide countertraction by lifting anteriorly.

As the dissection is deepened in one area it releases the rectum further out of the pelvis, and facilitates better traction and vision elsewhere. As dissection becomes impossible in one area, returning to an area that was previously difficult will often reveal it to have been opened up. Progress is made in this fashion until the dissection arrives at the top of the intersphincteric groove.

Unless an ileoanal pouch is being formed, the final part of the operation is carried out from the perineum. A purse-string suture is placed circumferentially close to the anus in order to prevent any contamination of the wound. A circum-anal incision is then made directly over the intersphincteric groove. A LoneStar retractor may then be inserted if available, and the intersphincteric plane is then followed proximally using diathermy to join on to the dissection from above. This join is easiest posteriorly. If the laparoscopic dissection anteriorly has not completely reached the upper border of the intersphincteric groove, then the final dissection of rectum off the prostate or vagina is most easily accomplished by delivering the specimen and using diathermy to dissect it free from above.

The perineal wound is closed in layers with a heavy dissolvable suture. This does not usually present any difficulty following an intersphincteric dissection as no pelvic floor has been resected, and the skin can be closed with an absorbable subcutaneous monofilament suture.

POUCH

An ileoanal pouch is the only option where a patient who has had, or is going to have, a proctocolectomy wishes to avoid a long-term stoma. In selected patients with ulcerative colitis (UC) it is a good option, but pouch failure requiring excision or permanent defunctioning may subsequently be required in 5%–10% of patients with a significant impact on quality of life (17,18). Surgery should therefore be reserved for those without significant other comorbidity, with good sphincter function, and who have been consented appropriately, including discussion of the alternative of a long-term ileostomy. Appropriate arrangements need to be made for long-term care, including management of complications that may occur late, and surveillance for malignancy in those with dysplasia in their proctocolectomy specimen or primary sclerosing cholangitis.

In indeterminate colitis, the risk of pouch excision or defunction is around 50% greater than in UC, and patients wishing to have an ileoanal pouch need to be appropriately counselled regarding the risks. The outcomes in Crohn's colitis are poor with more than half of patients requiring pouch excision or permanent diversion within 10 years and a pouch is contraindicated (19).

Surgery to create a pouch involves a colectomy, a proctectomy, and pouch formation, and finally reversal of any covering ileostomy. These steps may be carried out across two to three separate operations as a two-stage or three-stage pouch, or occasionally in a single operation. The colectomy and proctectomy are carried out as described above. It is vital for the long-term outcome of the pouch that the pouch-anal anastomosis is low enough – ideally 1–2 cm proximal to the dentate line. The rectal dissection should be continued into the upper part of the intersphincteric groove, and the rectum transected by linear stapler introduced via the right iliac fossa port, and the position of the stapler confirmed by digital rectal examination prior to firing. In a narrow pelvis a suprapubic port may be needed in order to position the cross stapler sufficiently distally on the rectum, especially if the initial right iliac fossa port has been placed laterally (20).

Once the rectum has been divided the specimen is removed from a Pfannenstiel or midline incision. This same incision is used to deliver the terminal ileum so that the pouch can be constructed *extracorporally*.

Mesenteric tethering in the distal ileal mesentery can prevent adequate pouch length. The ileocolic artery is frequently implicated and should be followed proximally to its junction with the superior mesenteric artery and divided here. The small bowel mesentery may then be mobilised anteriorly off the retroperitoneum as far as the third part of the duodenum. If additional length is still required then divisions of the anterior peritoneal leaf of the small bowel mesentery over the IMA can also be useful (21).

The pouch should be 15- to 20-cm long. The terminal ileum is folded back on itself to achieve this length while ensuring that the apex is the most dependent part and can reach the pubic symphysis without tension.

Stay sutures are used to tack the antimesenteric borders of the two limbs of the pouch together prior to stapling. A small enterotomy is then made at the apex of the pouch, two-thirds of the distance from the antimesenteric border to allow each half of the stapler to be inserted up a separate limb of the pouch. Three firings of a TLC75 will be required to create the entire pouch. Two small defects are occasionally left, one on each staple line, and these should be looked for and closed if present.

The pouch-anal anastomosis may either be stapled or hand-sewn. A hand-sewn per-anal anastomosis with mucosectomy gives less good function, but has the benefit of removing more of the mucosa. While this theoretically further reduces the malignancy risk and may be considered where the colectomy is carried out for dysplasia, the evidence for this is poor. It is also a useful technique to be able to fall back on where a stapled anastomosis is not technically possible, or the anastomosis needs re-fashioning.

The stapled anastomosis is carried out in a similar fashion to an anterior resection. The anvil of a circular staple gun is sutured into the enterotomy of the pouch with a purse-string suture. The pouch is then returned to the abdomen, the extraction wound closed, and pneumoperitoneum reestablished. The stapled anastomosis is carried out under direct vision, ensuring that there is no twist in the pouch, that the vagina has not been included in the staple line anteriorly, and that no small bowel is trapped under the free edge of the pouch mesentery as it comes down into the pelvis. A defunctioning ileostomy may be formed, taking care not to put the pouch-anal anastomosis under tension in doing so.

CROHN'S DISEASE

SURGERY FOR SMALL BOWEL DISEASE

PRE-OP

Surgery does not provide a cure for small bowel Crohn's disease – 70% of patients undergoing surgery for Crohn's will need further surgery in the future. The role of surgery is therefore in cases where medical management has failed, but will still be needed in 60%–70% of patients with Crohn's disease over their lifetime (22,23).

The most common reasons for surgery are small bowel strictures (24). These may have both a fibrotic and an inflammatory component. The inflammatory component is amenable to medical treatment, but the fibrosis is not. If obstructive symptoms, upstream bowel dilatation, or persistent weight loss persist in the absence of inflammation, or despite escalation of medical therapy, then surgery is indicated.

Endoscopy may be used to dilate accessible strictures in the terminal ileum. This is ideal for short strictures that the balloon can be passed through. As strictures become longer, or more proximal in the terminal ileum, endoscopic dilatation becomes more difficult. Recurrence after balloon dilatation is common, with most requiring more than one dilatation, and around half of patients needing surgery within the subsequent 4 years (25).

All patients due to have surgery for their Crohn's disease should have preoperative imaging. Magnetic resonance imaging (MRI) enterography is the best option, with good views of any small bowel disease and no radiation dose. The MRI is also useful for assessing the proximity of any inflammatory mass to the ureters or other organs. Where there is concern that the ureter may be involved, preoperative stenting of one or both ureters may reduce the risk of ureteric injury, and certainly reduces the risk of any ureteric injury going unrecognised during surgery. If MRI is not possible then either an x-ray contrast follow-through or CT may be useful alternatives.

In fistulating Crohn's disease, surgery is indicated either where entero-enteric fistulae have created malabsorption, or where there is symptomatic fistulation from bowel to other organs. Where there is an intra-abdominal collection alone this can potentially be managed conservatively, with radiological drainage of any collections up to 3 cm in diameter, followed by antibiotics, and subsequent immunosuppression once any sepsis is under control. If there is any deterioration in the patient's physiological state during this approach, or where the initial abscess is larger than 3 cm in diameter, surgery should be considered (26).

STRICTUROPLASTY

Stricturoplasty is effective at treating Crohn's small bowel strictures, with similar recurrence rates to resection, but allowing conservation of small bowel length (27). In practice it is relatively rare to find strictures that are suitable for simple stricturoplasty, and the more complex stricturoplasty procedures described for long strictures are not in common usage. The role of laparoscopy in stricturoplasty is purely to assess the small bowel, and identify the stricture. The stricture can then be delivered through a small extraction site, and stricturoplasty performed externally without the risks of abdominal contamination from attempting it laparoscopically.

ILEOCOLIC RESECTION

The most common site for small bowel Crohn's disease is in the terminal ileum, and this disease is normally too close to the ileocaecal valve to allow it to be preserved. Recurrent disease is usually at the anastomosis and also requires resection of a short portion of colon. Laparoscopic ileocolic resection is a safe alternative to open surgery, although few direct comparator studies have been done (28).

The aim of laparoscopy is to mobilise the affected segment of terminal ileum, caecum, and proximal ascending colon sufficiently that they can be delivered via the extraction incision. In difficult cases this incision often needs to be large to allow delivery of the inflammatory mass, and this allows some pragmatic decisions to be made about how much of the surgery is carried out laparoscopically. Certainly the anastomosis will be carried out externally, but it may be that some of the dissection can also be carried out more easily externally without any need to extend the incision further.

Three ports in the left lateral abdomen usually provide the best access to the right colon for mobilisation, and these can also be used to mobilise any adherent small bowel loops up from the pelvis. An additional right-sided port may be used so that an assistant can provide countertraction. Mobilisation of the right colon proceeds laterally to medially as described for colitis above. If enough length can be obtained for a safe anastomosis without mobilising the hepatic flexure, this may make any future resections easier as subsequent mobilisation will take place in undisturbed tissue planes. The terminal ileum is frequently adherent to the right pelvic side wall, and more proximal loops may be adherent deeper in the pelvis. These adhesions need careful division. Some areas may respond to blunt dissection, but this can easily result in serosal tears, and sharp dissection with scissors is the safest way to avoid small bowel injury. Any serosal tears require immediate repair. A steep Trendelenburg head down tilt will help with this mobilisation.

Once the bowel is mobilised a vertical transumbilical midline incision provides the easiest extraction site with good cosmesis. Proximal and distal resection margins can be established and the mesentery divided externally. Determining the proximal point of the resection is often a case of weighing the relative risks of leaving a segment of mildly abnormal small bowel *in situ*, of multiple short resections with several anastomoses, or a safe single resection that sacrifices more small bowel. The length of small bowel left behind after resection should be recorded, and with a transumbilical extraction incision it should be possible to run the small bowel from the DJ flexure to measure this.

Preoperative intra-abdominal abscesses, steroid usage, poor nutrition, positive histological margins, and prolonged disease duration have all been reported as risk factors for anastomotic leakage after Crohn's resection (29–32). Anastomotic-related complications may rise to 15% with one of these risk factors, and to 40% or more when more than one is present (31). In this situation a double-barrelled ileocolic stoma is a safer alternative to anastomosis, and it can be reversed once these risk factors have been addressed, and following endoscopic assessment of the peristomal mucosa.

No consistent differences between stapled and hand-sewn anastomoses have been demonstrated in the literature in terms of leak rate. Some have advocated the wider lumen of a stapled side-side anastomosis as being less likely to re-stenose, but there is no good evidence to support this. A hand-sewn end-to-end anastomosis results in less functional loss of bowel length, and will be easier to pass at subsequent endoscopy for management of recurrent disease. If a hand-sewn anastomosis is performed, then leaving two small metal clips attached to two of the sutures at the end of the procedure will aid identification of the anastomosis at any future imaging.

The anastomosis should be returned to the abdomen, the extraction site wound closed, and a final laparoscopy carried out to ensure the bowel is lying as intended and to wash out any residual blood in the peritoneal cavity.

SPECIAL CONSIDERATIONS

Fistulae

Where there is a fistula between two segments of bowel, the management depends primarily on whether both segments are exhibiting signs of active Crohn's disease, or whether the active inflammation is limited only to the side that has initiated the fistula. Fistulae often occur between adjacent loops of inflamed terminal ileum. These are best treated with *en bloc* resection of the affected area, with either two anastomoses, or if the loops are close by resecting the intervening small bowel and carrying out a single join.

Where inflamed small bowel has fistulated into apparently normal colon, then a choice must be made between simultaneous small and large bowel resections, or dissecting the small bowel free and resecting it, and repairing the residual colonic defect with a suture. Suture repair of a colonic defect is reasonable if the surrounding colon is not inflamed, and this may be carried out laparoscopically. If the situation is suspected preoperatively then the patient can be given oral mechanical bowel preparation, and then creating a double-barreled ileocolic sltoma will also effectively defunction this repair.

Fistulae to bladder or vagina can be treated by resection of a small cuff of the affected organ with the bowel resection and suture repair of the defect. When a colovesical fistula is repaired in this fashion, a urinary catheter and a pelvic drain should be left *in situ*. A cystogram should be performed prior to removal of the urinary catheter.

RECURRENT DISEASE

Recurrent surgery is common in Crohn's disease. The extent of previous surgery is a poor guide to the extent of intra-abdominal adhesions, and laparoscopic surgery may be possible even in those who have had multiple previous operations (33). Provided that pneumoperitoneum is achieved safely, nothing is lost by an initial laparoscopy followed by conversion if necessary.

In those with multiple previous operations, gaining initial pneumoperitoneum and port insertion may be difficult and there are various methods to achieve this. We prefer entry with a blunt 5-mm port level with the umbilicus lateral to the midclavicular line. Initial port insertion may lead to an area within omental adhesions and adherent loops of bowel from where it is not possible to see the abdominal wall adequately for safe subsequent port insertion. It may be possible to navigate the camera around these adhesions, potentially using it gently to carry out blunt dissection of adhesions from the abdominal wall, to an area where further port insertion is possible. Use of a 5-mm camera is invaluable here as it may be used in each new port as it is inserted to look back at an area of adhesions that were not previously visible.

The ureters are more at risk when there has been previous colonic mobilisation, especially if the anastomosis or any recurrent disease is sitting close to them. Up-to-date preoperative imaging is vital, and any suggestion that the ureters may be at risk should prompt consideration of preoperative ureteric stenting or catheterisation.

POST-OPERATIVE MANAGEMENT

Crohn's disease may recur following surgery, and the majority of patients who have had a resection will require further surgery in the future. Numerous strategies exist to delay recurrent disease, and it is important that these are employed.

The most important intervention for reducing recurrence is for smokers to stop smoking (34). A 12-week course of metronidazole delays recurrence for around 6 months on average, but when used for prolonged periods peripheral neuropathy is a risk, and patients should be advised to stop if they develop any of these symptoms. The evidence for benefit of a post-operative 5-ASA is poor. A thiopurine (such as azathioprine) reduces endoscopic recurrence rates, especially if combined with a short course of metronidazole, but the thiopurine needs to be continued in the long term (23). Anti-TNF therapy is more effective still, and again better outcomes are seen with longer-term use (35). Initial selection of therapy based on an individual's risk of recurrence, followed by endoscopic surveillance at 6 months with appropriate escalation of medical therapy if there is recurrent disease, has been shown to reduce reoperation rates (36). A multidisciplinary approach is needed post-operatively, and it is vital that this is provided to patients and that they are given follow-up appointments with gastroenterologists as well as in the surgical clinic.

SUMMARY

Laparoscopic surgery is practical in both ulcerative colitis and Crohn's disease. Colonic and rectal surgery in inflammatory bowel disease may be carried out in a similar fashion to the cancer operations described elsewhere in this book, but in most cases the mesenteric dissection does not need to be so extensive, and this allows alternative less radical approaches to colonic mobilisation.

In small bowel Crohn's disease laparoscopic surgery is primarily used to mobilise sufficient bowel to deliver the diseased segment through an extraction wound and allow extracorporal anastomosis. This may involve division of adhesions from previous operations, division of inflammatory adhesions from the Crohn's disease itself, or resection of parts of other involved organs where there is a fistula. In terminal ileal disease a limited mobilisation of the right colon is also required.

In both Crohn's and ulcerative colitis, perioperative planning and optimisation is vital if good results are to be achieved. In some patients surgery will be required without good optimisation, either because they require surgery in an emergency setting, or because their condition cannot be improved without resection of diseased bowel. In this situation a staged approach should be considered with any anastomosis of bowel delayed until the patient has fully recovered.

KEY POINTS

- Good perioperative management with optimisation of medical therapy within the multidisciplinary team is vital for good outcomes in laparoscopic IBD surgery.
- Colonic resections for IBD do not usually need to include extensive mesenteric resection, and as a result a lateral to medial mobilisation can be used.
- In small bowel resections for IBD, the role of laparoscopy is mainly to mobilise the affected bowel so it can be delivered externally for resection and anastomosis.

TAKE-HOME MESSAGE

Laparoscopic surgery offers real benefits to patients with IBD in both the elective and acute settings.

REFERENCES

1. Maartense S et al. Laparoscopic-assisted versus open ileocolic resection for Crohn's disease: A randomized trial. *Ann Surg* 2006;243:143–9; discussion 150–153.
2. Eshuis EJ et al. Long-term outcomes following laparoscopically assisted versus open ileocolic resection for Crohn's disease. *Br J Surg* 2010;97:563–8.
3. Spinelli A et al. Short-term outcomes of laparoscopy combined with enhanced recovery pathway after ileocecal resection for Crohn's disease: A case-matched analysis. *J Gastrointest Surg Off J Soc Surg Aliment Tract* 2013;17:126–32; discussion pp. 132.
4. Mowat C et al. Guidelines for the management of inflammatory bowel disease in adults. *Gut* 2011;60:571–607.
5. UK IBD Audit. *National audit report of inflammatory bowel service provision: National adult report.* London: Royal College of Physicians; 2014.

6. Turner D, Walsh CM, Steinhart AH, Griffiths AM. Response to corticosteroids in severe ulcerative colitis: A systematic review of the literature and a meta-regression. *Clin Gastroenterol Hepatol Off Clin Pract J Am Gastroenterol Assoc* 2007;5:103–10.

7. Molnár T et al. Long-term outcome of cyclosporin rescue therapy in acute, steroid-refractory severe ulcerative colitis. *United Eur Gastroenterol J* 2014;2:108–12.

8. Moskovitz DN et al. Incidence of colectomy during long-term follow-up after cyclosporine-induced remission of severe ulcerative colitis. *Clin Gastroenterol Hepatol Off Clin Pract J Am Gastroenterol Assoc* 2006;4:760–5.

9. Nelson R, Liao C, Fichera A, Rubin DT, Pekow J. Rescue therapy with cyclosporine or infliximab is not associated with an increased risk for postoperative complications in patients hospitalized for severe steroid-refractory ulcerative colitis. *Inflamm Bowel Dis* 2014;20:14–20.

10. Bernstein CN, Shanahan F, Weinstein WM. Are we telling patients the truth about surveillance colonoscopy in ulcerative colitis? *Lancet Lond Engl* 1994;343:71–4.

11. Choi C-HR et al. Forty-year analysis of colonoscopic surveillance program for neoplasia in ulcerative colitis: An updated overview. *Am J Gastroenterol* 2015;110:1022–34.

12. Blackstone MO, Riddell RH, Rogers BH, Levin B. Dysplasia-associated lesion or mass (DALM) detected by colonoscopy in long-standing ulcerative colitis: An indication for colectomy. *Gastroenterology* 1981;80:366–74.

13. Munie S, Hyman N, Osler T. Fate of the rectal stump after subtotal colectomy for ulcerative colitis in the era of ileal pouch-anal anastomosis. *JAMA Surg* 2013;148:408–11.

14. Waljee A, Waljee J, Morris AM, Higgins PDR. Threefold increased risk of infertility: A meta-analysis of infertility after ileal pouch anal anastomosis in ulcerative colitis. *Gut* 2006;55:1575–80.

15. Bartels SAL et al. Significantly increased pregnancy rates after laparoscopic restorative proctocolectomy: A cross-sectional study. *Ann Surg* 2012;256:1045–8.

16. da Luz Moreira A, Kiran RP, Lavery I. Clinical outcomes of ileorectal anastomosis for ulcerative colitis. *Br J Surg* 2010;97:65–9.

17. Berndtsson I, Lindholm E, Oresland T, Börjesson L. Long-term outcome after ileal pouch-anal anastomosis: Function and health-related quality of life. *Dis Colon Rectum* 2007;50:1545–52.

18. Fazio VW et al. Ileal pouch anal anastomosis: Analysis of outcome and quality of life in 3707 patients. *Ann Surg* 2013;257:679–85.

19. Brown CJ et al. Crohn's disease and indeterminate colitis and the ileal pouch-anal anastomosis: Outcomes and patterns of failure. *Dis Colon Rectum* 2005;48:1542–9.

20. Hemandas AK, Jenkins JT. Laparoscopic pouch surgery in ulcerative colitis. *Ann Gastroenterol* 2012;25:309–16.

21. Kirat HT, Remzi FH. Technical aspects of ileoanal pouch surgery in patients with ulcerative colitis. *Clin Colon Rectal Surg* 2010;23:239–47.

22. Bernell O, Lapidus A, Hellers G. Risk factors for surgery and postoperative recurrence in Crohn's disease. *Ann Surg* 2000;231:38.

23. De Cruz P, Kamm MA, Prideaux L, Allen PB, Desmond PV. Postoperative recurrent luminal Crohn's disease: A systematic review. *Inflamm Bowel Dis* 2012;18:758–77.

24. Peyrin-Biroulet L et al. Surgery in a population-based cohort of Crohn's disease from Olmsted County, Minnesota (1970–2004). *Am J Gastroenterol* 2012;107:1693–701.

25. Krauss E et al. Long term follow up of through-the-scope balloon dilation as compared to strictureplasty and bowel resection of intestinal strictures in Crohn's disease. *Int J Clin Exp Pathol* 2014;7:7419–31.

26. Feagins LA, Holubar SD, Kane SV, Spechler SJ. Current strategies in the management of intra-abdominal abscesses in Crohn's disease. *Clin Gastroenterol Hepatol Off Clin Pract J Am Gastroenterol Assoc* 2011;9:842–50.

27. Ozuner G, Fazio VW, Lavery IC, Milsom JW, Strong SA. Reoperative rates for Crohn's disease following strictureplasty. Long-term analysis. *Dis Colon Rectum* 1996;39:1199–203.

28. Dasari BV, McKay D, Gardiner K. Laparoscopic versus open surgery for small bowel Crohn's disease. In *Cochrane Database of Systematic Reviews* 2011, Issue 1. Art. No.: CD006956. Available at: http://onlinelibrary.wiley.com/doi/10.1002/14651858.CD006956. pub2/abstract

29. Alves A et al. Risk factors for intra-abdominal septic complications after a first ileocecal resection for Crohn's disease: A multivariate analysis in 161 consecutive patients. *Dis Colon Rectum* 2007;50:331–6.

30. Shental O, Tulchinsky H, Greenberg R, Klausner JM, Avital S. Positive histological inflammatory margins are associated with increased risk for intra-abdominal septic complications in patients undergoing ileocolic resection for Crohn's disease. *Dis Colon Rectum* 2012;55:1125–30.

31. Tzivanakis A et al. Influence of risk factors on the safety of ileocolic anastomosis in Crohn's disease surgery. *Dis Colon Rectum* 2012;55:558–62.

32. Yamamoto T, Allan RN, Keighley MR. Risk factors for intra-abdominal sepsis after surgery in Crohn's disease. *Dis Colon Rectum* 2000;43:1141–5.

33. Chaudhary B, Glancy D, Dixon AR. Laparoscopic surgery for recurrent ileocolic Crohn's disease is as safe and effective as primary resection. *Colorectal Dis Off J Assoc Coloproctology G. B. Irel* 2011;13:1413–6.

34. Sutherland LR, Ramcharan S, Bryant H, Fick G. Effect of cigarette smoking on recurrence of Crohn's disease. *Gastroenterology* 1990;98:1123–8.

35. Regueiro M, Kip KE, Baidoo L, Swoger JM, Schraut W. Postoperative therapy with infliximab prevents long-term Crohn's disease recurrence. *Clin Gastroenterol Hepatol Off Clin Pract J Am Gastroenterol Assoc* 2014;12:1494–502.e1.

36. De Cruz P et al. Crohn's disease management after intestinal resection: A randomised trial. *Lancet* 2015;385:1406–17.

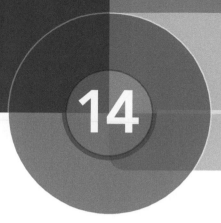

14

Laparoscopic ventral mesh rectopexy: A standardised modular approach

PETER ALEXANDER NEWMAN AND TONY DIXON

LEARNING OBJECTIVES

- Gain a greater understanding of a standardised approach to performing laparoscopic ventral mesh rectopexy.
- Understand and apply a standard modular and safe approach to performing laparoscopic ventral mesh rectopexy in females with a uterus, post-hysterectomy females, and male patients.
- Understand the principles of functional and anatomical pelvic floor disorders and the role of surgical intervention (C1-3, PL1).
- Consider appropriate surgical approaches taking into account history, examination, and investigation findings (PL2).
- Describe the equipment, devices, and materials needed (PL3).
- Demonstrate appropriate preparation and positioning of patient and equipment (PR1-5).
- Describe port placement for efficient and ergonomic operating (E1, IT12).
- Understand how to gain maximal exposure of the pelvis; dissect the lateral and anterior pelvic peritoneum; and demonstrate awareness of ureters, pelvic nerves, and relevant organs, for females with a uterus, hysterectomised females, and males (E2-3, IT1-2,5-7,9,13-14).
- Understand how to select and prepare the appropriate mesh, and placement and securing of mesh with an appropriate suture (IT16-17).
- Understand how to close the peritoneum and abdominal wall (IT18,19).
- Consider common intra-operative problems and pitfalls (IT 3,7-8).
- Describe expected post-operative recovery (C5).

This chapter should be used in conjunction with the Pelvic Floor Society published procedure-based assessment for laparoscopic ventral mesh rectopexy (see Appendix 14.1) (1).

INTRODUCTION

Laparoscopic ventral mesh rectopexy (LVMR) has gained in popularity by colorectal surgeons as a procedure for internal and external rectal prolapse. The fundamental principle of this operation is to correct morphological abnormalities of the posterior and middle compartments, while preserving neuromuscular function of the pelvic floor, the outcome of which is to improve the functional symptoms associated with prolapse. This operation is technically demanding and requires expert levels of skill and judgement in patient selection and laparoscopic pelvic surgical technique in order to achieve a high level of clinical and quality-of-life outcome improvements.

BACKGROUND

ANATOMY OF THE PELVIC FLOOR

The pelvic floor is complex consisting of deep and superficial myofascial structures supported by strong osteoligamentous attachments. Separating the lesser pelvis from the perineum is the pelvic floor that is pierced by urogenital and anorectal hiatuses. The puborectalis, pubococcygeus, and iliococcygeus form the levator ani which together with the coccygeus acts as a diaphragm; tonically contracted to support abdominopelvic viscera during changes in intra-abdominal pressure (2). Puborectalis tonicity maintains the anorectal angle allowing stool to fill within the rectum, during defecation reflex inhibition relaxes the puborectalis, straightening the angle, and aids expulsion. The superficial muscles include the internal and external anal sphincters, perineal body, and transverse perineal muscles, together these are largely responsible for controlling evacuation (3). Pelvic fascia is continuous with endoabdominal fascia deep to the peritoneum and sweeps over the pelvic floor and envelops the visceral organs. This fascia consists of loose areolar tissue (e.g. presacral space) and regions of thickened fibrous tissue surrounding neurovascular structures and providing mechanical support (e.g. hypogastric sheath) (4). Somatic innervation is provided by the anterior rami of the sacral nerve roots and autonomic innervation by S2-S4 via the inferior hypogastric plexus.

MECHANISM OF PELVIC SUPPORT

It is not just the muscles, tendons, and ligaments that provide support, the quality of the connective tissue fascia that envelops and invests the visceral organs as they penetrate the urogenital and anal hiatus plays a significant role. This extracellular matrix is rich in collagen type I providing tensile strength and III providing more elastic support (5), glycoprotein collagen forming cross-linkage between fibrils (6) and elastin (7). The vaginal suspensory axis is a collagen-rich thickening of this connective tissue running from the sacrum to the perineum, acting as a leash (8). Obstetric damage during delivery can cause overwhelming shearing forces that result in tears within the endopelvic fascia. The peri-cervical ring can be torn from the uterosacral ligaments (superiorly) or from the rectovaginal septum (inferiorly). Disruption to the connective tissue support results in areas of lower resting pressure into which organs will preferentially herniate during periods of increased intra-abdominal pressure. Histologically prolapsed tissue has a lower concentration of collagen (9), a lower collagen I:III ratio (10), and up to four times greater concentration of lytic proteases (11).

AETIOLOGY OF RECTAL PROLAPSE

External rectal prolapse (ERP) is a full thickness protrusion of the rectum through the anus involving all layers. Internal rectal prolapse (IRP) is rectal intussusception (RI) which can be graded according to the Oxford prolapse grade (OPG); from 1 (high rectorectal intussusception) through to 5 (ERP) (12). Rectal prolapse can occur independently or in association with other pelvic floor disorders (PFDs) such as solitary rectal ulcer, rectocele, enterocele, uterine or vaginal vault prolapse. Aetiology is unclear but associated with conditions that increase the intra-abdominal pressure and decrease the strength of support mechanisms (13).

The key events are aging, pregnancy, and vaginal delivery. Aging will disrupt the extracellular tissue matrix and decrease the effectiveness of muscular hypertrophy in response to stress (14). Pregnancy-related hormonal changes result in decreased collagen levels with subsequent softening of connective tissue (15). Vaginal delivery can tear the fascia, avulse the pelvic diaphragm from its origin on the levator tendon, and cause a stretch neuropathy of the pudendal nerve (8). Nulliparous women and men form a significant subset of those with rectal prolapse, up to 20%. Here the underlying mechanism is likely to be decreased quality of the connective tissue due to genetic factors (e.g. Ehlers-Danlos syndrome or benign joint hypermobility syndrome) aging, or behavioral factors such as smoking, eating disorders, and chronic straining (8).

During defecation increased intra-abdominal force is transmitted to the luminal contents of the rectum, which with a straightened ano-rectal junction allows expulsion. This force needs to be resisted in the pelvis by the rectum, uterus, and pelvis and hence channelled intra-luminally. The force vector will be inefficient as energy will be transmitted to herniating organs in preference to the luminal contents.

Anatomical features include diastasis of the levator ani, redundant sigmoid, loss of the vertical position of the rectum and sacral attachments, and a deep rectouterine or rectovesical recess (3). Performing a hysterectomy will reduce the pelvic support and the recurrence risk fails to diminish with each re-operative attempt (16).

PATIENT SELECTION AND OPTIMISATION

PATIENT ASSESSMENT

A thorough proctological history should be sought including assessment of symptoms such as a mass or bulge; when this occurs, spontaneous reduction or not, also inquire about functional components including incontinence of bowel and bladder, constipation, obstructive symptoms, bleeding, pain, and sexual function. Urological and gynaecological symptoms need assessment along with effect on quality of life. Validated symptom questionnaires such as the Cleveland Clinic Incontinence Score (CCIS), Wexner constipation score, and quality of life such as the Birmingham bowel and urinary symptoms questionnaire-22 (BBSQ-22) should be used at the time of initial assessment and during follow-up thereafter (17). Appropriate past medical, surgical, obstetric, and gynaecological history need taking into account. Often there is a significant psychological overlay, and understanding patient views and expectations is of paramount importance when considering further investigation and intervention.

All patients should have a pelvic floor examination of posterior and middle compartments supine, in the left lateral position, and while squatting. Endoluminal studies with or without biopsies to exclude colonic pathology should be performed as appropriate. Dynamic defecography and anorectal physiology studies in patients with concomitant symptoms of incontinence and constipation can help in consideration of appropriate surgical approach. Examination under anaesthesia with a circular anoscope that allows prolapsed tissue to 'drop' into view is useful in patients with clinical suspicion of prolapse but in whom the outpatient clinical assessment was equivocal (18). Laparoscopy to gauge and understand the pelvic floor anatomy may also be required prior to undertaking rectopexy.

As PFDs are complex and often involve different surgical specialities with limited high-quality evidence base for therapy, patients ideally need discussing in a pelvic floor multidisciplinary team meeting bringing together specialist surgeons, physicians, radiologists, specialist nurses, and physiologists. The aim of which should provide an individualised treatment care plan, an opportunity to be involved in clinical trials, continuity of care, and clear communication between primary, secondary, and tertiary care and with the patient (19).

SURGICAL APPROACH

The treatment of rectal prolapse is exclusively surgical, and multiple operations have been described. Approaches include perineal or abdominal, open or laparoscopic or robotic, varying degrees of mobilisation, with mesh or sutured rectopexy with or without colonic resection (13). A Cochrane Review of 15 randomised studies concluded that laparoscopic surgery was associated with lower morbidity (0% versus 21%, $p < .05$) and a shorter hospital length of stay (mean difference 2.35 days, $p < .01$), division of lateral ligaments was associated with a lower recurrence of prolapse (OR 15.35, CI 0.73–321.58) but a higher incidence of constipation (OR O.32, CI 0.08–1.23) and bowel resection resulting in less constipation (OR 0.14, CI 0.04–0.44) (20). The Prolapse Surgery: Perineal or Rectopexy (PROSPER) trial found no significant difference in outcomes between abdominal or perineal procedures or suture or resection rectopexy. This trial was limited with difficulty in recruitment and randomisation (21). Laparoscopic rectopexy was first described by Berman in 1992 (22) and LVMR was described in 2004 (23). LVMR has been shown to be safe and effective in the treatment of ERP, IRP, solitary rectal ulcer syndrome (SRUS), associated genital prolapse, mechanical obstruction, in elderly and male patients (24–29).

The principles of any surgical intervention should aim to correct the underlying abnormality rather than just the pathological effect. This is especially true for rectal prolapse surgery where understanding the anatomy and pathophysiology is key prior to undertaking corrective surgery. LVMR restores anatomy to the posterior and middle compartment by elevating the rectum, perineal body, cervix, and vaginal vault. The rectovaginal septum and rectovaginal (rectovesicular) recess are reconstructed and peritonealised correcting any rectocele or enterocele. LVMR is effective for controlling ERP and IRP causing faecal incontinence and obstructive defecation syndrome; indeed the worse the symptoms, the more effective the surgery and benefits are maintained in the medium to long term (23–29). Posterior rectopexy does not treat middle compartment prolapse and denervation surgery leads to unacceptably high rates of constipation up to 50% (23), whereas LVMR improves evacuatory function in 80%–84% (27) with infrequent new onset constipation (23). Full continence returns to 90% of those undergoing LVMR (27).

Surgeons have to adapt to the patient, pathology, and problem in front of them and LVMR is no different. This is a technically demanding operation working within the confines of the pelvic cavity often at the limit of laparoscopic instruments. The complexity of the operation is reflected in the learning curve of over 100 operations to ensure predictable functional outcomes (30). As with all operations good outcomes relate to surgery done correctly without cutting corners. We would recommend starting the learning curve under the guidance of a mentor, using the procedure-based assessment (Appendix 14.1), commencing with external rectal prolapse. Predictably more challenging patients are those with raised body mass index (BMI), the frail, those who had previous surgery with likely or known adhesions, and those with SRUS. This surgical approach, however, allows for correction of PFDs that may not have been planned for (e.g. posterior rectal prolapse or cystocele).

ADVANTAGES AND DISADVANTAGES OF LAPAROSCOPIC VENTRAL MESH RECTOPEXY

Advantages:

- Laparoscopic hence lower morbidity and reduced length of stay even in the elderly (28)
- Ventral mobilisation
- Prevention of long-term constipation seen in almost half of patients with a posterior rectopexy by retaining the autonomic nerve supply to the rectum (23)
- Reduced morbidity (e.g. avoid bleeding from pre-sacral venous plexus)
- Treatment of middle compartment
- Reinforcement of the rectovaginal septum and treatment of genital prolapse, rectocele, and enterocele, as posterior colporrhaphy and vaginal sacrocolpopexy are performed at the same time (particularly important in the post-hysterectomy female who has lost cardinal-uterosacral ligaments) (27)
- Treatment of anterior compartment
- Ability to perform anterior colporrhaphy and vaginal sacrocolpopexy with a second mesh, secured on top of the first (27)

Disadvantages:

- Mesh-related complications
- Risk of infection, fistulation, stricturing, and technical failure due to placement of foreign material within the body, not unique to LVMR (Polyester mesh has been shown to significantly increase mesh-related complications and should *not* be used.) (30)
- Protracted learning curve
- Demonstrated learning curve for clinical and quality-of-life outcomes of 80–100 cases; shown to be up to 150 operations for similar complex colorectal laparoscopic operations (31); mentoring, fellowships, and workshops important (30)
- Evidence base
- Lack of high-quality evidence regarding surgical interventions for rectal prolapse (17)

INDICATIONS AND CONTRAINDICATIONS

The consensus statement on ventral rectopexy classifies the indications into definitive and relative, and the contraindications into absolute and relative (17):

Definitive indication:

- External rectal prolapse where age should not preclude selection

Relative indication:

- High-grade internal rectal prolapse (OPG 3–4)
- Significant symptoms of obstruction defecation (ODS) or faecal incontinence (FI) that have failed to respond to conservative measures
- Complex rectocele or enterocele
- SRUS

Absolute contraindications:

- Pregnancy
- No demonstrable anatomical abnormality
- Severe intra-abdominal adhesions
- Active proctitis
- Psychological instability
- Anismus resistant to conventional treatment

Relative contraindications:

- Male (as more difficult and greater potential risks performing laparoscopic surgery in male pelvis, however good outcomes have been reported) (29)
- Body mass index >40 kg/m^2
- Endometriosis
- Pelvic radiotherapy
- Surgery for sigmoid diverticulitis
- Minimal bowel dysfunction

PREPARATION AND CONSENT

Preoperatively a full discussion with the patient explaining the potential benefits and risks of the operation needs to take place, including, if appropriate, inclusion in clinical research. An explanation of alternative therapies including no intervention must be explained. The patient will require time to consider options, be guided to accessing correct and up-to-date information, and have questions and concerns answered in order to make an informed decision. This may require a further outpatient appointment. If the patient has medical comorbidities, an anaesthetic review prior to operation should be sought.

All patients are given a phosphate enema, are risk assessed for thromboembolic events and prescribed thromboembolic deterrent (TED) stockings and low molecular weight heparin as appropriate; the administration of which is determined after the surgical procedure. Prophylactic antimicrobials are administered at induction; in our unit amoxicillin 1 g, metronidazole 500 mg, and gentamicin 5 mg/kg (ideal body weight) IV are given to non-penicillin allergic patients.

EXPOSURE

CORRECT THEATRE SETUP AND EQUIPMENT

The following equipment should be available:

- High-definition camera and monitor with the screen on the patient's left
- 30° laparoscope

- Ports – 10 mm umbilical, two 5 mm right iliac fossa
- Atraumatic bowel graspers
- Left and right laparoscopic needle holders
- Laparoscopic diathermy hook
- Laparoscopic scissors
- Vaginal Spackmann Cannula
- ProTack 5-mm Fixation Device
- Titanium-coated lightweight polypropylene mesh (20 × 4 cm; Tilene, PFM, Nuremburg, Germany)
- 3/0 Polydioxanone suture (PDS) on round-bodied one half circle needle (to secure mesh)
- 3/0 PDS on 'J' needle (to close 10-mm and 12-mm ports)
- 2/0 Absorbable V-Loc 180 on curved needle (to close peritoneum over mesh)
- 2/0 Polyethylene terephthalate (Ethibond) for posterior rectal prolapse repair
- 3/0 Polyglecaprone (Monocryl) on curved cutting needle (to close skin)

APPROPRIATE PATIENT POSITIONING

Patients are placed into the modified Lloyd-Davies on the operating table lying on a non-slip gel mat to allow significant Trendelenburg and lateral tilt positioning. The arms are wrapped with gel and incontinence pads. The legs are placed into Allen stirrups. All patients are catheterised. Intermittent pneumatic compression devices are placed on the lower limb. Hair removal is performed, and an electrosurgery split pad is placed on the thigh. A digital rectal examination or examination under anaesthesia with an anoscope is performed prior to the procedure. A World Health Organization surgical checklist is performed to ensure patient safety. The patient's abdomen from xiphisternum to pubis is prepared with alcoholic 2% chlorhexidine gluconate solution and allowed to evaporate prior to drape placement.

SAFE ACCESS TECHNIQUES

Pneumoperitoneum is established by placement of the 10-mm umbilical port using a modified Hasson technique. Once confirmed within the peritoneal cavity CO_2 insufflation is initiated with a maximum pressure of 12 cmH_2O and maximum flow rate of 20 L/min. Two 5-mm working ports are inserted in the right lower quadrant under direct visualisation with appropriate triangulation to allow for ergonomic positioning. One is placed low down and as lateral as possible, the other a handbreath superior to this at the level of the umbilicus just lateral to the rectus abdominus (Photo 14.1).

EXPOSURE OF THE OPERATING FIELD

An assistant competent in the use of a 30° laparoscope holds the camera for the duration of the procedure. A laparoscopic assessment of the peritoneal cavity is made to assess for any potential difficulties during the procedure, such as adhesions, diverticular disease, and bulky fibroid uterus. The stomach is also assessed and if distended the anaesthetist can place a nasogastric tube to aspirate the contents, which can be removed at the end of the procedure. The patient is placed in steep Trendelenburg position and the omentum and small bowel are delivered from the pelvis, a swab can be placed to prevent the small bowel reentering the operative field. The sigmoid colon is removed from the pelvis by grasping the appendix epiploic. Retraction of the sigmoid will aid dissection, and this can be performed by fixing two or more appendices

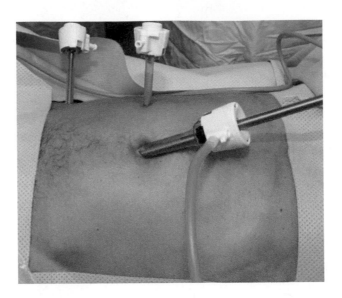

Photo 14.1 Port placement.

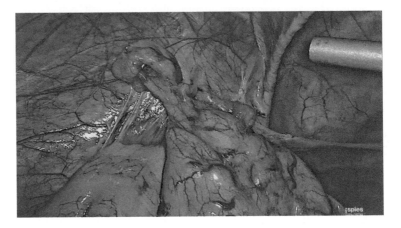

Photo 14.2 Retraction of the sigmoid by fixation of two appendices epiploicae using ProTack.

epiploicae onto the anterolateral left abdominal wall just superior to the pelvic brim with a few fixation devices using the ProTack (Photo 14.2). Optimal exposure is essential for safe and effective laparoscopic surgery, especially within a confined space like the pelvis. To aid vision and dissection the scrub nurse can retract the uterus anteriorly using the vaginal Spackman cannula and if necessary the uterus can be sutured to the anterior abdominal wall.

MOBILISATION

DISSECTION

Consistent with surgical principles the retracting hand does the majority of the work – displaying the correct tissue planes under the right amount of tension for the diathermy to

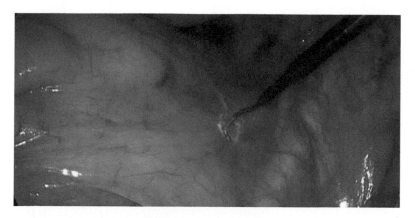

Photo 14.3 Incision to the right of the sacral promontory.

cauterise and divide the tissues in a safe and avascular fashion. With the upper rectum retracted cranially, anteriorly, and to the patient's left, the mesorectum is displayed. The peritoneum is opened superficially just to the right of the sacral promontory (Photo 14.3). This incision is continued caudally along the plane of the right outer border of mesorectum, down to the right side of the pouch of Douglas. Care is taken to avoid the right hypogastric nerve, gonadal vessels, ureter, and the deeper structures of the pelvic side wall.

FEMALE DISSECTION

At the level of the pouch of Douglas the peritoneal incision is continued from right to left over the ventral aspect of the rectum (Photo 14.4). The rectovaginal septum is incised, and dissection continues caudally in this plane facilitated by traction on the rectum cranially, the pneumoperitoneum, and vaginal Spackmann cannula. Dissection continues as inferiorly as possible, to the level of the levator plate and laterally to cardinal ligaments and pelvic side walls (Photo 14.5). The 30° laparoscope is invaluable in providing a clear view of the dissection plane by swinging the light lead to the 6 o'clock position. A second incision is made at the most cranial level of the pouch of Douglas in the midline (Photo 14.6). The peritoneum and underlying

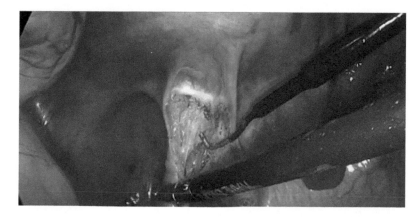

Photo 14.4 Incision continued from right to left.

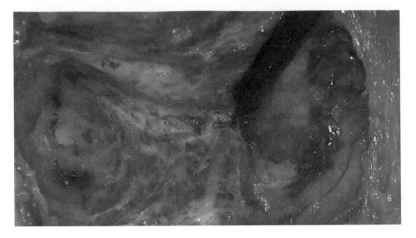

Photo 14.5 To the level of the pelvic floor.

fibroadipose tissue of the pouch of Douglas is dissected off the ventral rectum as these two incisions unite; a *pouchectomy* is thus performed and this tissue is removed through the 12-mm port (Photo 14.7). Any remaining anterior peritoneum or fibro-adipose tissue can be cleared. In symptomatic anterior compartment prolapse (e.g. complex cystocele or anterior enterocele), the vesicovaginal plane is incised and the bladder is carefully mobilised from the anterior vaginal wall. This dissection is the same for post-hysterectomised females.

MALE DISSECTION

Common anatomical features in males with rectal prolapse include tall slim men, wide gynecoid pelvis with widely spaced ischial spines, deep rectovesicle pouch, a mobile mesorectum, and paucity of Denonvilliers fascia (19). The dissection is the same as described above except that it is the plane between Denonvilliers fascia and seminal vesicles which is incised to allow dissection to the pelvic floor (Photo 14.8).

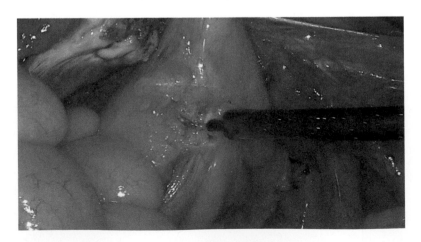

Photo 14.6 Incision at the cranial aspect of the pouch of Douglas.

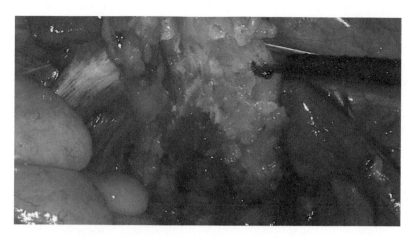

Photo 14.7 Pouchectomy.

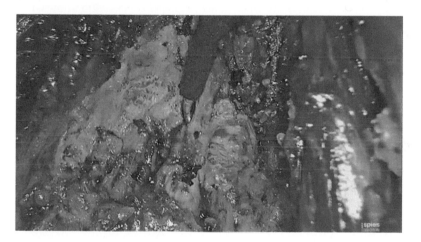

Photo 14.8 Dissection to the pelvic floor in a male.

MESH

MESH SELECTION

Mesh can be biological or synthetic. The consensus statement on ventral rectopexy recommends the use of titanium-coated lightweight polypropylene mesh (17). Standard polypropylene or poliglecaprone may stretch, heavy polypropylene can shrink, and both can result in recurrence of symptoms. Polyester mesh is associated with a significant increase in complications and hence should *not* be used (30). Biological mesh can be considered in younger patients, women of reproductive age, patients with a higher risk for mesh infection and fistulation, revisional surgery, contamination during surgery, diabetics, smokers, pelvic radiation, and inflammatory bowel disease.

MESH PLACEMENT IN FEMALE PATIENTS

The mesh is marked with indelible ink along the longitudinal axis in the midline; this aids orientation during suturing. The mesh is cut to size (approximately 20 × 4 cm) with a quarter-centimeter circle cut out of the left proximal corner to allow room for the upper rectum when the mesh is secured. The 3/0 PDS suture is placed in the midline at the distal end of the mesh extracorporeally, the mesh with the suture is then inserted into the peritoneal cavity through the umbilical port site. Using the laparoscopic needle holders a bite is taken through the inferiormost anterior fibrous tissue within the pelvis in the midline (Photo 14.9). The needle is then brought back through the mesh in the midline. The mesh is placed in the correct position, this can be aided by retracting on both limbs of the suture with the left hand, pulling the suture taught, and the mesh is gently brought into correct position, an intracorporeal surgeon knot is thrown, laid carefully, and suture cut. Several interrupted sutures, 1–2 cm apart, working caudocranially up the mesh in the midline (hence the importance of the indelible ink) should be placed and anchored to the ventral rectal wall (Photo 14.10). The technique used in our centre is to take a bite through the mesh, swing the laparoscope under the mesh, which provides a good view of the needle as it passes through the mesh and physically splints the mesh, preventing crumpling or rotation (Photo 14.11). Once under the mesh, an adventitial-muscular bite of the anterior rectal wall can be taken, then passed back through the mesh at which point the laparoscope is swung over the mesh (Photo 14.12). An intracorporeal surgeon knot is thrown, laid down correctly, and suture cut. This process is repeated to the level of the upper rectum. The lateral margins of the mesh are also secured to the pelvic side walls. An overview of the mesh in the pelvis is shown in Photo 14.13.

Finally, the plane between the peritoneum and the sacral promontory, the site of the first incision, is opened slightly and the mesh brought up to this point with gentle traction. The ProTack fixation device is used to fix the mesh on the sacral promontory, ensuring fixation into bone and avoiding the L5/S1 disc. Several tacks can be used to keep the mesh 'open' to prevent crumpling (Photo 14.14).

For those with significant posterior rectal prolapse a narrow 2-cm window is created in the mesorectum. This dissection is extended caudally for a few centimeters and an 2/0 polyethylene terephthalate (Ethibond) suture is placed and secured to the mesh at the level of the sacral promontory (Photo 14.15).

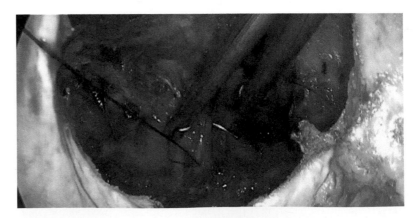

Photo 14.9 Bite taken through the inferiormost anterior fibrous tissue.

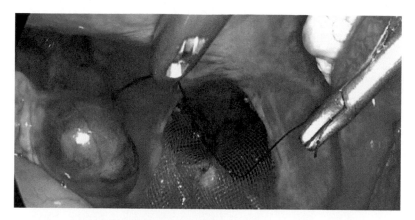

Photo 14.10 Mesh secured to anterior rectum in pelvis.

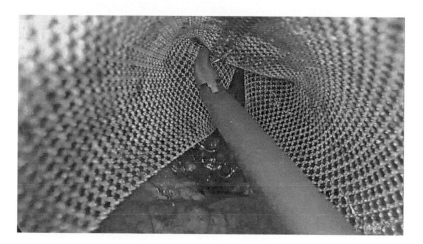

Photo 14.11 Laparoscope under the mesh splinting it and providing a good view of the needle.

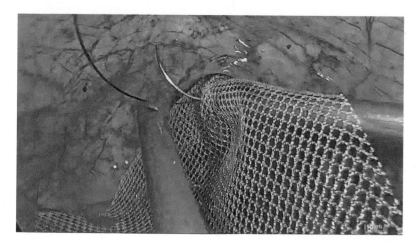

Photo 14.12 Laparoscope over the mesh once a bite is taken through the anterior rectal wall and back through the mesh.

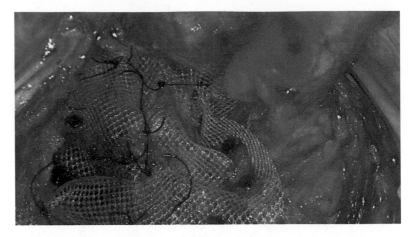

Photo 14.13 Mesh secured in pelvis (light lead at 6 o'clock looking towards pelvic floor).

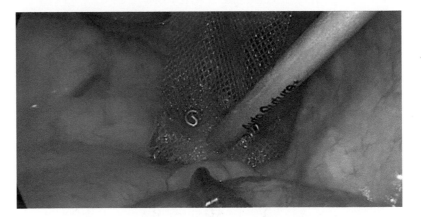

Photo 14.14 Mesh secured on sacral promontory with ProTack device.

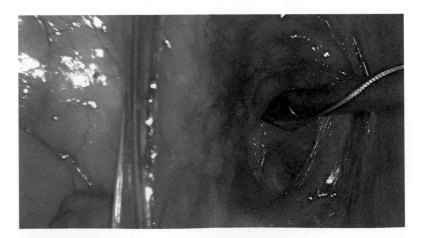

Photo 14.15 Placement of suture.

MESH PLACEMENT IN MALE PATIENTS

Mesh placement is the same as described for females (Photo 14.16).

CLOSURE

A 3/0 V-Loc with a welded loop is inserted through the umbilical port into the pelvis. Bites are taken of the peritoneum and the mesh to cover the mesh with peritoneum and obliterate potential space between the two. In females bites can be taken through the posterior vaginal wall, peritoneum, mesh, and anterior rectal wall (Photo 14.17). This reconstitutes the rectovaginal septum, as the vaginal wall is secured to the mesh a posterior colporrhaphy is performed, a neo-pouch of Douglas is formed, which is much shallower and prevents enterocele. This continues caudocranially until, at the site of the first incision, the peritoneum is closed over the fixation tacks.

Photos 14.18 to 14.20 show the pelvis at the completion of the procedure.

Haemostasis is ensured, the 5-mm ports are withdrawn under direct vision, then the umbilical port and the pneumoperitoneum is deflated. The 10-mm port is closed in standard fashion using a 3/0 PDS on a 'J'-shaped needle. Local anaesthetic (e.g. 0.5% bupivacaine) is applied to the wounds. Skin is closed with 3/0 polyglecaprone, and dressings or skin glue is applied. An examination under anaesthesia (EUA) should be performed to assess the rectopexy and if required a sutured mucopexy can be performed.

POST-OPERATIVE CONSIDERATIONS

The catheter is removed prior to the patient waking. A gauze tampon is placed in the vagina to provide support for the first 24 hours. Patients are managed with enhanced recovery principles with the aim of going home the day after surgery, although same-day discharge has been shown to be safe and feasible (32). The use of opiates should be discouraged due to their

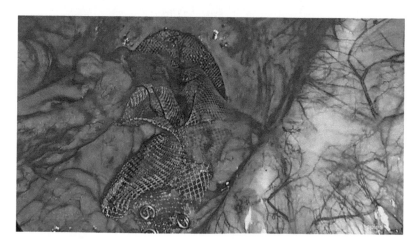

Photo 14.16 Placement of mesh in a male.

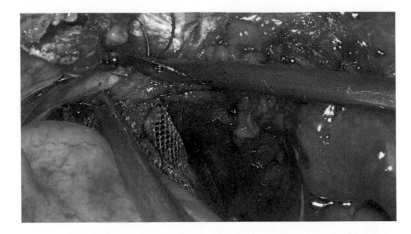

Photo 14.17 V-Loc suture taken through peritoneum, posterior vaginal wall, mesh, and anterior rectal wall.

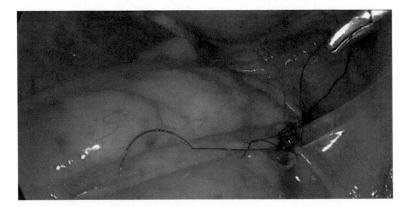

Photo 14.18 Female (with uterus) pelvis at end of procedure.

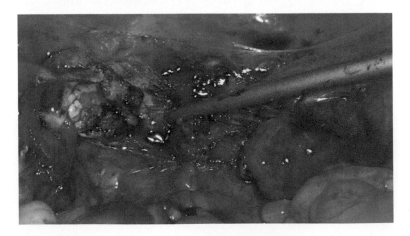

Photo 14.19 Female (post-hysterectomy) pelvis at end of procedure.

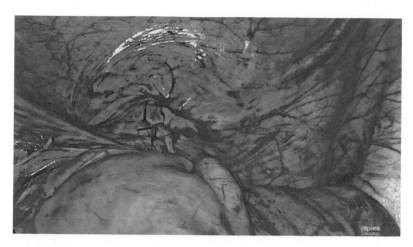

Photo 14.20 Male pelvis at end of procedure.

significant gastrointestinal side effect profile, alternative analgesics such as Gabapentin should be considered. If the patient has significant chronic pelvic pain a 24-hour ketamine infusion should be considered. Patients should be followed up long term with the completion of validated symptom and quality-of-life questionnaires.

COMPLICATIONS

Complications arise during all forms of surgical intervention. The most common complication is urinary retention post procedure (17). Specific complications to be mindful of include haemorrhage from the posterior vaginal wall, perforation of the rectum or vagina, urinary retention, worsening of symptoms or non-resolution of symptoms, and sexual dysfunction. Incorrect placement of the ProTack into the L5/S1 disc can result in spondylodiscitis (33). Mesh-related complications are a reality and include erosion 2%–3% through vagina, rectum, or bladder, infection, stricture of the rectum, and technical failure (i.e. incorrect placement or securing) (34). However, these patients do respond to revisional surgery carried out by an experienced operator with sustained functional outcomes (35).

Intra-operative perforation may occur. If this is in the vagina this can be repaired and the operation continued, if the rectum is perforated this will require immediate repair and defunctioning, enterotomies will require repair. In our experience it is rare for patients to develop adhesional obstruction, although there is a risk with fixation tacks that bowel may become caught resulting in obstructive symptoms. Many patients will develop a systemic response to the surgery and mesh, resulting in pyrexia; they will of course secrete serous fluid in reaction to the mesh and hence any imaging of these patients will invariably show fluid collection at the level of the mesh, which may be misinterpreted as an intra-abdominal source of sepsis. If mesh is infected this can be treated with antibiotics and the mesh allowed to fistulate through the vagina or rectum where it can be retrieved in a safer fashion via an EUA rather than a transabdominal approach.

SUMMARY

Laparoscopic ventral mesh rectopexy is a safe and effective operation for external rectal prolapse or internal rectal prolapse with ODS, FI, complex cystocele or enterocele, and SRUS. This is a technically demanding operation, and surgeons need to develop skills through mentorship, fellowships, and lab-based sessions outside the operating theatre. Using a standardised modular approach can help surgeons through the learning curve (36).

KEY POINTS

- Thorough clinical assessment is required with sound knowledge and understanding.
- PFDs are complex, and patients should be referred to and discussed at pelvic floor MDTs.
- LVMR addresses the underlying pathophysiological and anatomical abnormalities.
- LVMR has a proven safety and efficacy profile.
- LVMR is effective for ERP and IRP causing FI or ODS.
- Surgery is technically challenging with a prolonged learning curve.
- Using a modular approach with a mentor is advised.
- Take time to ensure the operation is done correctly.
- Mesh-related complications happen, but they do respond well to revisional surgery by an experienced operator.

TAKE-HOME MESSAGE

Laparoscopic ventral mesh rectopexy requires modular training and a multidisciplinary approach.

APPENDIX 14.1: PELVIC FLOOR SOCIETY PUBLISHED PROCEDURE-BASED ASSESSMENT FOR LAPAROSCOPIC VENTRAL MESH RECTOPEXY (1)

Procedure-based assessment: Laparoscopic ventral mesh rectopexy

I.	Consent	Rating	Comment
C1	Demonstrates sound knowledge of indications and contraindications including alternatives to surgery.		
C2	Demonstrates awareness of different surgical approaches and advantages and disadvantages.		
C3	Demonstrates sound knowledge of complications of surgery and rates of recurrence.		
C4	Explains the procedure to the patient/relatives/carers and checks understanding.		
C5	Explains likely outcome and time to recovery and checks understanding.		

II.	Preoperative planning	Rating	Comment
PL1	Demonstrates recognition of anatomical and pathological abnormalities, and their likely clinical relevance, and selects appropriate operative strategies/techniques to deal with these.		
PL2	Demonstrates ability to make reasoned choices of appropriate equipment, materials, or devices (e.g. mesh) taking into account appropriate investigations (e.g. proctograms).		
PL3	Checks materials, equipment, and device requirements with operating staff.		
PL4	Checks operative records; personally reviews investigations.		

III.	Preoperative planning	Rating	Comment
PR1	Checks in theatre that consent has been obtained.		
PR2	Gives effective briefing to theatre team.		
PR3	Ensures proper and safe positioning of the patient on the operating table.		
PR4	Demonstrates careful skin preparation.		
PR5	Demonstrates careful draping of the patient's operative field.		
PR6	Ensures general equipment and materials are deployed safely (e.g. diathermy).		
PR7	Ensures appropriate drugs are administered.		

IV.	Exposure and closure	Rating	Comment
E1	Demonstrates knowledge of optimum skin incision/portal/access.		
E2	Achieves an adequate exposure through purposeful dissection in correct tissue planes and identifies all structures correctly.		
E3	Uses graspers, diathermy, and other energy devices so as to minimise the risk of iatrogenic injury.		
E4	Completes a sound wound repair.		
E5	Protects the wound with dressings or glue.		

V.	Intra-operative technique: global (G) and task-specific items (T)	Rating	Comment
IT1 (G)	Follows an agreed-on, logical sequence or protocol for the procedure.		
IT2 (G)	Consistently handles tissue well with minimal damage.		
IT3 (G)	Controls bleeding promptly by an appropriate method.		
IT4 (G)	Demonstrates a sound technique of knots and sutures.		
IT5 (G)	Uses instruments appropriately and safely.		
IT6 (G)	Proceeds at appropriate pace with economy of movement.		
IT7 (G)	Anticipates and responds appropriately to variation, for example, anatomy.		
IT8 (G)	Deals calmly and effectively with unexpected events/complications.		
IT9 (G)	Uses assistant(s) to the best advantage at all times.		
IT10 (G)	Communicates clearly and consistently with scrub team.		
IT11 (G)	Communicates clearly and consistently with the anaesthetist.		

V.	Intra-operative technique: global (G) and task-specific items (T)	Rating	Comment
IT12 (T)	Safely obtains pneumoperitoneum and places ports in suitable positions.		
IT13 (T)	Ensures small bowel is safely delivered out of the pelvis, and the rectum is clearly exposed.		
IT14 (T)	Performs dissection of the lateral pelvic peritoneum and continues dissection anteriorly. Shows awareness of ureters, pelvic nerves and vagina in females, seminal vesicles in males.		
IT15 (T)	Appropriately uses traction and maintains field of view to facilitate dissection.		
IT16 (T)	Identifies the pelvic floor and performs insertion and suturing of mesh.		
IT17 (T)	Safely secures mesh to sacral promontory.		
IT18 (T)	Safely performs peritoneal closure.		
IT19 (T)	Performs abdominal wall closure.		
VI.	Post-operative management	Rating	Comment
PM1	Ensures the patient is transferred safely from the operating table to the bed.		
PM2	Constructs a clear operation note.		
PM3	Records clear and appropriate post-operative instruction.		
PM4	Deals with specimens (if appropriate). Labels and orientates specimens appropriately.		

REFERENCES

1. The Pelvic Floor Society. 2014. *Procedure Based Assessment—Laparoscopic Ventral Mesh Rectopexy*. [Online]. [Accessed 10 January 2016]. Available at: http://thepelvicfloorsociety.co.uk/pages.php?t=Training-&-Education&s=Training-and-Education&id=102

2. Moore KL, Dalley AF. 2006. *Clinically Oriented Anatomy*. 5th ed. Baltimore: Lippincott Williams and Wilkins.

3. Bordeianou L, Hicks CW, Kaiser AM, Alavi K, Sudan R, Wise PE. Rectal prolapse: An overview of clinical features, diagnosis, and patient-specific management strategies. *J Gastrointest Surg* 18(5):1059–69.

4. Ellis H, Mahadevan V. *Clinical Anatomy: Applied Anatomy for Students and Junior Doctors*. 12th ed. Chichester: Wiley-Blackwell, 2010.

5. Lammers K, Lince SL, Spath MA, van Kempen LC, Hendriks JC, Vierhout ME, Kluivers KB, 2012. Pelvic organ prolapse and collagen-associated disorders. *Int Urogynecol J* 2014;23(3):313–9.

6. Lin S, Tee Y, Ng S, Chang H, Lin P, Chen G. 2007. Changes in the extracellular matrix in the anterior vagina of women with or without prolapse. *Int Urogynecol J* 18(1):43–8.

7. Bai SW, Choe BH, Kim JY, Park KH. 2002. Pelvic organ prolapse and connective tissue abnormalities in Korean women. *J Reprod Med* 47(3):231–4.

8. Dixon AR. 2010. Pathophysiological approach to obstruction defecation. In I. Lindsey, K. Nugent, A.R. Dixon (Eds.) *Pelvic Floor Disorders for the Colorectal Surgeon*. Oxford: Oxford University Press, pp. 57–68.

9. Soderberg MW, Falconer C, Bystrom B, Malmstrom A, Ekman G. 2004. Young women with genital prolapse have a low collagen concentration. *Acta Obstet Gynecol Scand* 83(12):1193–8.

10. Jackson S, Avery NC, Tarlton JF, Eckford SD, Abrams P, Bailey AJ. 1996. Changes in metabolism of collagen in genitourinary prolapse. *Lancet* 347(9016):1658–61.

11. Moalli PA, Shand SH, Zyczynski HM, Gordy SC, Men LA. 2005. Remodelling of vaginal connective tissue in patients with prolapse. *Obstet Gynecol* 106(5 Pt 1):593–63.

12. Collinson R, Cunningham C, D'Costa H, Lindsey I. 2009. Rectal intussusception and unexplained faecal incontinence: Findings of a proctographic study. *Colorectal Dis* 11(1):77–83.

13. Rickert A, Kienle P. Laparoscopic surgery for rectal prolapse and pelvic floor disorders. *World J Gastrointest Endosc* 2015;**7**(12):1045–54.

14. Marzetti E, Leeuwenburgh C. Skeletal muscle apoptosis, sarcopenia and frailty in old age. *Exp Gerontol* 2006;41(12):1234–8.

15. Sangsawang B. Risk factors for the development of stress urinary incontinence during pregnancy in primigravidae: A review of the literature. *Eur J Obstet Gynecol Reprod Biol* 2014;178:27–34.

16. Clark AL, Gregory T, Smith VJ, Edwards R. Epidemiological evaluation of reoperation for surgically treated pelvic organ prolapse and urinary incontinence. *Am J Obstet Gynaecol* 2003;189(5):1261–7.

17. Mercer-Jones MA, D'Hoore A, Dixon AR, Lehur P, Lindsey I, Mellgren A, Stevenson AR. Consensus on ventral rectopexy: Report of a panel of experts. *Colorectal Dis* 2014;16(2):82–8.

18. Hompes R, Jones OM, Cunningham C, Lindsey I. What causes chronic idiopathic perineal pain? *Colorectal Dis* 2011;13(9):1035–39.

19. The Pelvic Floor Society. 2014. *QA and Standards*. [Online]. [Accessed 10th January 2016]. Available at: http://thepelvicfloorsociety.co.uk/pages. php?t=QA-&-standards&s=QA-&-Governance&id=101

20. Tou S, Brown SR, Nelson RL. Surgery for complete (full-thickness) rectal prolapse in adults. *The Cochrane Database of Systematic Reviews* 2015, Issue 11. Art. No.: CD001758.

21. Senapati A, Gray RG, Middleton LJ, Harding J, Hills RK, Armitage NC, Buckley L, Northover JM. PROSPER Collaborative Group. PROSPER: A randomised comparison of surgical treatments for rectal prolapse. *Colorectal Dis* 2013;15(7):858–8.

22. Berman IR. Sutureless laparoscopic rectopexy for procidentia: Technique and implications. *Dis Colon Rectum* 1992;35(7):689–93.

23. D'Hoore A, Cadoni R, Penninckx F. Long-term outcome of laparoscopic ventral rectopexy for total rectal prolapse. *Br J Surg* 2004;91(11):1500–5.

24. Randall J, Smyth E, McCarthy K, Dixon AR. Outcome of laparoscopic ventral mesh rectopexy for external rectal prolapse. *Colorectal Dis* 2014;16(11):914–9.

25. Collinson R, Wijffels N, Cunningham C, Lindsey I. Laparoscopic ventral rectopexy for internal rectal prolapse: Short-term functional results. *Colorectal Dis* 2010;12(2):97–104.

26. Badrek-Amoudi AH, Roe T, Mabey K, Carter H, Mills A, Dixon AR. Laparoscopic ventral mesh rectopexy in the management of solitary rectal ulcer syndrome: A cause for optimism? *Colorectal Dis* 2013;15(5):575–81.

27. Slawik S, Soulsby R, Carter H, Payne H, Dixon AR. Laparoscopic ventral rectopexy, posterior colporrhaphy and vaginal sacrocolpopexy for the treatment of recto-genital prolapse and mechanical outlet obstruction. *Colorectal Dis* 2008;10(2):138–43.

28. Wijffels N, Cunningham C, Dixon A, Greenslade G, Lindsey I. Laparoscopic ventral rectopexy for external rectal prolapse is safe and effective in the elderly. Does this make perineal procedures obsolete? *Colorectal Dis* 2011;13(5):561–6.

29. Owais AE, Sumrien H, Mabey K, McCarthy K, Greenslade GL, Dixon AR. Laparoscopic ventral mesh rectopexy in male patients with internal or external rectal prolapse. *Colorectal Dis* 2014;16(12):995–1000.

30. Mackenzie H, Dixon AR. Proficiency gain curve and predictors of outcome for laparoscopic ventral mesh rectopexy. *Surgery* 2014;156(1):158–67.

31. Miskovic D, Ni M, Wyles SM, Tekkis P, Hanna GB. Learning curve and case selection in laparoscopic colorectal surgery: Systematic review and international multicenter analysis of 4852 cases. *Dis Colon Rectum* 2012;55(12):1300–10.

32. Powar MP, Ogilvie JW Jr, Stevenson AR 2013. Day-case laparoscopic ventral rectopexy: An achievable reality. *Colorectal Dis* 15(6):700–6.

33. Propst K, Tunitsky-Bitton E, Schimpf MO, Ridgeway B. 2014. Pyogenic spondylodiscitis associated with sacral colpopexy and rectopexy: Report of two cases and evaluation of the literature. *Int Urogynecol J* 2014;25(1):21–31.

34. Evans C, Stevenson AR, Sileri P, Mercer-Jones MA, Dixon AR, Cunningham C, Jones OM, Lindsey I, 2015. A multicenter collaboration to assess the safety of laparoscopic ventral rectopexy. *Dis Colon Rectum* 58(8):799–807.

35. Badrek-Al Amoudi AH, Greenslade GL, Dixon AR. 2013. How to deal with complications after laparoscopic ventral mesh rectopexy: Lessons learnt from a tertiary referral centre. *Colorectal Dis* 2013;15(6):707–12.

36. Hemandas A, Flashman KG, Farrow J, O'Leary DP, Parvaiz A. 2011. Modular training in laparoscopic colorectal surgery maximizes training opportunities without clinical compromise. *World J Surg* 2011;35(2):409–14.

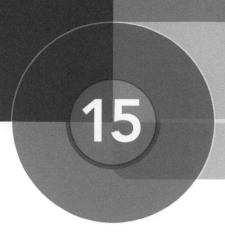

Robotic colorectal surgery

15

HENRY TILNEY AND MARK GUDGEON

LEARNING OBJECTIVES

- Explore the evidence behind the use of the robot with the potential advantages and disadvantages.
- Develop an appreciation of the technical approach to robotic total mesorectal excision (TME).

INTRODUCTION

Today's robotic surgical systems are capable of performing complex multivisceral surgery and function as 'master and slave' devices with the benefits of stereoscopic (three-dimensional) vision and scaled movements using wristed instruments permitting precise dissection in confined body cavities. The robotic platform in current use is the da Vinci system made by Intuitive Surgical, Inc. The latest refinement is the da Vinci Xi released in 2014.

While the most common procedure performed with the da Vinci Surgical System is radical prostatectomy, many other urological, gynaecological, cardiothoracic, paediatric and general surgical procedures have also been performed, and the list continues to grow. Only relatively recently has robotic colorectal surgery become popular. The procedures performed include right and left hemicolectomy, total mesorectal excision (TME), proctectomy and ileal pouch-anal anastomoses, and ventral mesh rectopexy. In the authors' opinion it is within the pelvis that the value of the robot lies and this issue is considered in more detail in the present chapter.

ROBOTIC RECTAL SURGERY

Surgery for rectal cancer is more challenging than colonic surgery because of the anatomical characteristics of the rectum lying within the rigid confines of the pelvis. The principle underlying TME is precise dissection in the avascular plane between the pre-sacral fascia and the fascia propria of the mesorectum to ensure a good quality specimen. This quality correlates closely with the oncological outcome (1,2). The ability of the da Vinci surgical system to offer a three-dimensional view with magnification, hand tremor filtering, fine dexterity and motion scaling suggests a potential technical surgical advantage over open or laparoscopic TME. The robotic instrument allows a single surgeon to create traction and countertraction in the narrow pelvic cavity, thereby exposing the ideal tissue planes for dissection.

EVIDENCE FOR ROBOTIC TME

There have been a number of studies published in the literature comparing robotic TME to laparoscopic TME, of varying quality and size. Most studies relating to robotic anterior resection have reported only initial experiences. The sample sizes have been very small and nearly all are non-randomised, apart from one small randomised study from South Korea (3). There have, however, been several large comparative series published (4–8). Larger, randomised studies are necessary to assess not only the feasibility and safety of the robotic system but also whether there are real benefits of the robotic system compared to conventional laparoscopic surgery, in terms of short-term surgical outcomes and long-term quality of life and oncological results. Tables 15.1 to 15.3 summarise the results of studies to date that have compared the outcomes between robotic and laparoscopic rectal resections.

Overall, few studies have shown substantial differences in short-term outcomes between robotic and laparoscopic resections (Table 15.2). Six studies have identified a significantly reduced length of stay with use of the robot (3,5,8–11). In addition four studies have reported a reduced incidence of conversion with the use of robotics compared to laparoscopic TME (8–11). These studies have shown robotic surgery to be at least as safe as, and oncologically equivalent to laparoscopic surgery (Table 15.3). There is a need for further exploration in large-scale randomised trials to determine whether robotic-assisted TME is superior in oncological and quality-of-life terms to laparoscopic and open surgery; the published results of the Robotic versus Laparoscopic Resection for Rectal Cancer (ROLARR) study are eagerly awaited (12).

THE DA VINCI SURGICAL SYSTEM

The robotic system consists of three main components:

Non-sterile: The console (Photo 15.1), which is the robot's user interface and comprises scissor handle–type 'master controls' that translate the surgeon's hand movement directly to the instrument tips including the 'wristing' angulation and rotation (Photo 15.2). There are foot pedals for camera control, disengaging instruments (clutch), focusing and the application of both monopolar and bipolar diathermy (Photo 15.3). The electronic tower holds the video processing system, light source and a monitor displaying the view from one 'eye' of the stereoscopic robotic camera.

Table 15.1 Overall characteristics of studies reporting outcomes of robotic rectal cancer surgery

Study	Author	Year	Institution	Years of study	Type of study	Number of patients		Procedures	
						Robotic	Lap	Robotic	Lap
1	Delaney et al. (14)	2003	Cleveland Clinic, OH	2001–2002	Case matched	6	6	R Hemi (2) Sigmoid resection (3) Rectopexy (1)	R Hemi (2) Sigmoid resection (3) Rectopexy (1)
2	D'Annibale et al. (15)	2004	Padova, Italy	2001–2003	Case matched	53	53	R Hemi 10 Ileccaecal 0 Transverse Colectomy 0 L Hemi 17 Sigmoid resection 11 AR 10 APER 1 Total colectomy 2 Hartmann's 1 Hartmann reversal 0 Rectopexy 1	R Hemi 13 Ileocaecal 1 Transverse colectomy 1 L Hemi 17 Sigmoid resection 4 AR 15 APER 0 Total colectomy 1 Hartmann's 1 Hartmann reversal 2 Rectopexy 0
3	Pigazzi et al.† (16)	2006	City of Hope National Medical Center, CA	2004–2005	Non-randomised, comparative	6	6	Low AR	Low AR

(Continued)

Table 15.1 (*Continued*) Overall characteristics of studies reporting outcomes of robotic rectal cancer surgery

Study	Author	Year	Institution	Years of study	Type of study	Number of patients		Procedures	
						Robotic	Lap	Robotic	Lap
4	Spinoglio et al. (17)	2008	Alessandria, Italy	2005–2007	Non-randomised, comparative	50	161	R Hemi 18 L Hemi 10 AR 19 APER 1 Transverse colectomy 1 Total colectomy 1	R Hemi 50 L Hemi 73 AR 26 APER 7 Transverse colectomy 2 Total colectomy 3
5	Baik et al.* (3)	2008	Seoul, South Korea	2006–2007	RCT	18	18	'Tumour-specific TME'	'Tumour-specific TME'
6	Baik et al.* (9)	2009	Seoul, South Korea	2006–2007	Non-randomised, comparative	56	57	Low AR	Low AR
7	Bianchi et al. (18)	2010	University of Milan, Italy	2008–2009	Non-randomised, comparative	25	25	AR 18 APER 7	AR 19 APER 6
8	Park et al.$ (7)	2011	Kyungpook National University Hospital, Korea	2007–2009	Non-randomised, comparative	52	123	AR 52	AR 123
9	Kim et al. (19)	2012	Yonsei University College, Seoul, Korea	2009	Prospective cohort study	30	39	AR 29 Hartmann's 1	AR 38 Hartmann's 1

(Continued)

Table 15.1 (Continued) Overall characteristics of studies reporting outcomes of robotic rectal cancer surgery

Study	Author	Year	Institution	Years of study	Type of study	Number of patients		Procedures	
						Robotic	Lap	Robotic	Lap
10	Baek et al. (6)	2012	Korea University, Anam Hospital, Korea	2007–2010	Non-randomised, comparative	154	150	AR 143 APER 11	AR 144 APER 4 Proctocolectomy and IPAA 2
11	Fernandez et al. (20)	2013	VA Medical Center, Houston, TX	2002–2012	Non-randomised, comparative	13	59	AR 5 APER 8	AR 44 APER 15
12	Kang et al. (5)	2013	Yonsei University College, Seoul, Korea	2007–2010	Retrospective matched cohort analysis	165	165	AR 164 APER 0 Hartmann's 1	AR 158 APER 6 Hartmann's 1
13	Saklani et al.^ (4)	2013	Yonsei University College, Seoul, Korea	2006–2010	Non-randomised, comparative	74	64	AR 72 APER 2	AR 61 APER 3
14	Park et al.$ (21)	2013	Kyungpook National University Hospital, Korea	2008–2011	Non-randomised, comparative	40	40	IS AR 40	IS AR 40
15	D'Annibale et al. (11)	2013	Rome, Italy	2004–2012	Non-randomised, comparative	50	50	AR 50	AR 50
16	Baek et al. (10)	2013	Seoul, South Korea	2007–2010	Non-randomised, comparative	47	37	AR 47	AR 37
17	Erguner et al. (22)	2013	Acibadem Maslak Hospital, Istanbul, Turkey	2008–2011	Non-randomised, comparative	27	37	AR 27	AR 37

(Continued)

Table 15.1 (*Continued*) Overall characteristics of studies reporting outcomes of robotic rectal cancer surgery

| Study | Author | Year | Institution | Years of study | Type of study | Number of patients | | Procedures | |
						Robotic	Lap	Robotic	Lap
18	Yoo et al. (23)	2014	Korea University Anam Hospital, Seoul, Korea	2006–2011	Non-randomised, comparative	44	26	AR 44	AR 26
19	Ielpo et al. (24)	2014	San Pablo University, Madrid, Spain	2010–2013	Non-randomised, comparative	56	87	AR 40 APER 15	AR 64 APER 20
20	Barnajian et al. (25)	2014	State University of New York	2012	Non-randomised, comparative	20	20	AR 15 APER 5	AR 15 APER 5
21	Levic et al. (26)	2014	Hvidovre Hospital, Copenhagen	2010–2012	Non-randomised, comparative	56	36	AR 32 APER 15 Hartmann's 9	AR 20 APER 12 Hartmann's 4
22	Tam, Abbass and Abbas (27)	2014	Kaiser Permanente, LA	2011–2013	Non-randomised, comparative	21	21	AR 12 APER 7 Proctocolectomy 2	AR 19 APER 2
23	Park et al.§ (28)	2014	Seoul, South Korea	2006–2011	Non-randomised, comparative	89	89	AR 89	AR 89
24	Koh et al. (29)	2014	Singapore	2008–2011	Non-randomised, comparative	19	19	AR 19	AR 19
25	Park et al.§ (8)	2015	Seoul, South Korea	2006–2011	Non-randomised, comparative	133	84	AR 133	AR 84

Notes: Robotic, robotic surgery; Lap, laparoscopic surgery; TME, total mesorectal excision; R Hemi, right hemicolectomy; L Hemi, left hemicolectomy; AR, anterior resection; APER, abdominoperineal excision of rectum; Ileocaecal, ileocaecal resection; †,*, ∧, $,§, Denote multiple publications by the same departments with likely duplication of reported outcomes.

Table 15.2 Short-term outcomes from studies reporting outcomes of robotic rectal cancer surgery

Study	Author	Conversion		Duration surgery (min)		Blood loss (mL)		LOS (days)		Anastomotic leak		Complications	
		Robotic	Lap	Robotic	Lap	Robotic	Lap	Robotic	Lap	Robotic	Lap	Robotic	Lap
1	Delaney et al. (14)	—	—	216.5 (170–274)	150 (116–165)	100 (50–350)	87.5 (50–200)	3 (2–5)	2.5 (2–7)	—	—	1 Atelectasis	1 Incisional hernia
2	D'Annibale et al. (15)	6 (2 to laparocopy, 4 to hand-assisted laparoscopy)	3	240 (±61)	222 (±77)	21 (±80)	37 (±102)	—	—	0	1	2 bowel injuries 1 CVA 1 wound infection	—
3	Pigazzi et al.† (16)	—	—	264 (192–318)	258 (198–312)	104 (50–318)	150 (50–300)	4.5 (3–11)	3.6 (3–6)	—	—	1 Prolonged ileus	1 Pelvic abscess
4	Spinoglio et al. (17)	2 (1 to laparoscopy, 1 to laparotomy)	4	383.8	266.3	—	—	7.74	8.31	2	—	1 Incisional hernia 1 Atelectasis 1 Wound infection 1 Phlebitis 1 CVA	—
5	Baik et al.* (3)	0	2	202.5 (149–315)	196.0 (114–297)	—	—	7 (5–10)	9 (6–12)	—	—	—	—
6	Baik e al.* (9)	0	6	178 (120–315)	179 (100–360)	—	—	5 (5–10)	6 (4–16)	1	4	'Serious complication' 5.4%	'Serious complication' 19.3%

(Continued)

Table 15.2 (*Continued*) Short-term outcomes from studies reporting outcomes of robotic rectal cancer surgery

Study	Author	Conversion		Duration surgery (min)		Blood loss (mL)		LOS (days)		Anastomotic leak		Complications	
		Robotic	Lap	Robotic	Lap	Robotic	Lap	Robotic	Lap	Robotic	Lap	Robotic	Lap
7	Bianchi et al. (18)	0	1	240 (170–420)	237 (170–545)	—	—	6.5 (4–15)	6 (4–20)	1	2	Wound infection 1 Stomal stenosis 1 Peritonitis 1	Wound infection 2
8	Park et al. (7)	0	0	232.6 (52.4)	158.1 (49.2)	—	—	10.4 (4.7)	9.8 (3.8)	5	7	Ileus: 1 Pelvic abscess: 1 Bleeding: 2 CVS problem: 1	ARF: 1 Wound problem: 1 AUR: 2 Ileus: 1 Pelvic abscess: 1 Bleeding: 2
9	Kim et al. (19)	—	—	—	—	—	—	—	—	—	—	IPSS score: 6.43 (5.27) IIEF score: 54.67 (14.27)	IPSS score: 7.95 (5.6) IIEF score: 51.55 (11.98)
10	Baek et al. (6)	0	0	285.2 (130–475)	219.7 (95–465)	167.8 (0–1500)	126.2 (0–1500)	11.1 (5–50)	10.8 (4–75)	17	18	Anastomotic bleed 4 Ileus 19 Other 10	Anastomotic bleed 2 Ileus 7 Other 14
11	Fernandez et al. (20)	1	10	528 (416–700)	344 (183–735)	157 (50–550)	200 (25–1500)	13 (29)	8 (45)	1	3	SSI 9 DVT 0 AUR 5 Mortality 0	SSI 26 DVT 1 AUR 18 Mortality 1

(*Continued*)

Table 15.2 (Continued) Short-term outcomes from studies reporting outcomes of robotic rectal cancer surgery

Study	Author	Conversion		Duration surgery (min)		Blood loss (mL)		LOS (days)		Anastomotic leak		Complications	
		Robotic	Lap	Robotic	Lap	Robotic	Lap	Robotic	Lap	Robotic	Lap	Robotic	Lap
12	Kang et al. (5)	1	3	309.7 ±115.2	277.8 ±81.9	133 ±192.3	140.1 ±216.4	10.8 ±5.5	13.5 ±9.2	12	17	SSI 1 Ileus 6 Other 4	SSI 2 Ileus 9 Other 6
13	Saklani et al. (4)	1	4	365.2 ±108.4	311.6 ±79.8	180 ±28.1	210 ±35.7	8 ±3.8	9.2 ±4.3	4	8	Ileus 2 SSI 1 Other 4	Ileus 3 SSI 0 Other 6
14	Park et al. (21)	0	0	235.5 ±57.5	185.4 ±72.8	45.7 ±40	59.2 ±35.8	10.6 ±4.2	11.3 ±3.6	3	2	Intra-abdo infection 17 AUR 1 Colon ischaemia 1	Intra-abdo infection 1 AUR 1 Colon ischaemia 1
15	D'Annibale et al. (11)	0	6	270 (240–315)	280 (240–350)	–	–	8 (7–11)	10 (8–14)	5	7	Morbidity 5	Morbidity 11
16	Baek et al. (10)	1	6	352.7 ±130.3	360.7 ±88.2	190.9 ±284.7	302.7 ±305.3	9 (7–14)	11 (9–18.5)	4	3	Abscess 2 SSI 1 Ileus 1 Other 1	Abscess 3 SSI 0 Ileus 2 Other 2
17	Erguner et al. (22)	0	0	280 (175–480)	190 (110–300)	50 (20–100)	125 (50–400)	4 (4–20)	5 (4–16)	0	3	Morbidity 3	Morbidity 8
18	Yoo et al. (23)	–	–	316.43 ±65.11	286.77 ±51.46	239.77 ±278.61	215.38 ±247.29	11.41 ±5.56	11.04 ±6.33	5	0	Ileus 8 AUR 4 Other 7	Ileus 4 AUR 1 Other 4

(Continued)

Table 15.2 (*Continued*) Short-term outcomes from studies reporting outcomes of robotic rectal cancer surgery

Study	Author	Conversion		Duration surgery (min)		Blood loss (mL)		LOS (days)		Anastomotic leak		Complications	
		Robotic	Lap	Robotic	Lap	Robotic	Lap	Robotic	Lap	Robotic	Lap	Robotic	Lap
19	Ielpo et al. (24)	2	10	309 ± 84	252 ± 90	280 ± 35.3	240 ± 53.7	13 ± 10.5	10 ± 3.6	4	3	4 Intra-abdo abscess 3 Wound infection 4 Ileus 4 Clavien >3	6 Intra-abdo abscess 5 Wound infection 6 Ileus 5 Clavien >3
20	Barnajian et al. (25)	0	2	240 (150–540)	180 (140–480)	125 (50–650)	175 (50–900)	6 (4–31)	7 (5–36)	—	—	2 Ileus 2 Pelvic abscess 2 Anastomotic stricture 1 Presacral bleeding 1 Asthma attack	1 Ileus 1 Urinary retention
21	Levic et al. (26)	3	0	247 (130–511)	295 (108–465)	50 (0–400)	35 (0–400)	8 (4–100)	7 (3–51)	6	3	Morbidity 12 (9–30)	Morbidity 10 (12–43)
22	Tam et al. (27)	1	0	260 (189–449)	240 (171–360)	150 (30–2000)	100 (50–1200)	6 (4–23)	5 (3–14)	0	3	ARF 2 UTI 4 Wound infection 1 SBO 1 Abdo wall hematoma 1 Pneumonia 1	ARF 3 UTI 1 Wound infection 1 SBO 1 Cardiac 2

(*Continued*)

Table 15.2 (Continued) Short-term outcomes from studies reporting outcomes of robotic rectal cancer surgery

Study	Author	Conversion		Duration surgery (min)		Blood loss (mL)		LOS (days)		Anastomotic leak		Complications	
		Robotic	Lap	Robotic	Lap	Robotic	Lap	Robotic	Lap	Robotic	Lap	Robotic	Lap
23	Park et al. (28)	0	5	208.6 ±54.8	202.7 ±76.1	55.8 ±119.4	73.2 ±157.1	8.4 ±3.8	10±6.3	—	—	Grade 1:5 Grade 2:1 Grade 3:3 Grade 4:0	Grade 1:8 Grade 2:4 Grade 3:8 Grade 4:3
24	Koh et al. (29)	1	5	**390** **(289–771)**	**225** **(130–495)**	—	—	7 (4–21)	6 (4–28)	0	2	Ileus 1 Neuropraxia 1 SSI 0 Bleed 1	Ileus 4 Neuropraxia 1 SSI 3 Bleed 0
25	Park et al. (8)	0	6	205.7 ±67.3	208.8 ±81.2	77.6 ±153.2	82.3 ±185.8	**5.86** **±1.43**	6.54 ±2.65	6	3	Grade 1:11 Grade 2:5 Grade 3:9 Grade 4:1 Grade 5:0	Grade 1:7 Grade 2:4 Grade 3:6 Grade 4:2 Grade 5:0

Notes: Robotic, robotic surgery; Lap, laparoscopic surgery; LOS, length of stay; UTI, urinary infection; ARF, acute renal failure; SBO, small bowel obstruction; SSI, surgical site infection; DVT, deep vein thrombosis; IPSS, International Prostate Symptom Score; IIEF, International Index of Erectile Function. Statistically significant results from individual studies are highlighted in bold. Figures for continuous outcomes represent median values with range in parentheses unless ± stated which denotes standard deviation.

Table 15.3 Oncologic outcomes from studies reporting outcomes of robotic rectal cancer surgery

Study	Author	LN Yield		DRM (cm)		TME Assessment			CRMI	
		Robotic	Lap	Robotic	Lap	Robotic	Lap		Robotic	Lap
1	Delaney et al. (14)	—	—	—	—	—	—		—	—
2	D'Annibale et al. (15)	17 (±10)	16 (±9)	—	—	—	—		—	—
3	Pigazzi et al.† (16)	14 (9–28)	17 (9–39)	3.8 (1.8–9)	3.5 (2.2–5)	—	—		—	—
4	Spinoglio et al. (17)	22.03	22.85	7.3	7.9	—	—		—	—
5	Baik et al.* (3)	18 (6–49)	22 (9–42)	4 (1–5.5)	3.5 (1.5–6.0)	Complete 17 Nearly complete 1	Complete 13 Nearly complete 5		—	—
6	Baik et al.* (9)	17.5 (4–43)	17 (4–53)	4 (1–7)	3 (1–9)	Complete 52 Nearly complete 4 Incomplete 0	Complete 43 Nearly complete 12 Incomplete 2		4	5
7	Bianchi et al. (18)	18 (7–34)	17 (8–37)	2 (1.5–4.5)	2 (1.8–3.5)	—	—		0	1
8	Park et al. (7)	19.4 (10.2)	15.9 (10.1)	2.8 (1.9)	3.2 (2.1)	—	—		1	3
9	Kim et al. (19)	—	—	2.79 (1.02)	2.86 (1.36)	Complete 29 Incomplete 1	Complete 37 Incomplete 2		2	1
10	Baek et al. (6)	—	—	—	—	—	—		—	—
11	Fernandez et al. (20)	16 ± 2	20 ± 2	—	—	Complete 9 Nearly complete 4 Incomplete 0	Complete 24 Nearly complete 8 Incomplete 1		0	1
12	Kang et al. (5)	15 ± 9.4	15.6 ± 9.1	1.9 ± 1.4	2 ± 1.7	—	—		7	11
13	Saklani et al. (4)	11.6 ± 6.9	14.7 ± 6.5	1.7 ± 1.4	2.2 ± 1.5	—	—		3	1

(Continued)

Table 15.3 (Continued) Oncologic outcomes from studies reporting outcomes of robotic rectal cancer surgery

Study	Author	LN Yield		DRM (cm)		TME Assessment		CRMI	
		Robotic	Lap	Robotic	Lap	Robotic	Lap	Robotic	Lap
14	Park et al. (21)	12.9	13.3	1.4 ± 0.9	1.3 ± 0.9	—	—	3	2
15	D'Annibale et al. (11)	16.5 ± 7.1	13.8 ± 6.7	3 ± 1.1	3 ± 1.6	—	—	0	6
16	Baek et al. (10)	10.6 ± 6.3	14.1 ± 10.4	1.1 ± 1.1	1.6 ± 2.3	—	—	1	3
17	Erguner et al. (22)	16 (3–38)	16 (3–31)	4 (3–8)	2.5 (0.5–5)	Complete 19 Nearly complete 0 Incomplete 0	Complete 12 Nearly complete 5 Incomplete 0	—	—
18	Yoo et al. (23)	13.93 ± 9.27	21.42 ± 15.71	1.33 ± 0.97	1.67 ± 3	—	—	4	5
19	Ielpo et al. (24)	10 ± 8	9 ± 4.8	—	—	—	—	2	2
20	Barnajian et al. (25)	14 (3–22)	11 (4–18)	2.5 (0.5 –5)	2.2 (0.1–5.5)	Complete 16 Near complete 1 Incomplete 3	Complete 19 Near complete 1 Incomplete 0	—	—
21	Levic et al. (26)	21 (7–83)	13 (3–33)	3 (0.5–8)	3 (0.5–7.5)	—	—	1	0
22	Tam, Abbass and Abbas (27)	17 (8–40)	15 (8–21)	3.9 (1–18)	5.5 (0.5–8)	—	—	0	1
23	Park et al. (28)	16 ± 9.1	17.6 ± 10.2	2.7 ± 1.9	2.9 ± 1.6	—	—	6	6
24	Koh et al. (29)	16 (4–24)	14 (5–27)	—	—	—	—	1	0
25	Park et al. (8)	16.34 ± 8.79	16.63 ± 10.24	2.75 ± 2.14	2.87 ± 1.63	—	—	9	6

Notes: Robotic; robotic surgery; Lap, laparoscopic surgery; LN, lymph node; DRM, distal resection margin; TME, total mesorectal excision; CRMI, circumferential resection margin involvement (tumour ≤1 mm from circumferential cut edge).

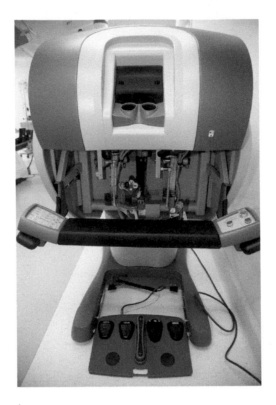

Photo 15.1 Robot console.

Sterile covered: The patient-side cart consists of a powered trolley holding three or four robotic arms, although the authors strongly recommend the use of the four-arm system (Photo 15.4). The scrub nurse is responsible for preparing the robot cart with specially designed transparent sterile covers. The stereoscopic scope, camera and light lead are also prepared in sterile fashion with a special disposable outer sleeve. When utilizing a hybrid approach

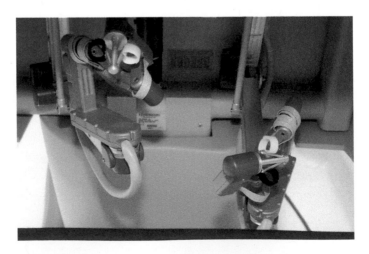

Photo 15.2 Surgeon controls: scissor grips.

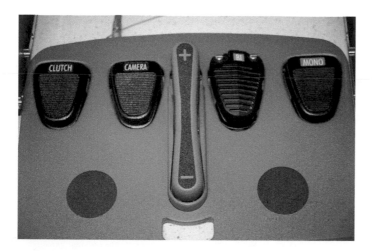

Photo 15.3 Surgeon controls: foot pedals.

with a laparoscopic mobilization of the splenic flexure and left colon it is preferable to defer draping the patient cart until after an initial laparoscopy has confirmed that use of the robot is appropriate. A second scrub nurse may then drape the arms of the cart while the colon is mobilized laparoscopically thereby maximizing efficiency when transitioning from laparoscopic to robotic surgery.

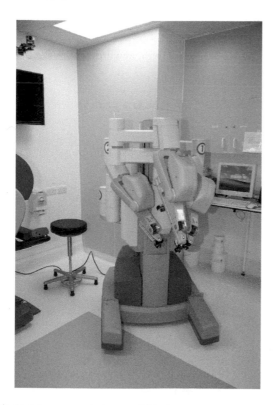

Photo 15.4 Patient side cart: four-arm robot, arms folded.

Sterile equipment: There is a range of dedicated robotic instruments including dissectors, graspers and retractors and many of these can be connected to monopolar and bipolar diathermy sources. Each disposable instrument has a life span of 10 procedures, in order to minimize the cost of disposables we recommend choosing 3 preferred instruments to complete the operation. The authors prefer the use of a diathermy hook or monopolar diathermy scissors ('Hot Shears') in the right-side operative port, Maryland or Fenestrated bipolar forceps in the primary left hand port and either a large grasping retractor or a Cadiere forceps in the secondary left hand port.

The central robotic camera arm is attached to a disposable 12-mm port when using the da Vinci S or Si. The other 3 arms are coupled to the metal 8 mm ports designed specifically for the disposable instruments.

EXPOSURE IN ROBOTIC SURGERY

CORRECT THEATRE SETUP AND POSITIONING OF THE ROBOT

The choice of robot docking position is entirely personal to the surgeon and will be influenced by experience both positive and negative in terms of ease of dissection, minimisation of arm clashes and instrument clashes. When using the robot solely for pelvic dissection we favor docking the patient cart between the legs. When a totally robotic approach is favored the patient cart is docked at an oblique angle over the upper part of the left thigh.

The setup involves manoeuvring the patient-side cart into position between the patient's legs. The central hub, trolley and camera arm of the robot should all be in line with the patient's midline. This enables the 'sweet spot' of the camera arm to be found with ease and without the camera arm getting in the way of the other instrument arms.

Once the camera arm is engaged with the umbilical port, the patient-side cart becomes locked and immobile. The remaining robotic arms are carefully positioned under clutch control to the proximity of the robotic ports. They are each then carefully manoeuvred and fixed to their respective ports using their clasp attachments, the arms are separated to allow free movement during dissection. The assistant is then responsible for insertion of camera and instruments under the careful instruction of the surgeon now sitting at the console. The camera is introduced first to allow for safe introduction of the other robotic instruments, in most cases the 0° scope is suitable for visual access. When difficulty is encountered the 30° scope can be used although the angled view using the da Vinci S and Si is fixed either 'down' or 'up' without the usual benefit of being able to rotate the lens to view the surgical field from varying angles.

Each arm is fitted in turn with an appropriate robotic instrument. The primary arm usually holds the scissors or hook dissector with monopolar diathermy attachment. The secondary arm usually holds Cadiere or Maryland bipolar diathermy graspers. The third arm holds a further grasper of the surgeon's choice: a longer grasper that doubles as a retractor is a useful instrument for this arm. The assistant can lift the rectum out of the pelvis using another laparoscopic grasper via the right upper quadrant 5-mm port that is attached to the nylon tape encircling the bowel at recto-sigmoid-junction. Thus three-point traction can be achieved facilitating precise dissection in the correct plane in a confined space. The dissection and operative view is under the control of the operating surgeon at the console. The assistant, standing to the patient's right side, is responsible for communicating with the surgeon problems related to 'clashing' of the robotic arms which can impair the range of movement of the robotic dissector, and being an active participant in the procedure by retracting the rectum with their left-hand instrument and using suction/irrigation to aspirate the diathermy plume via the 12-mm right iliac fossa port, through which a tonsil swab can also be introduced.

APPROPRIATE PATIENT POSITIONING

Patients undergo standard preoperative investigations, imaging and anaesthetic evaluation prior to surgery as in the case of open or laparoscopic rectal surgery. The patient is usually placed in a modified Lloyd-Davies position, hips slightly extended with knees flexed to between 70° and 90° and placed just greater than shoulder width apart. In our experience the use of a body-length gel mat in direct contact with the patient's skin keeps the patient safely on the operating table without the need for shoulder supports, avoiding the potential risk of nerve injury. Antithromboembolic stockings (unless contraindicated) and intermittent calf compression are routinely used in addition to an upper body warmer. Arms are wrapped at the patient's side and protected from the metalwork of the table, and the patient is catheterised.

SAFE ACCESS TECHNIQUE

The optimum port siting is the subject of much conjecture and many arrays of 'standardised' port sites are described. The authors' preferred setup has evolved from assessment of the published techniques and as a result of trial and error. The authors' favoured sites are recommended as follows.

A suprumbilical incision is made and a 12-mm port is inserted using an open Hassan technique to accommodate the camera lens tube. The new da Vinci Xi has a smaller camera lens tube that fits through an 8-mm port, this allows a greater versatility in positioning the camera during the case. The pneumo-peritoneum is established with an insufflation pressure set to between 12 and 15 cm of water. A 10-mm laparoscope is used for the mobilization of the splenic flexure and left colon during the hybrid approach. The procedure continues by insertion of the robotic 8-mm ports under direct vision via incisions positioned optimally to avoid clashing of the robotic arms, a minimum of at least 80 mm is recommended between ports. The robotic cannulae are marked with broad black bands that represent the fulcrums for angulation and these should lie just within the abdominal wall to allow effective movement and minimise post-operative pain.

An additional 12-mm port in the right iliac fossa 3–4 cm inferomedial to the anterior superior iliac spine (ASIS) is used for laparoscopic instrumentation and for assistant access during the robotic phase of the procedure. A 5-mm port is also placed in the right upper quadrant to allow the assistant to move the upper rectum from side to side and exert traction out of the pelvis as required during the rectal dissection and also to aid splenic flexure mobilisation.

Ports are sited so as to optimise triangulation of instruments, avoid clashing and provide maximum field of view. The camera port is therefore placed in the mid-position of the instrumental port site arc ideally just above the umbilicus so that the field of vision is centred on the midline. The primary operative robotic 8-mm port is placed 8–10 cm to the right along the arc from umbilicus to the right ASIS. The secondary operative robotic 8-mm port is placed in the corresponding position to the left. The tertiary operative robotic 8-mm port is placed 8–10 cm laterally to this along the same arc at a site roughly corresponding to the 12-mm laparoscopic assistant port opposite (Photo 15.1). For a small patient the second operating arm can be placed a few centimeters cranially in order to maintain optimum spacing between ports.

VASCULAR DISSECTION

SAFE DISSECTION OF THE VASCULAR PEDICLE

While mobilisation of the splenic flexure and left colon with high ligation of the inferior mesenteric artery and vein can be performed using the da Vinci system, the authors favour a hybrid approach with standard laparoscopy for the abdominal component of the operation followed by robotic rectal dissection where the true benefits of robotic surgery are felt to be demonstrated. The authors generally mobilise the splenic flexure when performing an anterior resection with TME and this is done at the start of the procedure.

MOBILISATION

MOBILISATION OF SPLENIC FLEXURE

As the authors' preference is to perform a standard laparoscopic left colon and splenic flexure mobilisation, including inferior mesenteric artery division, the procedure will not be reiterated here. At the end of colonic mobilisation, however, a nylon tape is passed around the rectosigmoid junction and tied using a modified Roeder knot. The knot is secured with 2 Hem-o-lok clips with a gap between the clips leaving space for a ratcheted grasper that is manipulated via the right upper quadrant port to allow the scrubbed assistant to retract and manipulate the rectum during rectal mobilisation.

MESORECTAL DISSECTION: ROBOTIC TME

The patient remains in a steep head down right lateral tilt in order to prevent the small bowel from falling into the pelvis. In the female patient with an intact uterus a straight-needled polypropylene suture is driven through the suprapubic skin through the fundus of the uterus and back through the suprapubic skin and tied over a swab to allow anterior exposure and retraction.

Sharp dissection using a hook or scissors attached to monopolar diathermy is preferred by the authors. The harmonic scalpel can be used but the benefits of 'wristed' movement is not available, thereby limiting its utility within the pelvis. The bloodless mesorectal plane between mesorectum and parietal presacral pelvic fascia is well demonstrated due to the enhanced view and by gentle anterior traction on the mesorectum using a tonsil swab held by a grasping instrument. The swab provides a blunt broad compression of the posterior mesorectum minimising the risk of fascial breach. It also absorbs small amounts of blood/tissue fluid.

The initial dissection starts to the right side (Photo 15.5), continues as far as the pelvic floor posteriorly and down the right side of the mesorectum, remembering that the sacral concavity arcs forward as dissection progresses, although this tends to be well demonstrated by the three-dimensional view. Once right-sided and posterior dissection has been completed, it is often only necessary to release the peritoneal attachments on the left side (Photo 15.6) as most of the left side of the mesorectum can be mobilised from the right. The peritoneum is opened laterally taking care not to inadvertently damage the inferior hypogastric nerve or ureter. The posterolateral dissection is taken down to a comfortable level where progress starts to become a little more difficult (Photo 15.7), and at this stage the anterior dissection is started.

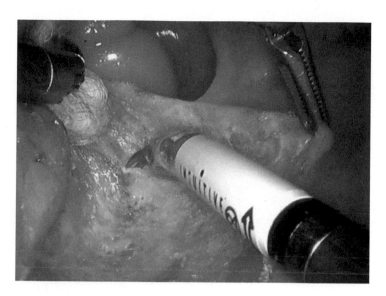

Photo 15.5 Initial dissection of right side of mesorectum.

The peritoneum is divided anterior to and above the reflection (Photo 15.8). The anterior dissection continues behind the seminal vesicles in the male at which point the Denonvilliers fascia is reached. The Denonvilliers fascia may exist in one or two layers: the anterior layer behind the prostate and the posterior layer in front of the anterior mesorectum. When two layers are present they fuse at the lower level of the prostate. At this point the fascia is divided to enter the plane in front of the mesorectum. At the lateral corners of Denonvilliers fascia the surgeon needs to be aware of the close proximity of the neurovascular bundles as these are easily damaged at this point. In the female patient the dissection continues down the

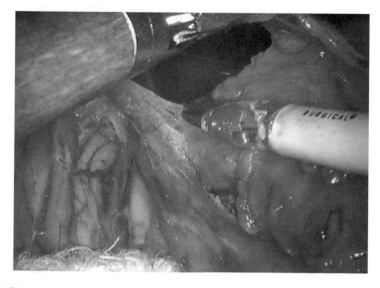

Photo 15.6 Dissection at the left pelvic brim.

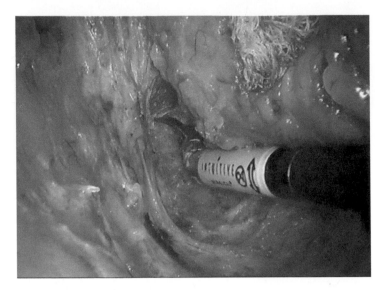

Photo 15.7 Low posterior dissection on left side.

rectovaginal septum to the pelvic floor. The mesorectum is often very thin at this level and easily breached.

The anterior dissection is perhaps the most challenging part of the operation and may require anterior retraction of the prostate in order to allow the dissection to proceed to the pelvic floor under direct vision. The mesorectal plane guides the surgeon along the pelvic floor to the rectal tube, which is encountered as it passes through the pelvic floor; at this point the dissection can continue into the intersphincteric plane if required. The surgeon switches from anterior to posterior to lateral as dictated by view and ease of access. Laterally the retraction

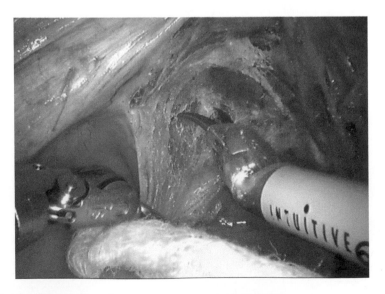

Photo 15.8 Initial anterior dissection.

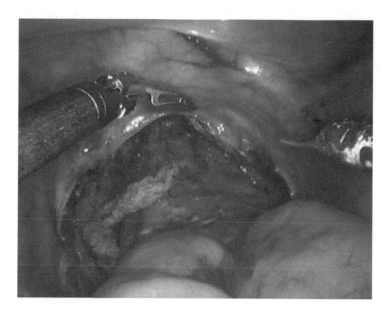

Photo 15.9 Fully mobilised rectum.

and three-dimensional view aids the identification and preservation of the inferior hypogastric plexus and nervi erigentes. A branch of the inferior hypogastric nerve passes medially to the rectum (previously known as the lateral ligament); this nerve is variable in thickness and will need to be divided. Occasionally, this nerve is accompanied by the middle rectal vessels. If progress is not being made in one area it is important to move to another. After the mesorectal dissection the peritoneum on the left side of the pelvis is divided to complete the TME. Finally any lower parts of the mesorectum are dissected from the pelvic floor to reveal a clean rectal tube. This can then be divided at the pelvic floor (Photo 15.9).

SAFE DISSECTION OF THE BOWEL: RECTAL TRANSECTION

A further nylon tape is tied around the rectal tube taking care that it is tightened well below the lower border of the tumour, occluding the lumen and allowing a distal rectal washout with a cytocidal solution of iodine and water. If a stapled anastomosis is to be performed there are two choices. The rectum can be divided with the robotic cutting instrument followed by the insertion of a purse-string suture using the robotic needle driver (13). Alternatively if there is space for a linear laparoscopic stapler, this can be inserted to divide in the standard laparoscopic fashion using an articulated 45-mm linear stapler cutter that is inserted via the 12-mm (right iliac fossa) port, after undocking of the robot. The distal nylon tape is helpful in positioning the rectal tube in the jaws of the stapler.

There are often difficulties getting a laparoscopic stapler into a tight male pelvis and it is vital not to compromise the distal resection margin because of inadequate instrumentation. Although robotic staplers are becoming available for the newest evolutions of robots, if in doubt it is better to enlarge the Pfannenstiel incision and apply an alternative narrow stapling device manually as commonly used in open surgery. These staplers can be manipulated laparoscopically providing a seal is established to prevent leakage of the CO_2 pneumoperitoneum.

ANASTOMOSIS

SAFE EXTRACTION OF SPECIMEN

A 5–7 cm suprapubic transverse incision is made and a self-retracting dual ring-reinforced wound protector is utilised to facilitate specimen extraction.

ANASTOMOSIS

The left colon is divided at a point of convenience providing a good blood supply based on the marginal artery, and sufficient length to reach the pelvic floor without tension. Some surgeons may also favour the fashioning of a colo-pouch. A circular stapler anvil is then inserted in the proximal colon and secured with a purse string suture. Caps are available to seal the site of the wound protector to allow re-establishment of pneumoperitoneum and an anastomosis is then fashioned with the circular stapling device. The anastomosis can be air-leak tested, but this is usually unnecessary as it is the author's routine practice to defunction all TME coloanal or low colorectal anastomoses with a loop ileostomy. It is our practice to examine the anastomosis digitally to exclude obvious flaws.

ADVANTAGES AND DISADVANTAGES

TECHNICAL ADVANTAGES

Laparoscopic colorectal surgery is technically very demanding and the learning curve is often long, particularly for pelvic dissection. There is considerable restriction of movement with standard laparoscopic instruments and these movements are compromised somewhat by dependence on the fulcrum effect of the instruments having to pass via ports through the abdominal wall.

The robot 'wristed' instruments have seven degrees of freedom that are particularly help-ful in the confined space of the pelvis. The ports are simply a means of access rather than an integral part of instrument movement, as with standard laparoscopy. The robot eliminates tremor and scales down movements made at the surgeon console, enhancing the accuracy of dissection.

The image of the operative field provided by high-definition camera systems in laparoscopic surgery is now excellent. Depth of field has to be interpreted by the surgeon and may adversely affect performance. The high-definition three-dimensional view provided by the robotic optics is vastly superior to the high-definition two-dimensional views produced by standard lapa-roscopic cameras and display monitors. The camera is held perfectly still avoiding the risk of assistant fatigue and reducing disorientation of the operating surgeon.

These advantages allow for more precise, meticulous, sharp dissection of clearly identified tissue planes resulting in less blood loss and reduced surgical trauma. These benefits are likely to shorten the learning curve for minimally invasive TME and reduce the chance of the need to convert to standard open procedure and its attendant disadvantages.

Robotic TME may demonstrate improvements in specimen quality and pelvic nerve preser-vation, with consequent oncological and quality-of-life benefits, but it is important to empha-sise that this is purely conjecture until the results of clinical trials such as ROLARR, designed to specifically investigate robotic TME, become available.

DISADVANTAGES

The main disadvantage is the complete lack of tactile feedback from the instruments. This can potentially lead to tissue damage both in and out of the field of view. The second drawback is the time-consuming procedure of the docking and undocking of the robotic cart from the patient. If significant bleeding occurs robotic instruments cannot be changed quickly to deal with the problem and the undocking process may lead to greater blood loss before control is achieved either laparoscopically or by open surgery, although all robotic surgeons should be comfortable with performing a rapid undocking should the need arise.

Another disadvantage is the duration of surgery. This applies to the setup ('docking') and the procedure itself. With progression up the learning curve the operating times will reduce, but until mastery is achieved they will always be longer than with standard laparoscopic surgery or open surgery. This has implications for list planning, service provision and training of juniors in the future.

The da Vinci system is expensive. This applies not just to the initial outlay for the robot but also to the annual servicing costs and the cost of consumables.

These disadvantages must be weighed against the potential benefits of unrivaled views of the anatomy, reduced blood loss through accurate dissection of the tissue planes and potentially improved nerve preservation and quality of the TME specimen. Overall reduction in conversion to open surgery, with a consequent reduction in length of hospital stay, may help to offset the cost implications.

THE FUTURE

Robotic surgical technology is constantly evolving and given time it is likely that costs will fall and the systems will become less bulky. There is potential to improve the quality of minimally invasive mesorectal dissection and we believe this is another step of progress in the surgical treatment of rectal cancer. Cross-stapling the low rectum in a narrow pelvis remains a challenge with the minimal access staplers currently available; however, robotic purse-string suturing may help overcome these difficulties in the short term until robotic staplers become widely available.

Robotic rectal cancer surgery has been evaluated through an international collaboration in a worldwide multicentre randomised controlled trial of robotic versus laparoscopic TME – the ROLARR trial – whose main outcome measures are rates of conversion to open surgery. Secondary measures are quality of resected specimen, positivity of resection margins, local recurrence, quality of life, pelvic nerve function and health economics analysis. The preliminary results are expected soon.

KEY POINTS

- An increasing number of studies are looking at robotic surgery, but the marginal but potentially vital gains accrued such as reduced conversion rates and pelvic nerve preservation are challenging to demonstrate.
- It provides fantastic views and access deep in the pelvis facilitating the challenge of low pelvic dissection in the male pelvis.
- Cost currently makes widespread robotic adoption prohibitive but will inevitably come down as technology evolves.

TAKE-HOME MESSAGE

- As technology reduces costs and improves ease of use, robotic surgery will provide an unrivaled platform for precision surgery.

REFERENCES

1. Nagtegaal ID, van de Velde CJ, van der Worp E, Kapiteijn E, Quirke P, van Krieken JH. Cooperative clinical investigators of the Dutch colorectal cancer group. Macroscopic evaluation of rectal cancer resection specimen: Clinical significance of the pathologist in quality control. *J Clin Oncol* 2002, Apr 1;20(7):1729–34.
2. Heald RJ, Husband EM, Ryall RD. The mesorectum in rectal cancer surgery—The clue to pelvic recurrence? *Br J Surg* 1982 Oct;69(10):613–6.
3. Baik SH, Ko YT, Kang CM, Lee WJ, Kim NK, Sohn SK et al. Robotic tumor-specific mesorectal excision of rectal cancer: Short-term outcome of a pilot randomized trial. *Surg Endosc* 2008 Jul;22(7):1601–8.
4. Saklani AP, Lim DR, Hur H, Min BS, Baik SH, Lee KY, Kim NK. Robotic versus laparoscopic surgery for mid-low rectal cancer after neoadjuvant chemoradiation therapy: Comparison of oncologic outcomes. *Int J Colorectal Dis* 2013 Dec;28(12):1689–98.
5. Kang J, Yoon KJ, Min BS, Hur H, Baik SH, Kim NK, Lee KY. The impact of robotic surgery for mid and low rectal cancer: A case-matched analysis of a 3-arm comparison—Open, laparoscopic, and robotic surgery. *Ann Surg* 2013 Jan;257(1):95–101.
6. Baek SJ, Kim SH, Cho JS, Shin JW, Kim J. Robotic versus conventional laparoscopic surgery for rectal cancer: A cost analysis from a single institute in Korea. *World J Surg* 2012 Nov;36(11):2722–9.
7. Park JS, Choi GS, Lim KH, Jang YS, Jun SH. S052: A comparison of robot-assisted, laparoscopic, and open surgery in the treatment of rectal cancer. *Surg Endosc* 2011 Jan;25(1):240–8.
8. Park EJ, Cho MS, Baek SJ, Hur H, Min BS, Baik SH et al. Long-term oncologic outcomes of robotic low anterior resection for rectal cancer: A comparative study with laparoscopic surgery. *Ann Surg* 2015;261(1):129–37.
9. Baik SH, Kwon HY, Kim JS, Hur H, Sohn SK, Cho CH, Kim H. Robotic versus laparoscopic low anterior resection of rectal cancer: Short-term outcome of a prospective comparative study. *Ann Surg Oncol* 2009 Jun;16(6):1480–7.
10. Baek SJ, Al-Asari S, Jeong DH, Hur H, Min BS, Baik SH, Kim NK. Robotic versus laparoscopic coloanal anastomosis with or without intersphincteric resection for rectal cancer. *Surg Endosc* 2013 Nov;27(11):4157–63.
11. D'Annibale A, Pernazza G, Monsellato I, Pende V, Lucandri G, Mazzocchi P, Alfano G. Total mesorectal excision: A comparison of oncological and functional outcomes between robotic and laparoscopic surgery for rectal cancer. *Surg Endosc* 2013 Jun;27(6):1887–95.
12. Collinson FJ, Jayne DG, Pigazzi A, Tsang C, Barrie JM, Edlin R et al. An international, multicentre, prospective, randomised, controlled, unblinded, parallel-group trial of robotic-assisted versus standard laparoscopic surgery for the curative treatment of rectal cancer. *Int J Colorectal Dis* 2012 Feb;27(2):233–41.
13. Prasad LM, deSouza AL, Marecik SJ, Park JJ, Abcarian H. Robotic pursestring technique in low anterior resection. *Dis Colon Rectum* 2010 Feb;53(2):230–4.

14. Delaney CP, Lynch AC, Senagore AJ, Fazio VW. Comparison of robotically performed and traditional laparoscopic colorectal surgery. *Dis Colon Rectum* 2003 Dec;46(12):1633–9.

15. D'Annibale A, Morpurgo E, Fiscon V, Trevisan P, Sovernigo G, Orsini C, Guidolin D. Robotic and laparoscopic surgery for treatment of colorectal diseases. *Dis Colon Rectum* 2004 Dec;47(12):2162–8.

16. Pigazzi A, Ellenhorn JD, Ballantyne GH, Paz IB. Robotic-assisted laparoscopic low anterior resection with total mesorectal excision for rectal cancer. *Surg Endosc* 2006 Oct;20(10):1521–5.

17. Spinoglio G, Summa M, Priora F, Quarati R, Testa S. Robotic colorectal surgery: First 50 cases experience. *Dis Colon Rectum* 2008 Nov;51(11):1627–32.

18. Bianchi PP, Ceriani C, Locatelli A, Spinoglio G, Zampino MG, Sonzogni A et al. Robotic versus laparoscopic total mesorectal excision for rectal cancer: A comparative analysis of oncological safety and short-term outcomes. *Surg Endosc* 2010 Nov;24(11):2888–94.

19. Kim JY, Kim NK, Lee KY, Hur H, Min BS, Kim JH. A comparative study of voiding and sexual function after total mesorectal excision with autonomic nerve preservation for rectal cancer: Laparoscopic versus robotic surgery. *Ann Surg Oncol* 2012 Aug;19(8):2485–93.

20. Fernandez R, Anaya DA, Li LT, Orcutt ST, Balentine CJ, Awad SA et al. Laparoscopic versus robotic rectal resection for rectal cancer in a veteran population. *Am J Surg* 2013 Oct;206(4):509–17.

21. Park SY, Choi GS, Park JS, Kim HJ, Ryuk JP. Short-term clinical outcome of robot-assisted intersphincteric resection for low rectal cancer: A retrospective comparison with conventional laparoscopy. *Surg Endosc* 2013 Jan;27(1):48–55.

22. Erguner I, Aytac E, Boler DE, Atalar B, Baca B, Karahasanoglu T et al. What have we gained by performing robotic rectal resection? Evaluation of 64 consecutive patients who underwent laparoscopic or robotic low anterior resection for rectal adenocarcinoma. *Surg Laparosc Endosc Percutan Tech* 2013 Jun;23(3):316–9.

23. Yoo BE, Cho JS, Shin JW, Lee DW, Kwak JM, Kim J, Kim SH. Robotic versus laparoscopic intersphincteric resection for low rectal cancer: Comparison of the operative, oncological, and functional outcomes. *Ann Surg Oncol* 2015;22(4):1219–25.

24. Ielpo B, Caruso R, Quijano Y, Duran H, Diaz E, Fabra I et al. Robotic versus laparoscopic rectal resection: Is there any real difference? A comparative single center study. *Int J Med Robot* 2014 Sep;10(3):300–5.

25. Barnajian M, Pettet D, Kazi E, Foppa C, Bergamaschi R. Quality of total mesorectal excision and depth of circumferential resection margin in rectal cancer: A matched comparison of the first 20 robotic cases. *Colorectal Dis* 2014 Aug;16(8):603–9.

26. Levic K, Donatsky AM, Bulut O, Rosenberg J. A comparative study of single-port laparoscopic surgery versus robotic-assisted laparoscopic surgery for rectal cancer. *Surg Innov* 2015;22(4):368–75.

27. Tam MS, Abbass M, Abbas MA. Robotic-laparoscopic rectal cancer excision versus traditional laparoscopy. *JSLS* 2014 Jul;18(3):e2014.00020.

28. Park EJ, Kim CW, Cho MS, Kim DW, Min BS, Baik SH et al. Is the learning curve of robotic low anterior resection shorter than laparoscopic low anterior resection for rectal cancer? A comparative analysis of clinicopathologic outcomes between robotic and laparoscopic surgeries. *Medicine (Baltimore)* 2014 Nov;93(25):e109.

29. Koh FH, Tan KK, Lieske B, Tsang ML, Tsang CB, Koh DC. Endowrist versus wrist: A case-controlled study comparing robotic versus hand-assisted laparoscopic surgery for rectal cancer. *Surg Laparosc Endosc Percutan Tech* 2014 Oct;24(5):452–6.

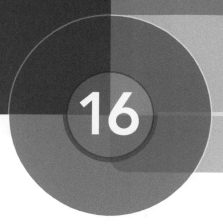

Single incision laparoscopic colorectal surgery

16

TALVINDER SINGH GILL

LEARNING OBJECTIVES

- Examine the history, evidence, and advantages related to single incision laparoscopic colorectal surgery.
- Understand the steps of different colorectal procedures along with the difficulties encountered and the solutions of those.
- Compare SILCS with the multiport laparoscopic surgery and use this in clinical practice.

INTRODUCTION

Many technical advances have taken place for laparoscopic colorectal surgery in the last few years. Higher-definition viewing systems and advancements in technical skills have pushed the boundaries for more development. It was a natural progression from multiport laparoscopic surgery to less ports or single-port surgery and natural orifice transluminal endoscopic surgery (NOTES). In the United Kingdom, surgeons are at different levels of their learning curve for performing laparoscopic colorectal surgery. A new technique that requires more advanced laparoscopic skills is likely to be popular only when most surgeons are near the peak of their learning curve.

The technique of NOTES for colorectal procedures is still in the early stages of development, but interest is growing in single incision laparoscopic colorectal surgery (SILCS). A few centres are routinely performing most colorectal procedures by this technique now. The worldwide popularity of this attractive technique has rapidly grown, as proven by the increase in the number of publications over the past few years (1).

Single incision laparoscopic surgery has got more relevance for colorectal surgery because there is usually the need to make an incision to take the specimen out of the abdominal cavity. Some patients require stoma placement and in that situation the whole procedure can be carried out through the anticipated stoma site. Those patients who already have a stoma and require restoration of bowel continuity can have the procedure through the stoma site.

Smaller studies are suggesting that by this technique, reduction of parietal incisions and surgical stress are likely to correlate with lower post-operative pain, fewer port site complications, a better morbidity profile, shorter hospital stay, and reduced cost while also providing a better cosmetic result (2). Lately, numerous studies have aimed to demonstrate the real benefits of SILCS over conventional laparoscopic surgery regarding short-term outcomes and appropriateness for oncological resections (3). However, conclusive advantages and long-term results need to be confirmed by large-scale, randomised controlled trials (RCTs).

HISTORY AND EVIDENCE

The first single incision laparoscopic surgery was reported in the field of gynaecology when Clifford Wheeless reported the first 400 cases of tubal ligation in 1969 (4). Since then this has been a standard procedure worldwide to do tubal ligation for female sterilization. In 1991, Pelosi reported total hysterectomy with bilateral salpingo-oophorectomy, the first complex extirpative procedure using the single incision laparoscopic technique (5).

The first general surgical operation by this technique was reported by Pelosi in 1992 when he reported a case series of appendicectomies in 25 patients (6). Cholecystectomy by SILS was first reported in 1997 in a letter to the editor by Navarra and colleagues (7). Piskun and Rajpal reported in 1999 that he performed a SILS cholecystectomy on 10 patients by placing two trocars through a common umbilical incision and using transabdominal sutures to manipulate the gallbladder (8).

Mostly interest was renewed again in 2008 when almost all surgical specialties started to explore its use on a wider scale. At the same time, the first major colorectal procedure was reported as a right hemicolectomy (9,10). In the next few years, it was reported that almost all colorectal procedures can be safely done with this technique (11,12).

Initially some case reports and then small case series were published to confirm the feasibility and safety of SILCS for different colorectal procedures. Comparative series have shown some advantages of SILCS over conventional laparoscopic surgery for colorectal procedures (13). Generally these series have shown less blood loss, shorter operating time, early bowel function, less post-operative pain, and shorter hospital stay. A meta-analysis of 14 comparative series including 1155 patients in 2012 showed no difference in operating time, conversion rate, and post-operative adverse events, but less blood loss, smaller incision, shorter hospital stay, and early bowel function were seen in the SILCS group (14).

Three small randomised controlled trials comparing SILCS with conventional laparoscopic colorectal surgery have been published so far. The Italian trial recruited 16 patients in each group and reported similar results for SILCS as compared to a traditional laparoscopic approach (15). The trial from Hong Kong recruited 23 patients in each group and reported reduced wound pain in the early post-operative period and shorter hospital stay (5 [4–6] versus 4 [3–4] days; $p < .01$] (16). Recently another randomised pilot study from Denmark recruited 20 patients with rectal cancer in each group and reported reduced post-operative pain for patients having single incision laparoscopic rectal surgery (17). Four randomised controlled trials related to SILCS, including one in the United Kingdom at University Hospital of North Tees and two in Korea, are presently recruiting patients.

A recent systematic review and pooled analysis of 34 comparative series including 3174 patients showed that there was no difference in operative time, mortality, and morbidity including anastomotic leak, re-operation, pneumonia, wound infection, and port-site hernia. The SILCS group had statistically significant advantages reflected by a reduction in estimated blood loss (WMD = −47.94 mL; p = .003), time to return of bowel function (WMD = −1.11 days; p = .03), and length of hospital stay (WMD = −1.9 days; p < .0001) (3).

TECHNIQUE

Single incision laparoscopic colorectal surgery is performed either through the umbilicus, through a potential stoma site, or through a previously constructed stoma site. An incision of 3–6 cm is made over the skin and abdominal wall and the peritoneal cavity is opened. The length of the incision usually depends on the size of the specimen that needs to be taken out after the procedure. A disc of skin is excised at a premarked stoma site and a cruciate incision over the rectus sheath is made to gain access to the peritoneal cavity in cases where surgery is planned through a potential stoma site. A port with multiple holes outside and an intra-peritoneal ring is put in place. Various types of commercial multichannel ports from different companies are available for use. Some surgeons use a glove port in which laparoscopic ports can be passed through different fingers of a hand glove put over a wound protector. There are few modifications in the access, for example, some surgeons use single skin incision and then put usual laparoscopic ports side by side through the abdominal wall.

Apart from access, the rest of the procedure is performed in a similar way as conventional laparoscopic colorectal surgery. There are a few technical differences while performing single incision laparoscopic surgery due to all instruments entering the peritoneal cavity through a small hole in a parallel direction without having an advantage of triangulation. Due to the small space around instruments, it does not allow free and wide movement of instruments. The instruments push against each other and the laparoscope as well. It gets difficult to maintain an optimal view when instruments are clashing due to crowding of the space. All the instruments and viewing scope have to keep the same relation and coherence all the time. The scope needs to be in the middle and operating instruments on either side of the scope, and this relation should be maintained at all times during the procedure.

PROCEDURES

RIGHT HEMICOLECTOMY

Right hemicolectomy (RHC) is relatively easy and is a good procedure to start to learn SILCS. Access is gained through the umbilicus by making a 3- to 5-cm incision (Photo 16.1) and insert-ing a multichannel port through that (Photos 16.2 and 16.3).

Slight head down with minimal tilt to the left side is a good position to start the proce-dure. Perform laparoscopy and start the procedure by putting omentum and transverse colon upwards, below the liver. Move the ileal loops towards the pelvis and to the left side.

Find the ileocaecal junction and lift it to see ileocolic vessels and a groove below these. Make an incision through the peritoneum in this grove along the vessels. Move the grasper towards the proximal side of these vessels and start dissection in that grove.

Find a plane between mesocolon and retroperitoneum by lifting the ileocolic vessel and mesocolon with a grasper in the left hand. Continue dissection on the medial side in front of the duodenum and decide the site of ligation of the ileocolic vessel near its origin. After dividing

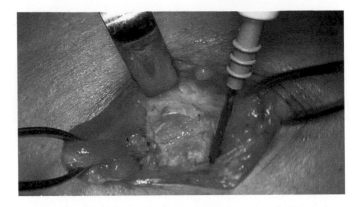

Photo 16.1 Access through umbilicus by 3- to 5-cm incision.

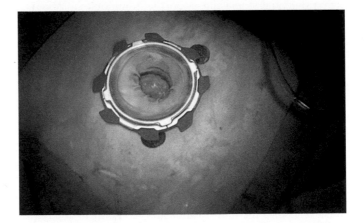

Photo 16.2 Base of port is placed through the incision in umbilicus.

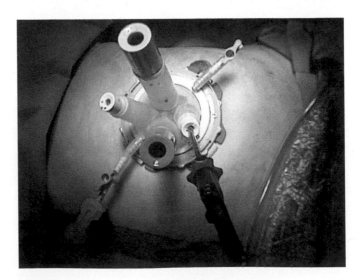

Photo 16.3 Multichannel single port device (Octoport).

the ileocolic vessels, continue dissection upwards to find and ligate the right colic vessels and the right branch of middle colic vessel if required.

Divide the mesocolon fully and divide omentum at the same level. Divide peritoneal attachments of hepatic flexure and lateral attachment of right colon to free it completely.

A functional end-to-end ileocolic anastomosis is performed with appropriate stapling devices after taking the specimen out through the port site.

SIGMOID COLECTOMY AND LEFT HEMICOLECTOMY

Left hemicolectomy or sigmoid colectomy is done by putting a port through an incision of 3–5 cm in the umbilicus.

Start with a tilt of the operating table towards the right and head down position. Small bowel loops are stacked towards the right upper quadrant of the abdomen.

Grasp the distal sigmoid colon with left-hand grasper and pull it outside the pelvis upwards and anteriorly. Maintain this traction and in stepwise fashion grasp the middle part of the mesocolon.

Make an incision over peritoneum at the level of the sacral promontory and extend it towards the proximal part of the inferior mesenteric artery (Photo 16.4). Find a plane behind the inferior mesenteric artery (IMA) between mesocolon and retroperitoneum and continue dissection towards the lateral side.

Define the appropriate level and divide the IMA after ligation or clip application (Photos 16.5 and 16.6). Continue dissection upwards and to the lateral side to separate mesocolon from Toldt fascia over the left kidney.

There is no need to look for retroperitoneal structures like ureter or gonadal vessels if retroperitoneal fascia is intact.

Dissection can be continued in front of the pancreas to enter the lesser sac. Divide the inferior mesenteric vein on the lateral side of the duodenal-jejunal flexure (Photo 16.7).

Divide the lateral peritoneal attachment of sigmoid and descending colon (Photo 16.8). Change the position of the operating table to head up and more tilt to the right side if there is need for splenic flexure mobilisation. Dissect the omentum from the distal transverse colon and continue towards the left colon. Extend the dissection from descending colon upwards and medially above the splenic flexure of the colon to free it completely.

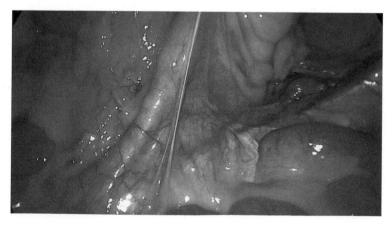

Photo 16.4 View of inferior mesenteric artery before dissection.

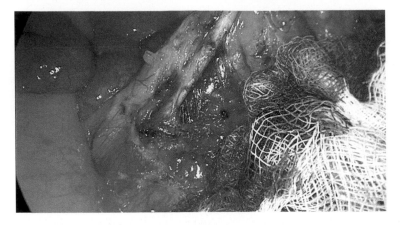

Photo 16.5 Dissection of inferior mesenteric artery for high ligation of the vessel.

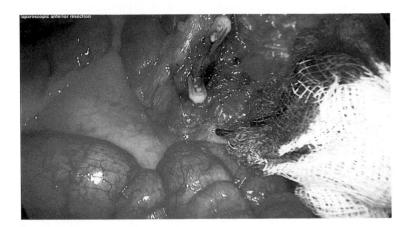

Photo 16.6 Division of inferior mesenteric artery near its origin after putting clips.

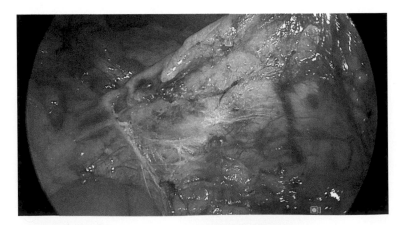

Photo 16.7 Dissection of inferior mesenteric vein and ready for ligation.

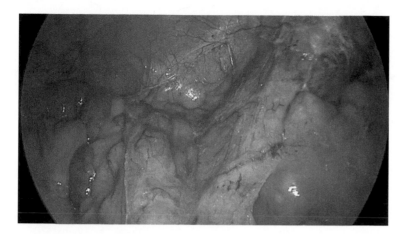

Photo 16.8 Lateral mobilisation of left colon.

Divide the rectosigmoid area at the required level after dividing the mesocolon or mesorectum and deliver out the specimen through the port site.

End-to-end or side-to-end colorectal anastomosis is constructed using a circular stapling gun through the anus as it is done in multiport laparoscopic surgery.

ANTERIOR RESECTION

The left colon is mobilised as described in left hemicolectomy. The rectum is mobilised in the total mesorectal excision plane by diathermy hook while keeping traction by holding at an appropriate level with the left hand (Photos 16.9 and 16.10). Care is taken to preserve pelvic nerves. Continue dissection to the required level and in case of partial mesorectal excision (high anterior resection), divide the mesorectum with harmonic ace or other energy instrument at appropriate level. Obliterate the rectum above the level of transection for rectal wash out before division of it with a laparoscopic linear cutting stapler gun (Photo 16.11). Anastomosis with circular stapler is done after removing specimen from port site (Photos 16.12–16.15). For low anterior resection, continue dissection down to the pelvic floor and divide the anorectal

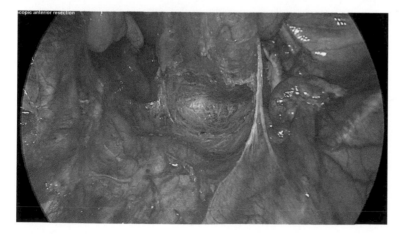

Photo 16.9 Posterior rectal dissection in tissue plane behind mesorectal fascia.

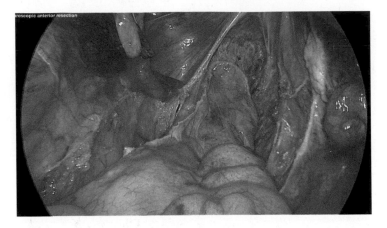

Photo 16.10 Dissection of rectum on lateral sides and anteriorly.

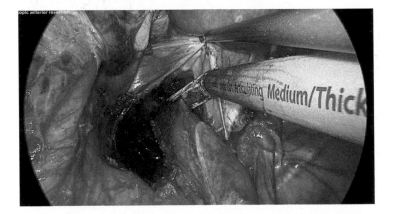

Photo 16.11 Division of lower rectum using a linear cutter stapling gun.

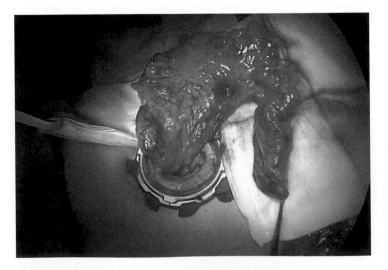

Photo 16.12 Specimen of rectum and sigmoid colon is taken out from the port site.

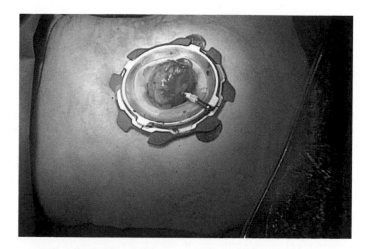

Photo 16.13 Colon end is prepared with anvil of a circular stapler gun.

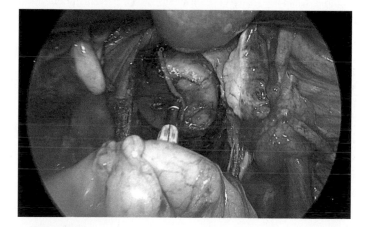

Photo 16.14 Side-to-end colorectal anastomosis is being performed.

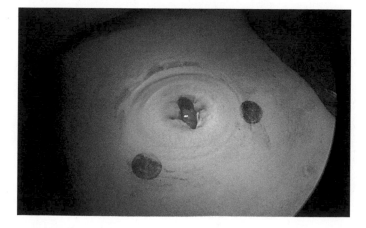

Photo 16.15 Final appearance at the end of anterior resection through the umbilicus.

junction. A 5-mm port can be used in the lower part of the left side of the abdomen to help retraction in difficult cases, and this can be used to leave a drain in the pelvis.

TOTAL COLECTOMY

Total colectomy with end ileostomy for inflammatory bowel disease (IBD) is performed through potential ileostomy site in the right iliac fossa. Cut the disc of skin with underlying subcutaneous fatty tissue. Make a cruciate incision over the anterior rectus sheath, separate rectus muscle fibers, and open the peritoneum to insert a multichannel port through this (Photo 16.16).

Start dissection from the left side and continue in anticlockwise fashion towards the caecum. The left colon is mobilised as described for left hemicolectomy but all the vessels can be divided at the most convenient level. For the transverse colon dissection, change the position of the patient to reverse Trendelenburg and separate the omentum from the transverse colon completely to preserve it. Divide the transverse mesocolon near the colon with a harmonic scalpel or any energy device to seal smaller branches of the middle colic vessels.

Mobilise the hepatic flexure from above and the lateral attachments of right colon, caecum and terminal ileum by standing in between the legs of the patient. Then, continue division of the mesocolon near the right colon. Divide the rectosigmoid junction at the pelvic brim and take the specimen out through a port site (Photo 16.17). Fashion an ileostomy with a 3-cm spout at the port site (Photo 16.18). Total colectomy with ileorectal anastomosis is performed

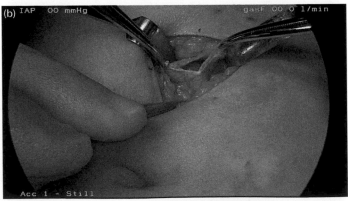
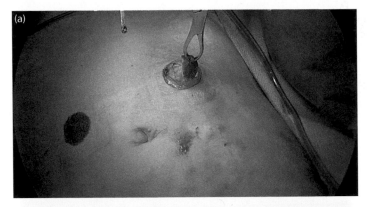

Photo 16.16 Total colectomy through potential ileostomy site. (a) Disc of skin cut at ileostomy site and (b) peritoneum opened for insertion of port.

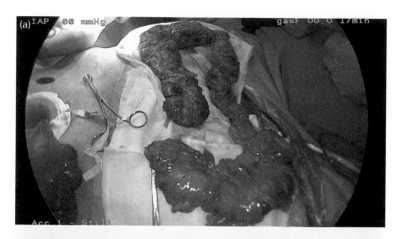

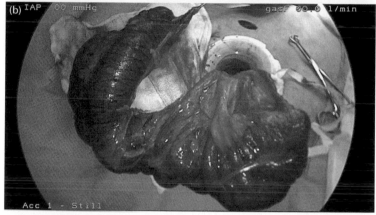

Photo 16.17 Total colectomy specimen out through a port site. (a) Removed in two parts, left and transverse colon and (b) right colon.

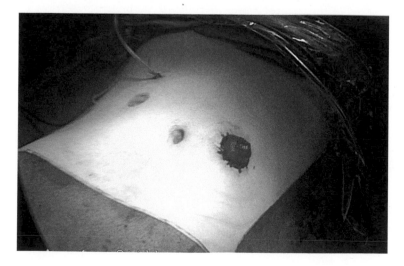

Photo 16.18 Ileostomy with a 3-cm spout at the port site.

by inserting a mutichannel port through the umbilicus. Depending on the indication of the surgery, one can decide the level of division of the vessels.

PROCTOCOLECTOMY OR PROCTECTOMY AND ILEAL POUCH

Patients requiring ileal pouch surgery are usually young. Completion of surgery through an ileostomy or potential ileostomy site is an attractive option for them (Photo 16.19). A multichannel port is inserted through the anticipated ileostomy site. Whole colon and rectum are mobilised as described before or the ileostomy and small bowel are mobilised (Photo 16.20). Care is taken to divide the anorectal junction by mobilising it fully so that no part of the rectum is left behind. The specimen is removed through the port site and a 20-cm J-pouch is constructed from the

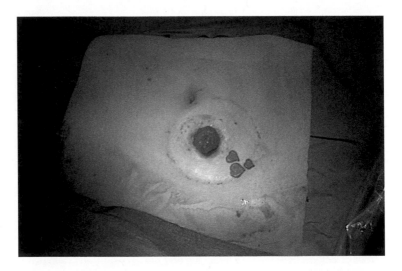

Photo 16.19 Pouch surgery through an ileostomy.

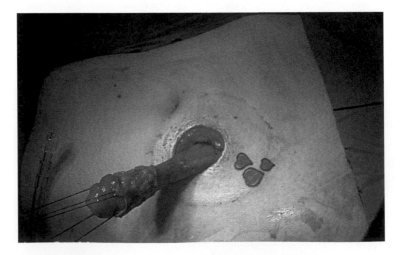

Photo 16.20 Mobilisation of ileostomy.

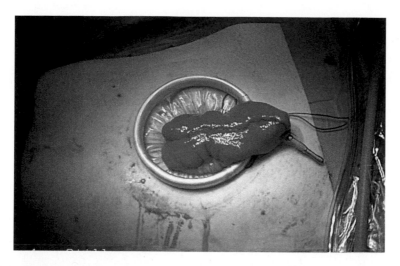

Photo 16.21 Formation of a 20-cm J-pouch.

terminal ileum (Photo 16.21). Ileal pouch anal anastomosis is done with circular stapler and a loop ileostomy is fashioned at port site.

HARTMANN REVERSAL

Reversal of Hartmann procedure through colostomy site by this technique was first described as a case series of five patients in 2011, and I would like to call it a North Tees technique of reversal. The end colostomy (Photo 16.22) is fully mobilised from skin and abdominal wall (Photo 16.23). The anvil of circular stapler gun is inserted after excising the end of colostomy and colon end is put back inside abdomen with the anvil. A multichannel port is inserted through the colostomy site (Photo 16.24). All adhesions to anterior abdominal wall are divided (Photo 16.25). Small bowel loops are taken out of the pelvis after dividing adhesions. Rectal stump is defined and assessed to confirm that a circular stapling gun through the anus will reach to the end of it. The

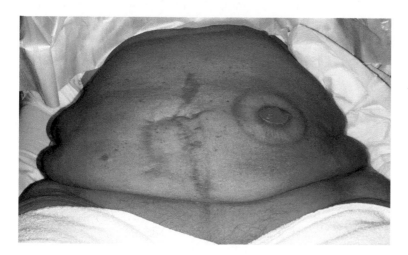

Photo 16.22 End colostomy note midline scar from open Hartmann.

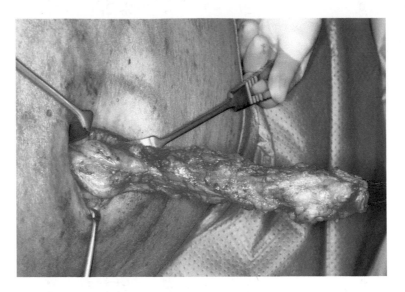

Photo 16.23 Colon mobilised at site of colostomy.

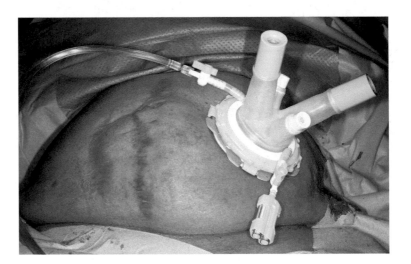

Photo 16.24 A multichannel port is inserted through the colostomy site.

left colon is mobilised and adhesions to omentum and small bowel loops are divided. Stapled colorectal anastomosis is done once the surgeon is happy with the length of the mobilised colon (Photo 16.26). The stoma site is then closed with appropriate sutures.

EMERGENCY COLORECTAL SURGERY

This technique is very useful for emergency procedures, and it is easy to deal with most of the problems related to the small bowel. Band adhesions, stricture, or tumour causing small bowel obstruction can be managed safely by this technique, and there is no need for laparotomy in these cases. Hartmann procedure for perforated sigmoid colon is feasible. Emergency total

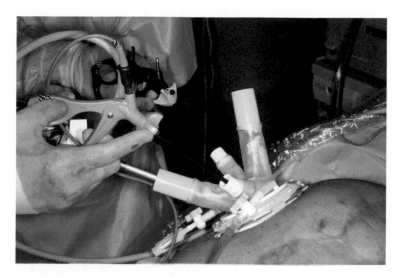

Photo 16.25 Small bowel adhesions divided.

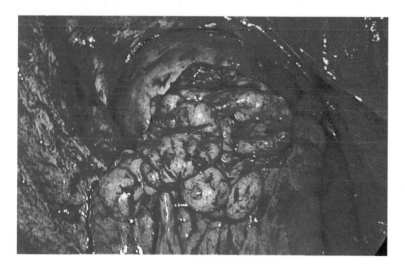

Photo 16.26 Stapled colorectal anastomosis.

colectomy for patients with inflammatory bowel disease who have failed medical treatment is a rewarding procedure by this technique.

SURGERY FOR INFLAMMATORY BOWEL DISEASE

IBD patients are relatively younger and many of these might require multiple operations. SILCS is particularly useful for this group of patients as they are more likely to appreciate cosmetic benefits along with all other advantages of this technique. In my opinion all surgeons operating on patients with inflammatory bowel disease should consider training in SILCS. Small bowel stricturoplasty, small bowel resection, ileocaecal resection, and segmental colonic resection are easily done through umbilicus by this technique. Total colectomy and proctocolectomy with ileal pouch are done through the ileostomy site with faster recovery and better functions.

ADVANTAGES

SILCS has some distinct advantages over conventional laparoscopic surgery. There is reduced risk of injury to abdominal organs or vessels during port insertion. Major injury to different structures during insertion of first port has been a concern with conventional laparoscopic surgery in the past. Comparative series are suggesting that post-operative pain is likely to be less with SILCS. I have noticed that early post-operative pain is significantly reduced after left-sided resections, total colectomy, proctocolectomy, and reversal of Hartmann procedure. Generally one might assume that operating time would be longer in SILCS but that has not been the case. Mostly it has been reported as similar or shorter operating time. In conventional laparoscopic surgery some extra time is taken to gain access through multiple ports and to close these port sites at the end of the operation. Bowel function returns quickly after SILCS, and along with reduced pain this has resulted in early recovery and shorter hospital stay. Cosmetic benefits are significant as there is no obvious scar in most patients. Scar is usually hidden in natural scar of the umbilicus. There is some suggestion that the risk of incisional hernia is also less in patients having SILCS.

CHALLENGES AND TIPS

SILCS is a relatively new technique and its use in colorectal surgery started only about 6 years ago. It is a more advanced laparoscopic surgery so conventional laparoscopic skills are necessary before one starts SILCS. There are some challenges that need special attention.

IN-LINE VISION

Grasping forceps, dissecting instruments, and camera entry through same place all make orientation of organs or anatomy slightly different compared to multiport laparoscopic procedures. Extra care is required to be certain that there is no important structure just behind the one you are dealing with at the moment. It is important to use 30°-view laparoscope and look either side of the important structure by pushing scope in and out before dividing it. The chances of an injury to the surrounding structures and off-camera injury are low with in-line vision and this type of view. An experienced laparoscopic surgeon does not take much time to adapt to this view.

CROWDING OF INSTRUMENTS

The movement of any instrument in a small space at the access point can move the scope and disturb the field of view. Clashing of instruments at the entry point is a big problem for the surgeon as well as the camera-holding assistant.

It is extremely important to keep the camera in the middle and grasping forceps and dissecting instruments on either side of it. The conscious efforts of both surgeon and assistant are required to keep this relationship of instruments maintained at all times. At the same time it is very important that the viewing screen is in front of the surgeon. The surgeon, camera assistant, and viewing screen should move together to keep this relation maintained when changing the operating field. I think this is the most important step in the technique of SILCS.

PROBLEMS WITH RETRACTION

Traction and countertraction along with appropriate retraction are very important for dissection in laparoscopic surgery. Due to the limitation of the number of access ports and space around instruments, it is not possible to use separate graspers for all these actions.

An extra instrument for retraction can be used through the fourth port sometimes but generally one should learn to perform the procedure without this. For example when dissecting greater omentum from transverse colon you should hold the omentum and lift it up and the weight of the colon will act as countertraction to reveal the plane of dissection between colon and omentum.

The quality of open surgery has improved after laparoscopic surgery due to magnified view and realization and necessity of dissection into tissue planes. This is even more highlighted in SILCS and the surgeon has to be precise in dissection to follow the natural tissue planes all the time.

LOSS OF TRIANGULATION

Conventional laparoscopic teaching is that two working ports in the hands of a surgeon should meet almost at a right angle at the target area and camera should be in between of these. This is not possible while doing SILCS as instruments and scope run almost parallel to each other. The range of movement is restricted due to this and one has to take smaller steps to complete the task.

KEY POINTS

- Single incision laparoscopic colorectal surgery is an advanced laparoscopic technique that gives additional benefits to patients in the form of reduced pain, shorter hospital stay, and better cosmesis.
- It is possible to perform most colorectal procedures by this technique, but the surgeon will require some additional skills apart from the usual laparoscopic skills.
- Younger patients with inflammatory bowel disease are likely to benefit more by single incision laparoscopic colorectal surgery.

TAKE-HOME MESSAGE

- SILCS is safe and feasible for most colorectal procedures and can be easily learned by laparoscopic colorectal surgeons.

REFERENCES

1. Waters JA, Rapp BM, Guzman MJ, Jester AL, Selzer DJ, Robb BW, Johansen BJ, Tsai BM, Maun DC, George VV. Single-port laparoscopic right hemicolectomy: The first 100 resections. *Dis Colon Rectum* 2012;55:134–9.
2. Chambers WM, Bicsak M, Lamparelli M, Dixon AR. Single incision laparoscopic surgery (SILS) in complex colorectal surgery: A technique offering potential and not just cosmesis. *Colorectal Dis* 2011;13:393–8.

3. Markar S, Wiggins T, Penna M, Paraskeva P. Single-incision versus conventional multiport laparoscopic colorectal surgery—Systematic review and pooled analysis. *J Gastrointest Surg* 2014;18:2214–27.

4. Wheeless CR. A rapid, inexpensive and effective method of surgical sterilization by laparoscopy. *J Reprod Med* 1969;3(5):65–9.

5. Pelosi MA, Pelosi MA 3rd. Laparoscopic hysterectomy with bilateral salpingo-oophorectomy using a single umbilical puncture. *N J Med* 1991;88:721–6.

6. Pelosi MA, Pelosi MA 3rd. Laparoscopic appendectomy using a single umbilical puncture (minilaparoscopy). *J Reprod Med* 1992 Jul;37(7):588–94.

7. Navarra G, Pozza E, Occhionorelli S, Carcoforo P, Donini I. One-wound laparoscopic cholecystectomy. *Br J Surg* 1997 May;84(5):695.

8. Piskun G, Rajpal S. Transumbilical laparoscopic cholecystectomy utilizes no incisions outside the umbilicus. *J Laparoendosc Adv Surg Tech A* 1999 Aug;9(4):361–4.

9. Remzi FH, Kirat HT, Kaouk JH, Geisler DP. Single-port laparoscopy in colorectal surgery. *Colorectal Dis* 2008;10:823–6.

10. Bucher P, Pugin F, Morel P. Transumbilical single incision laparoscopic sigmoidectomy for benign disease. *Colorectal Dis* 2010;12:61–5.

11. Geisler D, Kirat H, Remzi F. Single-port laparoscopic total proctocolectomy with ileal pouch-anal anastomosis: Initial operative experience. *Surg Endosc* 2011;25:2175–8.

12. Borowski D, Kanakala V, Agarwal A, Tabaqchali M, Garg D, Gill T. Single-port access laparoscopic reversal of Hartmann operation. *Dis Colon Rectum* 2011;54:1053–6.

13. Kanakala V, Borowski DW, Agarwal AK, Tabaqchali MA, Garg DK, Gill TS. Comparative study of safety and outcomes of single-port access versus conventional laparoscopic colorectal surgery. *Tech Coloproctol* 2012;16:423–8.

14. Yan-Ming Zhou, Lu-Peng Wu, Yan-Fang Zhao, Dong-Hui Xu, Bin Li. Single incision versus conventional laparoscopy for colorectal disease: A meta-analysis. *Dig Dis Sci* 2012;57:2103–12.

15. Huscher CG, Mingoli A, Sgarzini G, Mereu A, Binda B, Branchini G, Trombetta S. Standard laparoscopic versus single-incision laparoscopic colectomy for cancer: Early results of a randomized prospective study. *Am J Surg* 2012;204:115–20.

16. Poon JT, Cheung CW, Fan JKM, Lo OSH, Law WL. Single-incision versus conventional laparoscopic colectomy for colonic neoplasm: A randomized, controlled trial. *Surg Endosc* 2012;26:2729–34.

17. Bulut O, Aslak KK, Levic K, Nielsen CB, Rømer E, Sørensen S, Christensen IJ, Nielsen HJ. A randomized pilot study on single-port versus conventional laparoscopic rectal surgery: Effects on postoperative pain and the stress response to surgery. *Tech Coloproctol* 2015 Jan;19(1):11–22.

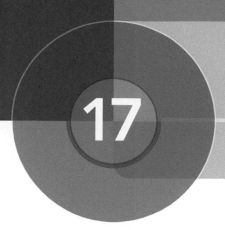

Transanal total mesorectal excision

17

STEVEN J. ARNOLD AND JOEP KNOL

LEARNING OBJECTIVES

- Understand the differences in technique and anastomosis for transanal versus abdominal dissection of the rectum, along with potential pitfalls when approaching the total mesorectal excision (TME) plane from below.

INTRODUCTION

Total mesorectal excision has long been established as the gold standard for treating rectal cancer, with the aim of achieving clear distal and circumferential margins, while removing the tumour and its lymphovascular drainage, in one embryological package (1). Outcomes from surgery following these oncological principles, particularly local recurrence, have been significantly improved over the years (2). Surgical technique has been modified during this time, from conventional open surgery, through laparoscopic techniques, and on to more recent advances with robotic surgery, in order to achieve the same oncological result, but there are inherent difficulties with any of these approaches when performing the pelvic dissection from above.

Even experienced rectal surgeons acknowledge that dissection of the mesorectal envelope can be challenging in certain patients, with the narrower male pelvis, visceral obesity, and distal tumours all widely recognised to add potential complexity to an already challenging group of patients (3). Technical challenges faced in such patients include difficulties in retraction and lighting to allow adequate exposure, imprecision in clearly identifying and then preparing the distal resection margin, and minimal access stapling devices that are not designed to operate at a 90° angle, deep in the confines of the pelvis, thereby promoting the use of multiple firings, which can lead to an increased leak rate (4,5).

Minimal access techniques have improved the outcomes in colonic cancer with low conversion rates and shorter hospital stays in experienced hands, while still achieving equivalent oncological outcome, but there is still a degree of uncertainty of the advantages of these techniques in rectal cancer surgery where the patient may still end up with a stoma, with a prolonged hospital stay (6). The multinational Colorectal cancer Laparoscopic or Open Resection (COLOR II) trial reported that outcomes from laparoscopic surgery were similar to those from open surgery, with equivalent rates of mortality and morbidity (7). Lower intra-operative blood loss from the laparoscopic group was offset by a longer operative time, but both groups had a relatively high positive circumferential resection margin of 10%. This may be a reflection of the difficulties already discussed of dissecting deep in the pelvis via an abdominal approach. More recently, two large multinational randomised controlled trials have reported, which may support this theory further (8,9). The Australasian ALaCaRT trial randomised 475 patients to open or laparoscopic surgery (8); a similar number were randomised in the North American ACOSOG Z6051 trial (462 patients) (9). Both trials reported simultaneously, with similar results and conclusions. In addition to a significantly longer operating time, there was a (non-significant) trend to a lesser proportion of mesorectal specimens being intact in the laparoscopic surgery group. Both trials concluded by saying they could not demonstrate non-inferiority for the laparoscopic approach to rectal cancer.

Transanal TME surgery has developed through a combination of differing surgical techniques, in an attempt to address at least some of the problems mentioned. The principles of TME surgery are rigidly maintained, but have evolved, blending the resurgent transanal endoscopic microsurgery (TEMS) and the established transabdominal transanal (TATA) technique to allow a bidirectional approach to the rectal dissection. As early as 2007, it was reported about the feasibility of performing this 'natural orifice' surgery on a human cadaver (10), and 3 years later came the first report of a human patient undergoing successful surgery using this method (11). At the time of writing, there has been wide interest in this technique, with various case series being reported (12–16), although the total number of cases in the literature is still very small, the largest series reporting on just 56 patients (15).

EXPOSURE

CORRECT THEATRE SETUP

Ideally, the operating room (OR) setup includes two laparoscopic towers (each with its own insufflator, camera, and monitor), one for the transabdominal part and another one for the transanal part of the procedure (Figure 17.1). Although a single surgical team can perform all parts of the technique in a sequential manner, simultaneous operating is to be preferred. This allows a more timely operation, but also facilitates the most difficult part of the procedure in the mesorectal dissection, with a more efficient way to achieve traction and countertraction from simultaneous abdominal and transanal operators.

APPROPRIATE PATIENT POSITIONING

The patient is placed in the Lloyd-Davies position for both the laparoscopic and transanal portions of the procedure, and the arms are protected and wrapped beside the patient. The procedure is performed under general anaesthesia and prophylactic antibiotics are given at induction. Standard bowel preparation is given the day before surgery.

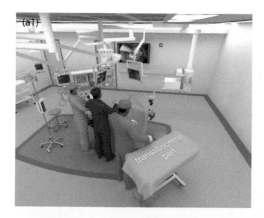
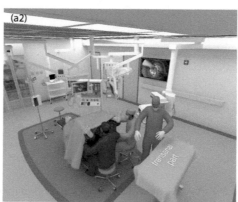
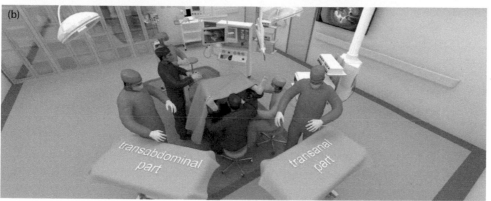

Figure 17.1 Schematic of operating theatre setup for transanal TME; transabdominal and transanal portions of the procedure can be performed sequentially (a1–a2) or simultaneously (b).

TECHNIQUE

TRANSABDOMINAL TECHNIQUE

The transabdominal portion is performed laparoscopically using a four-port technique (10-mm port above the umbilicus, 5-mm ports in the left and right flank, and right iliac fossa). A 30° 10-mm camera is used for optimal visualisation. For splenic flexure mobilisation, an additional 5-mm port may be placed in the upper abdomen in line with the surgeon's preference. If an abdominal extraction site is to be used, the left flank trocar incision can be enlarged and protected for specimen extraction or a small Pfannenstiel/suprapubic incision can be used.

A low threshold should be used to perform splenic flexure mobilisation, and many surgeons will do this routinely. By their nature, these operations often necessitate a low anastomosis, and no tension must be present when this is formed. Splenic flexure mobilisation is performed as the initial step in a standardised fashion (17).

The patient is then placed in steep Trendelenburg and either sequential or synchronised transabdominal and transanal procedures performed. From the abdomen, mesorectal mobilisation is performed until the seminal vesicles or rectovaginal septum anteriorly. It is preferable to identify hypogastric nerves, iliac vessels, seminal vesicles, or rectovaginal septum from the

abdominal site, in order to standardise technique. Some surgeons will continue further posteriorly while there is good access, and this is probably more important in sequential operating.

TRANSANAL TECHNIQUE

The initial sequence of the transanal dissection will depend to some extent on the height of
the tumour in the rectum. If the tumour is very low (within 2 cm of the anorectal junction
[ARJ]) and a coloanal anastomosis is to be performed, then an open dissection is commenced.
Commercially available retractors with adjustable hooks are useful for opening the buttocks
and displaying the perianum in order to assist with this step. Conventional monopolar diathermy is used to incise the bowel circumferentially at an appropriate height, even performing
a limited intersphincteric dissection when necessary. The same retractor at the anal verge can
help to introduce the flexible platform. During the procedure the retractor can be removed
or tension on the elastic bands can be released, as they become surplus to requirements and
this can limit the potential for trauma. A standard 30° laparoscopic camera and conventional
laparoscopic instruments are used. Many surgeons find that using a longer (bariatric) camera
allows less clustered instruments when performing the transanal surgery. Through the flexible platform, three trocars are introduced; one for introduction of the laparoscope and two
additional working ports. Most devices allow these to be rotated to facilitate intrapelvic access.

The start of the procedure depends on the level of the tumour. There is a difference between
starting the procedure for lesions within 2 cm from the ARJ, or for lesions higher up.

When lesions are located within 2 cm from the ARJ the procedure is begun with an intersphincteric dissection, continuing for approximately 2–3 cm. A purse-string suture is then
placed to close the rectal lumen, using a strong Prolene suture. Alternatively a purse-string
suture can be placed but not secured until after the mucosa is incised, and the initial dissection
commenced.

The flexible access platform can then be introduced into the anus and secured appropriately,
to continue the transanal dissection. When lesions are located more proximally, the flexible
platform can be introduced from the start.

The placement of a 2-0 Prolene purse-string suture may be considered the initial step of
the transanal technique (Photo 17.1). It is placed from within the rectum to seal closed the
lumen, distal to the tumour, and to mark the distal resection margin. The purse-string stitch
serves several functions. It is important to create an efficient use of the pneumopelvis, and

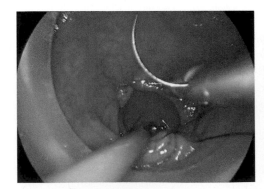 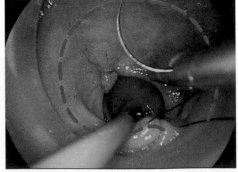

Photo 17.1 Placement of rectal purse-string. Note the dotted line indicating the accurate
circumferential placement of the stitch below the lower edge of the tumour.

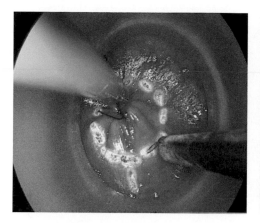
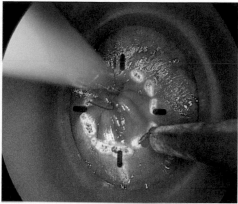

Photo 17.2 Diathermy marking of rectal mucosa to guide initial dissection. The contrast picture shows the distal rectal excision margin.

avoid distension of the proximal colon, but also to avoid soiling from above, particularly with regard to cells shed from the tumour surface. A thorough wash-out of the distal rectal stump is also permitted during the procedure, in order to try and combat infection and any loose tumour cells. The pneumopelvis is then created using a standard laparoscopic insufflator or an Airseal-platform with a target pressure of 8–12 mm Hg, with a 2–5 L/min CO_2-flow.

Before commencing dissection, it is the author's preferences to mark the rectal mucosa circumferentially, using a conventional diathermy hook, just distal to the secured purse-string stitch (Photo 17.2).

This guides the initial incision, and avoids getting too close to the suture, with the risk of breaking it. A full thickness incision of the rectal wall should be started at the posterolateral aspect, at either the 5 or 7 o'clock position. Incising posteriorly (6 o'clock) is more difficult, as the operator is then trying to cut into the dense fibers of the anococcygeal ligament.

Using the hook diathermy, a full thickness incision of the entire rectal wall is completed (Photos 17.3 and 17.4). Recognising this is a key step in the procedure, as it avoids dissecting too deep from the start (with potential damage to the pelvic side wall structures and presacral fascia) and allows the pressure of the pneumopelvis to facilitate dissection in the 'Holy Plane' during the rest of the procedure.

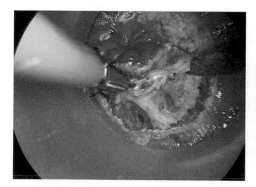
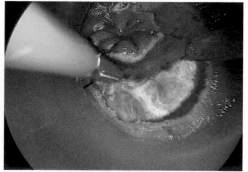

Photo 17.3 Diathermy hook dissection of the mesorectum, with yellow contrast showing entry into the correct mesorectal plane.

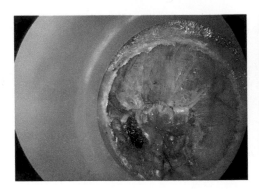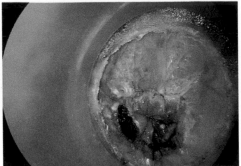

Photo 17.4 Circumferential entry into the correct mesorectal plane, highlighted in yellow.

Here on in, the dissection proceeds in a standardised manner. Starting posteriorly, dissection is carried out perpendicularly through the rectal wall to the mesorectal fascia. This requires quite a steep turn posteriorly in order to excise the whole mesorectum (16).

If the turn is not adequate, there is a risk of a mesorectal remnant being left behind, which may cause a local recurrence in future. Depending on the angulation of the curve of the sacrum and coccyx, this may be anything from 70° to 100° downward and backward to excise the mesorectum completely. Dissection then continues up through the TME dissection plane in the retrorectal space between the mesorectal fascia and the parietal pelvic fascia, which contains the pelvic autonomic nerves. When keeping the anterior side intact it acts as a guide to allow both working instruments a natural 'bridge' to work under. Anterior dissection is then performed in the rectovaginal septum or in the rectoprostatic plane, continuing ventral or dorsal to Denonvilliers fascia. It is considered easier to operate in the dorsal plane below Denonvilliers fascia. This helps to protect the neurovascular bundles, which lie anterolaterally to it, and may be damaged by surgical dissection in this plane. However, if the tumour is anteriorly situated and penetrating the bowel wall, it may be clinically necessary to dissect above Denonvilliers fascia, in order to achieve optimum tumour clearance, albeit with an increased risk of neurovascular injury.

Lateral dissection is purposely left to last because prior dissection of the posterior and anterior planes helps to differentiate the mesorectum from the lateral side wall at that level, and consequently from the neurovascular bundles that traverse close to the inside of the puborectal sling. If the lateral dissection is carried out too early, one can easily stray too lateral, into the pelvic side wall, as the natural tissue planes appear to encourage wider than necessary dissection. When the lateral dissection is nearing completion, the peritoneal cavity is entered from below, often anteriorly, and the pneumoperitoneum is established in continuity with the pneumopelvis. Any remaining tissue bridges are divided, to complete the dissection; in a synchronised dissection this can be done from both sides, and the last part of the lateral dissection can be facilitated by traction from both the abdominal and transanal surgeons.

The specimen is then extracted transanally or through the abdomen, depending on surgeon choice. It is imperative that the specimen is handled with great care in order not to damage the mesorectal envelope. Bulky tumours are probably best extracted via an abdominal incision with an appropriate wound protector, with a large enough incision to extract the specimen without any tension or traction. Some surgeons would advocate using the premarked ileostomy site for extraction, although this may not be suitable for larger specimens for reasons already discussed. Smaller specimens may be delivered per-anally through the access platform, or a freshly inserted wound protector. Once the rectum is delivered, either abdominally or anally, then the proximal division can take place, often utilising a stapling device to seal the cut end of the bowel.

ANASTOMOSIS

To reconstruct the bowel, a straight, end-to-side or J-pouch anastomosis is created, using either a hand-sewn technique with interrupted 3-0 dissolvable sutures, or a stapled technique.

We prefer a hand-sewn technique when the rectal stump is very short or a colo-anal anastomosis is to be fashioned. This may be the case after an initial intersphincteric dissection for a very low tumour, or when there are dense adhesions to surrounding tissues as sometimes seen in the lowest part of the rectovaginal septum. In all other cases a stapled technique can be used.

Two slightly different stapled anastomoses are described. Commercial staplers are available with extra-long pins on the anvil, and are often marketed for stapled haemorrhoidopexy procedures. These have an inherent advantage, with the longer pin being much easier to pass through the anal canal and connect with the staple gun.

For this technique, the anvil is initially tied into the proximal bowel using a Prolene 2-0 purse-string suture, just as in conventional surgery. A second purse-string suture is then placed circumferentially around the rectal stump, and this is tied once the anvil has been introduced through it, and joined to the pin of the circular stapler, prior to closing and then firing the gun (Figure 17.2).

If a regular circular stapler is to be used, the anvil is secured conventionally to the proximal bowel for anastomosis, with a Prolene purse-string. A catheter or tube drain (cut appropriately)

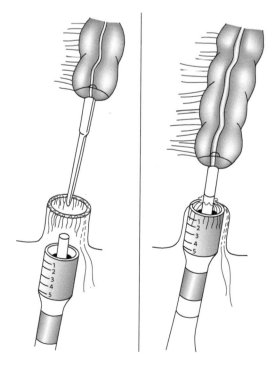

Figure 17.2 Stapled anastomosis using haemorrhoid stapler and long anvil.

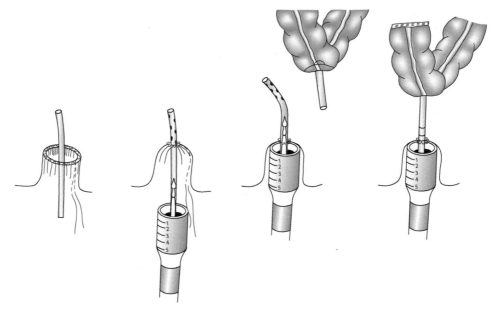

Figure 17.3 Conventional circular stapler with normal anvil, and attached drain to facilitate per-rectal passage of gun spike through lower rectal purse-string.

is attached to the advanced (open) pin of the stapler device. The second, distal purse-string on the rectal stump is then placed, and the drain used as a guide to introduce the pin through the rectal stump accurately and allow the distal purse-string to be tied.

The drain can then be detached from the abdominal side, and the anvil then secured on the pin of the gun prior to closure and firing (Figure 17.3).

The anastomosis can be checked with a rectoscope, digital examination, or by performing an air-leak insufflation test. Once the surgeon is happy with the anastomosis, then a defunctioning loop ileostomy is created, bringing the bowel out at the premarked spot.

OVERALL PERFORMANCE

POTENTIAL PITFALLS

Recognition of the anatomy of the pelvis when approached from below can be unfamiliar and challenging, especially when the operator is inexperienced with the technique. Transanal dissection has the potential for the operative plane to be continued either too deep, in the pelvic side wall or behind the pre-sacral fascia, or too shallow, close to the muscle tube, and it is crucial to recognise when dissection is not proceeding in the correct plane in order to perform good-quality TME surgery and avoid damaging pelvic structures.

AVOID DISSECTION TOO FAR POSTERIORLY

Although an initial steep posterior turn is important to avoid coning in on the specimen from below, it is important to avoid going too far posterior and running into the endopelvic/presacral fascia (Photo 17.5). Dissection is easier if commenced at the 5 or 7 o'clock positions,

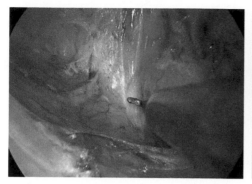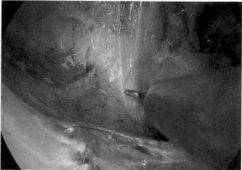

Photo 17.5 Showing dissection in correct TME plane, but with earlier error (highlighted in green) demonstrating dissection in incorrect plane behind presacral fascia.

as this avoids the anococcygeal ligament. It also allows easier recognition of the loose areolar tissue of the 'Holy Plane' from below, and the denser anococcygeal ligament, which lies posteriorly, can then be dissected when the lateral spaces of the TME plane have been opened on either side.

AVOID DISSECTION TOO FAR LATERALLY

When dissecting the lateral side, the lateral extensions of Waldeyer fascia tend to guide the dissection plane lateral to the TME plane, and into the pelvic side wall. It is quite easy to peel off the side wall and the associated neurovascular bundle, because it seems to be the perfect plane; this is accentuated by the fact that traction is used on the specimen, pulling it to the medial side in order to improve exposure. It's important to recognise this wrong plane of dissection, which can lead to neurovascular damage with an increased risk of bleeding and impaired functional outcome (Photo 17.6).

To circumvent this, first posterior, then anterior dissection planes should be established, as described, defining the TME envelope with the correct plane either side of the lateral aspects. Gentle medial traction then allows identification of the correct lateral plane, between the anterior and posterior dissections, and the lateral pelvic sidewall can be avoided.

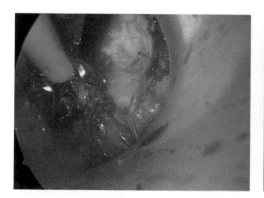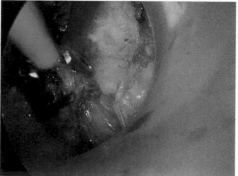

Photo 17.6 Incorrect plane of initial dissection in pelvic side wall (green highlight), with subsequent correction to medial TME plane.

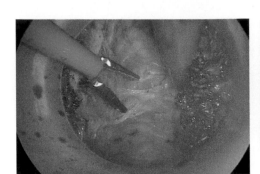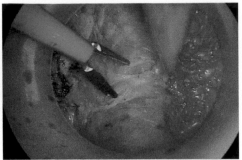

Photo 17.7 TME dissection plane with bulk of mesorectal specimen (highlighted purple) still attached on contralateral side.

AVOIDING DISSECTION IN AN ASYMMETRICAL WAY

When the correct plane of dissection is found, the temptation may be to continue in the same direction as long as adequate exposure allows. While this will result in operative progress, it can lead to subsequent difficulties. If one side of the specimen is dissected too much, the meso-rectum will still be tethered on the contralateral side. This allows the specimen to tilt slightly, adding to the difficulty of dissecting the other side (Photo 17.7). There may also be a tendency for the access platform to angulate, despite being anchored on the perineum, which may further impede contralateral access. To avoid this, it is considered important to perform the dissection from below in a symmetrical way, thereby encouraging adequate circumferential access.

KEY POINTS

- This technique has arisen due to the difficulties of access with conventional abdominal approaches to TME.
- Correct theatre setup and equipment are vital.
- The purse-string stitch is absolutely crucial in the technique.
- Be aware of pitfalls, especially 'wrong plane' surgery.
- Audit and record your results – this is a new technique with a relative paucity of clinical data/outcomes.

TAKE-HOME MESSAGE

Transanal TME shows promise in facilitating the difficult lower end dissection in TME surgery but should only be carried out by suitably trained surgeons who audit their outcomes on the national Transanal Total Mesorectal Excision Database.

REFERENCES

1. Heald RJ, Husband EM, Ryall RDH. The mesorectum in rectal cancer surgery—The clue to pelvic recurrence? *Br J Surg* 1982;69:613–6.

2. Heald RJ, Moran BJ, Ryall RDH, Sexton R, MacFarlane JK. Rectal cancer: The Basingstoke experience of total mesorectal excision, 1978–1997. *Arch Surg* 1998;133:894–9.

3. Heald RJ. A new solution to some old problems: Transanal TME. *Tech Coloproctol* 2013 Jun;17(3):257–8.

4. Ito M, Sugito M, Kobayashi A, Nishizawa Y, Tsunoda Y, Saito N. Relationship between multiple numbers of stapler firings during rectal division and anastomotic leakage after laparoscopic rectal resection. *Int J Colorectal Dis* 2008 Jul;23(7):703–7.

5. Kawada K, Hasegawa S, Hida K, Hirai K, Okoshi K, Nomura A, Kawamura J, Nagayama S, Sakai Y. Risk factors for anastomotic leakage after laparoscopic low anterior resection with DST anastomosis. *Surg Endosc* 2014 Oct;28(10):2988–95.

6. Cartmell MT, Jones OM, Moran BJ, Cecil TD. A defunctioning stoma significantly prolongs the length of stay in laparoscopic colorectal resection. *Surg Endosc* 2008 Dec;22(12):2643–7.

7. van der Pas MH, Haglind E, Cuesta MA, Fürst A, Lacy AM et al. Laparoscopic versus open surgery for rectal cancer (COLOR II): Short-term outcomes of a randomised, phase 3 trial. *Lancet Oncol* 2013 Mar;14(3):210–8.

8. Stevenson ARL, Solomon MJ, Lumley JW, Hewett P, Clouston AD et al. Effect of laparoscopic-assisted resection vs. open resection on pathological outcomes in rectal cancer. *JAMA* 2015;314(13):1356–63.

9. Fleshman J, Branda M, Sargent DJ, Boller AM, George V et al. Effect of laparoscopic-assisted resection vs open resection of stage II or III rectal cancer on pathological outcomes. *JAMA* 2015;314(13):1346–55.

10. Whiteford MH, Denk PM, Swanstrom LL. Feasibility of radical sigmoid colectomy performed as natural orifice translumenal endoscopic surgery (NOTES) using trans-anal endoscopic microsurgery. *Surg Endosc* 2007;21:1870–4.

11. Sylla P, Rattner DW, Delgado S, Lacy AM. NOTES trans-anal rectal cancer resection using trans-anal endoscopic microsurgery and laparoscopic assistance. *Surg Endosc* 2010;24:1205–10.

12. Fernández-Hevia M, Delgado S, Castells A, Tasende M, Momblan D, Díaz Del Gobbo G, DeLacy B, Balust J, Lacy AM. Transanal total mesorectal excision in rectal cancer: Short-term outcomes in comparison with laparoscopic surgery. *Ann Surg* 2015;261(2):221–7.

13. Atallah S, Martin-Perez B, Albert M, deBeche-Adams T, Nassif G, Hunter L, Larach S. Transanal minimally invasive surgery for total mesorectal excision (TAMIS-TME): Results and experience with the first 20 patients undergoing curative-intent rectal cancer surgery at a single institution. *Tech Coloproctol* 2014 May; 18(5):473–80.

14. Velthuis S, Nieuwenhuis DH, Ruijter TE, Cuesta MA, Bonjer HJ, Sietses C. Transanal versus traditional laparoscopic total mesorectal excision for rectal carcinoma. *Surg Endosc* 2014 Dec; 28(12):3494–9.

15. Tuech JJ, Karoui M, Lelong B, De Chaisemartin C, Bridoux V, Manceau G, Delpero JR, Hanoun L, Michot F. A step toward NOTES total mesorectal excision for rectal cancer: Endoscopic transanal proctectomy. *Ann Surg* 2015 Feb; 261(2):228–33.

16. Knol JJ, D'Hondt M, Souverijns G, Heald B, Vangertruyden G. Transanal endoscopic total mesorectal excision: Technical aspects of approaching the mesorectal plane from below—A preliminary report. *Tech Coloproctol* 2015;19(4):221–9.

17. Knol JJ, Wexner SD, Vangertruyden G. Laparoscopic mobilization of the splenic flexure: The use of color-grading as a unique teaching tool. *Surg Endosc* 2015 Mar; 29(3):734–5.

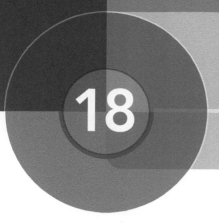

Future developments in laparoscopic colorectal surgery

18

SHAFAQUE SHAIKH AND DAVID JAYNE

LEARNING OBJECTIVES

- Better understand the limitations of current laparoscopic and minimally invasive surgical systems.
- Appreciate the different ways that new technologies can improve surgical performance and patient outcomes.
- Consider the likely direction of future innovation in surgical practice.

INTRODUCTION

The application of laparoscopy to treat colorectal disease in the late 1990s was a major sea-change in surgical approach. By substituting small 'key-hole' incisions for a large laparotomy wound, surgical access trauma was reduced, enabling patients to recover quicker with less pain and fewer complications. Initial uptake was slow due to unfamiliarity, increased technical difficulty, long learning curves, and lack of suitable instruments. Subsequent technological innovation, combined with structured training programmes (1), has seen a steady dissemination of laparoscopic colorectal surgery, with penetration rates now approaching 50% in the United Kingdom. Despite this progress, several challenges remain: laparoscopic instruments lack the dexterity and tactile feedback of the human hand; visualisation of the surgical field is in two dimensions without depth of field; an open incision is more often than not required for specimen retrieval; and surgical site (as opposed to surgical access) trauma is unaffected.

In this chapter, the technological innovations that aim to overcome challenges of current laparoscopic surgery will be discussed, including advances in laparoscopic instrumentation and imaging, the use of robotic assistance, novel endoluminal and hybrid approaches, and image-guided surgery.

Many of the recent technological advances in laparoscopic surgery have been incremental, building on established laparoscopic technology but adding a component that addresses a particular challenge. These incremental advances will be considered separately below.

ENERGY DEVICES

Reliable and safe means of achieving haemostasis are of paramount importance in laparoscopic surgery because of the light-absorbing effects of haemoglobin. Traditional monopolar and bipolar energy devices still have a role and are preferred by some surgeons due to their precision and familiarity to open surgery. But the risk of iatrogenic injury to neighboring structures is increased through direct or capacitive coupling, and this risk is increased with longer instruments, narrower trocars, thinner insulation, and higher voltages.

Bipolar diathermy works on the principle of combining both the active and receiving electrodes into a single instrument allowing for a lower voltage to deliver the same coagulative effect. The alternating current does not pass through the patient but is distributed through the target tissue reducing the risk of capacitive coupling (2). Bipolar electrosurgical instruments can seal vessels up to 3 mm in diameter.

Recent technological advancements have enabled the development of electrothermal bipolar vessel sealing devices that can safely seal vessels up to 7 mm in diameter, thus providing quicker, more consistent, and efficient haemostasis. Vessel sealing devices employ burst pressures and tissue-sensing technology that fuse tissue collagen to form a permanent seal (3). These devices can seal vessels with supraphysiologic burst pressures comparable to those obtained with clips or ligatures (4). Two popular bipolar vessel sealing devices are the PlasmaKinetics sealer (Gyrus Medical, Maple Grove, Minnesota) and the LigaSure sealing device (Valleylab, Boulder, Colorado) (5). The Caiman (Aragon, Palo Alto, California) is another device, similar to the LigaSure, but claims a smaller thermal spread and quicker operating time due to its bigger jaw with sealing lengths of up to 50 mm at a time (6).

Another exciting development was the introduction of the ultrasonic coagulating shears, which uses a high-frequency vibrating blade (55,000 cycles/sec) to generate heat and produce a coagulum seal effective for vessels between 3 and 5 mm in diameter (3). Several variants of ultrasonic shears are available, including the Harmonic scalpel, Harmonic ACE, and more recently HARMONIC ACE + 7 (Ethicon, Johnson & Johnson) (7), the Sonicision cordless dissector (Covidien, Minneapolis) (8), and the SonoSurgX ultrasonic surgical system (Olympus, Tokyo, Japan) (9).

The ENSEAL Device (Ethicon, Johnson & Johnson) (10) offers some incremental advancements, including a flexible articulating shaft to facilitate perpendicular sealing and an independent lower jaw for spot coagulation. The Thunderbeat (Olympus, Tokyo, Japan) (11) is a versatile device that has integrated bipolar and ultrasound technology enabling reliable haemostasis and rapid dissection within the same instrument.

Current developments in this area include minimising lateral thermal spread, decreasing haemostasis time, improved ergonomics, and cordless devices (12).

SMOKE ELIMINATION SYSTEMS

One problem common to all laparoscopic coagulating and cutting devices is the release of smoke or tissue vapor, which obscures optical vision and requires the frequent liberation of plume from the peritoneal cavity. There is also a theoretical risk of tumour implantation along port sites if the vapor plume contains viable cancer cells. Several smoke elimination systems are commercially available. Some are relatively simple in design, consisting of tubing attached to a filter that is connected to a trocar. The filter is usually a matrix of activated charcoal and ultra-low penetration air (ULPA) grade hydrophobic glass microfibers. Other technologies are more elaborate and include enhanced port technology, such as the PneuVIEW XE (Lexion Medical Technology) (12) and the Ultravision (Asalus, Cardiff, United Kingdom) (13), which uses electrostatic precipitation to produce continuous collection of airborne particles.

HUMIDIFICATION

Carbon dioxide insufflation is potentially damaging to the peritoneal lining, causing desiccation, acidification, and hypothermia (14). A systematic review of the effect of humidified and warm carbon dioxide on patients after laparoscopic procedures has shown benefits in terms of reduced post-operative pain, analgesic requirements, and maintenance of normothermia (15). However, there was no measurable benefit on clinical outcomes, such as length of hospital stay.

The Humigard system (Fisher & Paykel) provides controlled humidification and warming of the gas insufflation by means of an insulated and heated insufflation tube and the MR860 surgical humidifier, which continually adjusts to deliver optimal humidity (16). Another such device is the Insuflow (Lexion), which has the added advantage of combining anti-fog solution (FRED) to minimise lens fogging (17,18).

FRICTIONLESS PORT SYSTEMS

The use of laparoscopic ports introduces friction to the passage of instruments that in turn reduces the tactile feedback to the operating surgeon. Several strategies have been tried to overcome this problem, including the use of low-friction materials, such as silicon, for manufacture of the port valves. A neat solution is the Airseal (SurgiQuest) (19), which combines a valve-free trocar for frictionless surgery with stable pneumoperitoneum and continuous smoke elimination. This system is reported to be particularly beneficial in transanal endoscopic surgery, eliminating the 'bellows' effect of traditional insufflation.

FLEXIBLE INSTRUMENTS AND CAMERAS

FLEXIBLE INSTRUMENTS

One of the limitations of laparoscopic surgery is the poor design of the instruments, which lack freedom of movement and dexterity of the instrument tip. Innovation in this area has been driven by the enthusiasm for single incision laparoscopic surgery (SILS) and natural orifice transendoluminal surgery (NOTES), where articulating instruments become a necessity to achieve angulation for retraction and dissection. A variety of articulating instruments are now available for laparoscopic surgery and SILS and include instruments like ENSEAL G2 Articulating Tissue Sealers, ECHELON FLEXTM ENDOPATH Endocutter (Ethicon, Johnson & Johnson) (20), and the Goldfinger retractor (Artisan Medical, Medford, New Jersey) (21).

Several manufacturers have concentrated on the development of flexible platforms for laparoscopic surgery. This includes the SPIDER system (22), which allows multiple instruments to be used through a single incision with a design that accommodates a range of flexible instruments through articulating instrument delivery tubes (IDTs) and working channels (Photo 18.1).

Articulating instruments are an active area of research and several mechanical designs have been proposed, an example of which is the parallel kinematic system that offers three degrees of freedom with a larger working space (23). Another exciting concept is the modular orientation tool proposed by Vaida et al. (24), which comprises three components that permit various configurations that may be applied to several laparoscopic instruments of varying sizes providing increased degrees of freedom without the need to redesign the instrument.

FLEXIBLE CAMERA SYSTEMS

The rigidity of the straight laparoscopes and their fixed field of vision limits the ability to see the whole of the surgical field (i.e. it takes away the panoramic 'birds-eye' view of open surgery). Furthermore, the development of novel techniques such as SILS and NOTES relies heavily on the availability of more versatile camera systems.

One such system is Stryker's IDEAL EYES HD 5-mm articulating laparoscope (25), which features an angled handle and friction-assist control levers that enable placement and fixation of the articulating tip with great precision.

While flexible endoscopes are also currently in use as substitutes to laparoscopes in NOTES procedures, research is directed towards the development of deployable video cameras delivering more stable, high-definition (HD) and versatile vision (26).

A recent advancement is the development of the magnetic anchoring and guidance system (MAGS) camera (Karl Storz Endoscopy, Culver City, California) as an alternative solution (27).

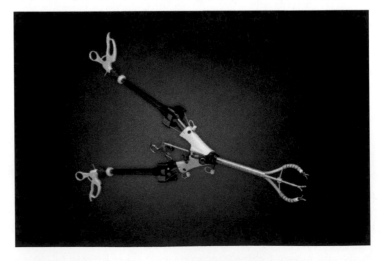

Photo 18.1 The SPIDER System's design accommodates a range of flexible instruments through articulating instrument delivery tubes (IDTs) and working channels. (From http://www.transenterix.com/spider/)

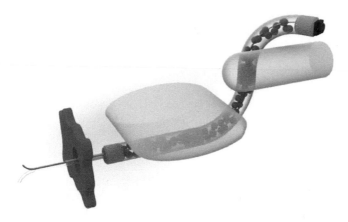

Photo 18.2 The core-snake is a low-cost system. The Core-Snake granules lock it into its rigid state, and holding a 180° bend. The flexibility and variable stiffness of the camera system allows surgeons to navigate to areas of interest and lock the camera in the position. (From Jiang A, et al. The Core-Snake, the Variable Stiffness Laparoscopic Camera. https://www.academia.edu/3776067/The_Core-Snake_the_Variable_Stiffness_Laparoscopic_Camera.)

Preclinical testing has shown promising results with the MAGS platform providing an unrestricted range of motion, improved triangulation, and freedom from instrument conflicts. This may provide a superior alternative to the conventional laparoscopic platform once it is fully developed.

Another novel technology under development is the Core-Snake which is a low-cost flexible laparoscopic camera (28). Essentially, the system consists of 10-mm diameter robot capable of altering its body stiffness via granular jamming – granular jamming is a phenomenon where a multitude of particles normally act like a fluid, but lock into a solid-like state when an external stress is applied, as commonly seen in rice or coffee bags (Photo 18.2). Thus, the Core-Snake is naturally compliant and can be pushed into position by the surgeons' laparoscopic tools, to be locked in position when a differential between the internal and external pressure is applied by a vacuum.

3D CAMERA SYSTEMS

Lack of a three-dimensional (3D) view to the operating field contributes to the laparoscopic learning curve and increases operating time in complex laparoscopic procedures. 3D vision is purported to improve dexterity and operator experience. The first commercial use of 3D optics was in the da Vinci Surgical System (Intuitive Surgical, Sunnyvale, California), but stand-alone 3D vision systems have subsequently been developed. These include the EndoSite 3Di Digital Vision System developed by Viking Systems (La Jolla, California), which couples a 3D view with an ergonomic head-mounted display, allowing improved spectral depth perception with the use of traditional laparoscopes. The system consists of a stereo digital scope (dual 3CCD optical channel) attached to a 3D data-processing unit, which conveys information to a head-mounted display, which consists of dual 800 × 600 miniature liquid crystal display (LCD) screens (29). The limited literature available suggests an improvement in performance times and accuracy for both expert and inexperienced operators (30).

HAPTIC INSTRUMENTS

Loss of haptic feedback is a problem in laparoscopic surgery (31) and potentially more so in robotic surgery. It limits fine tissue handling and makes assessment of tissue quality difficult to appreciate. Instead, a greater reliance has to be placed on visual cues (32). Whether a lack of tactile feedback predisposes to increased tissue injury (33) is uncertain and to date has not been substantiated in the literature (30). In robotic surgery, it has been suggested that the restoration of 3D vision may compensate for the absence of haptic feedback (34–36).

RETRACTION PLATFORMS

Good exposure of the operative field is an essential requirement of any operation. This can be difficult to achieve in laparoscopic surgery where the operating space of the enclosed abdomen can be restrictive and the operator is reliant on the skills of an assistant. A number of fixed position retraction devices are available that facilitate exposure of the surgical field. They do not obviate the need for repositioning and thus add to the operating time if repeated readjustments are needed. They also find more utility in procedures limited to a single quadrant (like liver and gynaecological procedures) and are thus not particularly helpful in colorectal procedures. One such device is the DASH system (37), which consists of a malleable sponge that can be molded into the required shape and positioned to retract soft tissue. It has the additional advantage of absorbing fluids, keeping the operative field dry (38).

Futuristic retraction platforms employing robotic retraction may provide greater benefits and be more intuitive to the operator's needs but are still in development. In the robotic device proposed by Tortora et al., a serial kinematic chain is employed with a magnetic base, allowing it to be passed down another port and attached to the abdominal wall obviating the need for an extra retraction port (39). The main function of this device is to retract tissue allowing its manipulation by other tools. The device has two degrees of freedom with a pitch-actuated joint and an end-effector with an opening/closing mechanism for the gripper that allows retraction of grasped tissue towards the abdominal wall. The robot is magnetically anchored to the abdominal wall and hence can be used multidirectionally.

ROBOTIC-ASSISTED LAPAROSCOPIC SURGERY

Robotic-assisted surgery is not new to clinical practice, with the first da Vinci system being used in 1999. Originally aimed at the cardiothoracic market, the da Vinci soon found a niche in radical prostatectomy and was applied to colorectal surgery in 2002 (40). Since then, the use of robotic-assisted colorectal surgery has continued to expand globally, despite criticism about its lack of clear cost-effectiveness (41), and has increasingly focused on anterior resection for rectal cancer. Many single-institution studies testify to the safety and efficacy of robotic rectal cancer surgery, and several systematic reviews have documented comparable results to conventional laparoscopy, but with reduced conversion rates to open surgery (42,43) and possibly better preservation of post-operative bladder and sexual function (44).

The advantages of robotic assistance appear to be fourfold: (a) the operating surgeon is in a comfortable position, remote from the operating table, with complete control over the laparoscopic camera, one operating instrument, and two retracting instruments – his reliance on a trained assistant is minimised; (b) the operating instruments are fully articulating with Endowrist technology that provides 7° freedom of movement to aid operative dexterity; (c) the operating field is stable and provides an immersive pseudo 3D image of the operative field with depth perception; and (d) the digital interface between the operating surgeon and the robotic effectors allows for computer assistance (zoom magnification, image stabilisation, tremor elimination) and integration of other digital technologies (fluorescence imaging, radiological imaging).

Robotic assistance appears to be the future evolution of laparoscopic surgery with its technological advantages overcoming many of the limitations of conventional laparoscopy (see Chapter 15). But, robotic surgery has struggled to gain universal acceptance, due mainly to the considerable capital cost of the da Vinci system that makes it difficult to justify its routine use in the absence of any rigorous data on cost-effectiveness. However, other cheaper robotic systems are progressing to market, which will no doubt end the current Intuitive monopoly and open up market competition. The DLR Miro system developed by the Institute for Robotics and Mechatronics at the German Aerospace Centre (45) (Photo 18.3) consists of a 7DoF robotic surgical manipulator incorporating position and torque sensors providing haptic feedback. It can be used as a single robotic arm or in combination as a multi-robot platform (MicroSurge) (46).

The Amadeus robotic surgical system (Titan Medical Inc., Canada) (47), bears similarities to the da Vinci system. It is promoted as a four-armed robotic surgical platform with enhanced vision systems, force feedback, and telecommunication features that enable long distance robotic surgery. There is little public information regarding the specifics of the system or how far it is from commercialisation. The University of Technology in Eindhoven are developing 'Sophie'; Surgeon's Operating Force-feedback Interface Eindhoven (48). This master-slave platform consists of a remote operating workstation, and a robotic base unit that is clamped to the operating table and accommodates three 4DoF manipulators, allowing for changes in patient position without the need to de-dock/re-dock the robot. A potential advantage is in the cost, which is expected to be considerably cheaper than the da Vinci system.

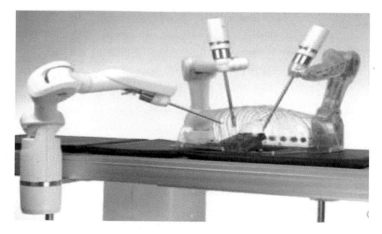

Photo 18.3 The DLR Miro robotic system: the robotic arms can be separately secured to the operating table for use in isolation or as a multi-robot platform. (From Hagn U et al. *Ind Robot* 2008;35(4):324–36.)

REDUCING SURGICAL TRAUMA

Although robotic systems bring much needed technological assistance, they continue to rely on a multiport laparoscopic approach and, as such, do little to reduce the extent of surgical trauma, which is so important to improving patient outcomes. Several innovations have focused on extending the capabilities of laparoscopic surgery, taking it from 'minimally invasive' to 'minimally traumatic'. In colorectal surgery, this development is supported by a need to alter current practices to reflect changes in disease presentation. The introduction of the NHS National Bowel Cancer Screening Programme is having a marked effect on the stage of presentation of colorectal cancer presentation: almost 50% of cancers are now diagnosed as early (Duke's stage A), in comparison to 10% in historical cohorts (49). As such, the risk of metastatic disease is reduced and in the future the need for radical resection with extended lymphadenectomy will no longer be necessary for many cancers. In addition, the population is aging and with this comes an inevitable increase in the number of elderly, frail patients who develop colorectal cancer and are less able to tolerate the insult of radical surgery. The development of 'minimally traumatic' techniques is therefore not only desirable but also a necessity. Below, we look at some of the recent innovations that address the challenges of surgical trauma.

SINGLE INCISION LAPAROSCOPIC SURGERY (SILS)

The main advantage of SILS is reported to be less post-operative pain and a better cosmetic outcome achieved by the reduction of surgical access trauma; the intra-abdominal operation remains the same. This undoubtedly translates into a technically more challenging operating experience for the surgeon. However, with the development of curved instruments, better quality ports, and increasing experience, SILS has carved a niche role for itself in the management of benign conditions like inflammatory bowel disease, especially in the younger patients (50,51).

The major drawbacks of SILS are a lack of triangulation, frequent instrument collisions, and poor visualisation making the operation technically more challenging (52). The combination of SILS and robotics may help to overcome some of the limitations. In particular, the ability to re-assign the operator controls to opposite hands overcomes the difficulties of operating with 'crossed instruments' (53). However, there is a trade-off as the current system of curved robotic instruments does not allow for the use of advanced energy sources, such as the harmonic scalpel. Nevertheless, the limited experience with robotic SILS suggests that it may have clinical application (54) (see Chapter 16).

NATURAL ORIFICE TRANSLUMINAL ENDOSCOPIC SURGERY (NOTES)

Natural Orifice Transluminal Endoscopic Surgery (NOTES) is more ambitious and seeks to eliminate external incisions altogether by utilising natural orifices (vagina, rectum, urinary bladder, stomach) to gain intraperitoneal access. Although successful in animal models, NOTES brings a range of new challenges. These include safe access to and visualisation of the peritoneal cavity, safe closure of the viscotomy, challenges with suturing/stapling devices, tumour seeding and infection risk, and training requirements. Because of this, its use to date has been confined to the research arena with only limited human application in simple laparoscopic procedures, such as appendicectomy (55).

TRANSANAL ENDOSCOPIC MICROSURGERY (TEMs) AND TRANSANAL MINIMALLY INVASIVE SURGERY (TAMIS)

TEMs is an attempt to reduce the morbidity of a major rectal resection by excising early lesions using a transanal rather than transperitoneal approach. A European consensus conference (56) concluded that TEMs is an established approach for local excision of early rectal cancer and is in widespread use; there is, however, a need for better level 1 evidence to support its implementation.

Transanal minimally invasive surgery–total mesorectal excision (TAMIS-TME) is a promising new technique that adopts a totally new approach to laparoscopic TME (see Chapter 17). An access device is placed into the anal canal and attached to an insufflator. Standard laparoscopic instruments can be inserted to perform a 'retrograde' dissection in the TME planes, if necessary combined with conventional laparoscopic guidance from the abdomen. The limited initial experience with this technique suggests that it may have advantages in terms of the quality of the TME specimen and reduced damage to the neurovascular bundles (57–60).

HYBRID LAPARO-ENDOSCOPIC SURGERY

Hybrid laparoscopic-endoscopic techniques are being explored as a minimally invasive option to avoid major resectional surgery for benign polyps that are difficult to remove with conventional colonoscopy. A variety of approaches have been tried with varying success. Essentially, conventional laparoscopic surgery is used to mobilise the colon and present the polyp for endoluminal resection using snare diathermy. The procedure can be monitored laparoscopically, and in the event of bowel perforation an immediate repair can be undertaken. So far, data are limited but the feasibility of the technique has been established even if it is not amenable for all lesions. One of the main difficulties is distinguishing benign from malignant disease in large polyps prior to local endoluminal resection (61).

FLUORESCENCE DIAGNOSTICS AND IMAGE-GUIDED SURGERY

BACKGROUND

The evolution of laparoscopic surgery towards less invasive and less traumatic interventions will only be possible with accompanying advances in diagnostic capabilities. For example, before embarking on a hybrid laparo-endoscopic procedure for an early cancer it is necessary to know with some certainty whether there are lymph node metastases. Current radiological imaging lacks the sensitivity and specificity to accurately predict lymph node metastases (62) and therefore other means of detection are necessary. In this regard, laparoscopic surgery has an advantage: the light source can be readily modified to provide illumination across the visible spectrum. In particular, fluorescence imaging is currently being explored in applications that include fluorescent lymph node mapping, fluorescence-guided surgery, and fluorescence angiography.

FLUORESCENT LYMPH NODE MAPPING

Around 30% of patients with colorectal cancer have nodal disease (63). The presence of regional lymph node metastasis is a strong predictor of outcome in colorectal cancer and guides adjuvant therapy (64). In this context, the sentinel lymph node, being the first lymphatic station in a given lymph drainage area, is crucial and has been shown to be of strategic significance, influencing extent of lymph node dissection as well as prognosticating risk of recurrence (65,66).

Current techniques for the detection of sentinel lymph nodes in colorectal cancer remain imperfect with a low sensitivity and specificity. Several patient- and disease-related factors contribute to the problem, including body mass index, centre-experience, aberrant drainage sites, and the presence of skip lesions (67). While there are problems with current techniques involving blue dye and radioisotopes, the use of fluorescent markers may hold more promise. Photodiagnostic tracers have been shown to accumulate in malignant cells enabling the detection of small cell aggregates in lymph nodes (68). Recent interest has centred on the use of indocyanine green and near-infrared imaging for sentinel lymph node mapping with reasonable sensitivity (69–71).

FLUORESCENCE-GUIDED SURGERY

In the future, as the pattern of colorectal disease changes with a shift to earlier stage disease, it will become increasingly important to tailor the extent of surgical resection to the biology of the disease. Several strategies for targeted intra-operative cancer diagnosis are under investigation. These include the use of bioactive fluorochromes, antigen recognition molecules labeled with fluorescent molecules, and nanoparticle fluorescent molecule delivery systems. Probably the mostly widely used in clinical practice are photosensitisers that can be administered systemically and emit fluorescence when stimulated with light of a specific wavelength. Such techniques are gaining popularity in certain areas of cancer surgery, with most experience in neurosurgery for glioblastoma (72) and urology for transitional cell carcinoma of the bladder (73). The most popular photosensitiser in clinical practice is the prodrug, 5-aminolevulinic acid. When administered orally, it is preferentially taken up by cancer cells and metabolised to the natural fluorophore, protoporphyrin IX. Use of a laparoscope emitting blue light (Storz D-light laparoscope) excites the photosensitiser, which emits a characteristic pink/red fluorescence that delineates the cancer from normal tissue. In glioblastoma surgery it has been shown to increase complete tumour resection, progression-free survival, and overall survival (74), while in bladder surgery it has shown to reduce recurrence and number of follow-up procedures in non-muscle-invasive disease (75). The use of fluorescence diagnostics in colorectal cancer surgery has been limited but a Medical Research Council/Efficacy and Mechanism Evaluation/ National Institute for Health Research clinical study is underway to determine the feasibility of a similar approach in mapping tumour-specific lymph node disease (76). Other strategies for fluorescence diagnosis and disease localisation are being explored and will undoubtedly translate into clinical practice in the near future, or in combination with other modalities, such as radioisotope and magnetic resonance imaging contrast-enhanced imaging.

FLUORESCENT PERFUSION ANGIOGRAPHY

Fluorescence perfusion angiography is another area in laparoscopic surgery that is attracting a lot of attention. Indocyanine green is used as an intravascular fluorescent marker to assess anastomotic perfusion and thereby prevent anastomotic leak. Clinical data are limited but the

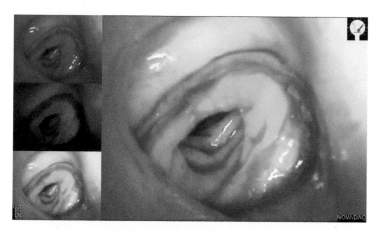

Photo 18.4 ICG fluorescence angiography. Transanal view demonstrating white light, near-infrared, and combined mode (left panel), and combined mode with fluorescence perfusion proximal and distal to the anastomotic line (right). (Courtesy of Novadaq, Ontario, Canada. http://www.novadaq.com.)

results of a recent U.S. multicentre study are encouraging: in a prospective, non-randomised study involving 147 patients undergoing anterior resection the leak rate following assessment of ICG tissue perfusion was only 1.4%, which compares favourably to leak rates of 10%–15% in historical controls (77) (Photo 18.4).

SUMMARY

Laparoscopic surgery has come a long way since its introduction to colorectal surgery in the late 1990s. The technique has evolved with a better understanding of the nuances of the surgical approach, aided by incremental developments in instrument and devices technology. Robotic assistance was introduced as the next paradigm shift in laparoscopic surgery, but to date, at least in colorectal surgery, it has not gained universal recognition; the undoubted technological advantages of the robot have not translated into clinical benefit in terms of demonstrable cost-effectiveness. The next era of laparoscopic surgery will likely involve the greater use of fluorescence and multimodal imaging, with strategies for intra-operative diagnostics and disease staging. This will open the door to personalised surgery where minimally traumatic interventions can be aligned to the underlying disease process, ensuring maximal preservation of normal function and minimising unnecessary surgical trauma. We are entering an exciting period in laparoscopic surgery, where advances in technology and biodiscovery are being integrated to produce intelligent solutions for future suffers of colorectal disease.

KEY POINTS

- The appropriate use of technology can facilitate laparoscopic and minimally invasive surgery to increase surgical skill and improve patient outcomes.
- Technological innovations that will play an increasingly important role in minimally invasive surgery include robotic assistance, fluorescent and multispectral imaging, and devices to facilitate endoluminal interventions.
- Technological advances in diagnostic capabilities and therapeutic interventions are the key to future personalised surgery.

TAKE-HOME MESSAGE

- 'It is not the strongest of the species that survives, nor the most intelligent that survives. It is the one that is the most adaptable to change'. Charles Darwin

REFERENCES

1. Lapco. Available at: http://www.lapco.nhs.uk
2. Harrell AG, Kercher KW, Heniford BT. Energy sources in laparoscopy. *Semin Laparosc Surg* 2004;11:201–9.
3. Campagnacci R, de Sanctis A, Baldarelli M, Rimini M, Lezoche G, Guerrieri M. Electrothermal bipolar vessel sealing device vs. ultrasonic coagulating shears in laparoscopic colectomies: A comparative study. *Surg Endosc* 2007;21:1526–31.
4. Newcomb WL, Hope WW, Schmelzer TM, Heath JJ, James Norton H, Lincourt AE, Todd Heniford T, Iannitti DA. Comparison of blood vessel sealing among new electrosurgical and ultrasonic devices. *Surg Endosc* 2009;23:90–96.
5. Medtronic. *Vessel Sealing*. Available at: http://www.covidien.com/surgical/products/vessel-sealing
6. Society of Laparoendoscopic Surgeons. Available at: http://laparoscopy.blogs.com/prevention_management_3/2010/10/laparoscopic-vessel-sealing-devices.html
7. Ethicon. http://www.ethicon.com/healthcare-professionals/products/advanced-energy
8. Medtronic. *Ultrasonic Dissection*. Available at: http://www.covidien.com/surgical/products/ultrasonic-dissection
9. Olympus. *SonoSurg X: Ultrasonic Instrument*. Available at: http://www.olympus.nl/medical/en/medical_systems/products_services/product_details/product_details_10121.jsp
10. Ethicon. *ENSEAL G2 Articulating Tissue Sealers*. Available at: http://www.ethicon.com/healthcare-professionals/products/advanced-energy/enseal/enseal-g2-articulating#!science-and-technology
11. Olympus. *Olympus to Launch THUNDERBEAT*. Available at: http://www.olympus-global.com/en/news/2012a/nr120321thunderbeate.jsp
12. Lexion. Available at: http://www.lexionmedical.com/technologies/
13. www.alesi-surgical.com
14. Volz J, Köster S, Spacek Z, Paweletz N. The influence of pneumoperitoneum used in laparoscopic surgery on an intraabdominal tumor growth. *Cancer* 1999 Sep 1;86(5):770–4.
15. Sajid MS, Mallick AS, Rimpel J, Bokari SA, Cheek E, Baig MK. Effect of heated and humidified carbon dioxide on patients after laparoscopic procedures: A meta-analysis. *Surg Laparosc Endosc Percutan Tech* 2008 Dec;18(6):539–46.
16. Fisher & Paykel. *HumiGard System*. Available at: https://www.fphcare.co.uk/surgical/lap-therapy/humigard-system/
17. Lexion. Available at: http://www.lexionmedical.com/technologies/
18. Nezhat C, Morozov V. A simple solution to lens fogging during robotic and laparoscopic surgery. *JSLS* 2008;12:431.
19. SurgiQuest. Available at: http://www.surgiquest.com
20. Ethicon. *Introducing the New Harmonic Focus+ Shears*. Available at: http://gb.ethicon.com/healthcare-professionals

21. Artisan Medical. *Goldfinger Retrator 5mm.* Available at: https://www.artisanmed.com/products/goldfinger-retractor-5mm

22. http://www.transenterix.com/spider/

23. Rose A, Schlaak HF. A parallel kinematic mechanism for highly flexible laparoscopic instruments. *IFMBE Proc* 2009;22(8):903–6.

24. Vaida C, Plitea C, Pisla D, Gherman B. Orientation module for surgical instruments—A systematical approach. *Meccanica* 2013;48:145–158.

25. Stryker. Available at: http://www.stryker.com/enus/products/Endoscopy/Laparoscopy/Laparoscopes/ArticulatingLaparoscopes/index.htm

26. Chang VC, Tang SJ, Swain CP, Bergs R, Paramo J, Hogg DC, Fernandez R, Cadeddu JA, Scott DJ. A randomized comparison of laparoscopic, flexible endoscopic, and wired and wireless magnetic cameras on *ex vivo* and *in vivo* NOTES surgical performance. *Surg Innov* 2013 Aug;20(4):395–402.

27. Arain NA, Cadeddu JA, Best SL, Roshek T, Chang V, Hogg DC, Bergs R, Fernandez R, Webb EM, Scott DJ. A randomized comparison of laparoscopic, magnetically anchored, and flexible endoscopic cameras in performance and workload between laparoscopic and single-incision surgery. *Surg Endosc* 2012 Apr;26(4):1170–80.

28. Jiang A et al. The Core-Snake, the Variable Stiffness Laparoscopic Camera. https://www.academia.edu/3776067/The_Core-Snake_the_Variable_Stiffness_Laparoscopic_Camera

29. Bhayani SB, Link RE, Varkarakis JM, Kavoussi LR. Complete da Vinci versus laparoscopic pyeloplasty: Cost analysis. *J Endourol* 2005 Apr;19(3):327–32.

30. van der Meijden OAJ, Schijven ÆMP. The value of haptic feedback in conventional and robot-assisted minimal invasive surgery and virtual reality training: A current review. *Surg Endosc* 2009;23:1180–90.

31. Bholat OS, Haluck RS, Kutz RH, Gorman PJ, Krummel TM. Defining the role of haptic feedback in minimally invasive surgery. *Stud Health Technol Inform* 1999;62:62–6.

32. Wagner CR, Soupoulos N, Howe RD. The role of force feedback in surgery: Analysis of blunt dissection. *10th Symposium on Haptic Interfaces for Virtual Environment and Teleoperator Systems (HAPTICS)*, Orlando, FL, 24–28 March 2002, pp. 68–74.

33. Bethea BT, Okamura AM, Kitagawa M, Fitton TP, Cattaneo SM, Gott VL, Baumgartner WA, Yuh DD. Application of haptic feedback to robotic surgery. *J Laparoendosc Adv Surg Tech A* 2004;14:191–5.

34. Falk V, Mintz D, Grünenfelder J, Fann JI, Burdon TA. Influence of three-dimensional vision on surgical telemanipulator performance. *Surg Endosc* 2001;15:1282–8.

35. Badani KK, Bhandari K, Tewari A, Menon M. Comparison of two-dimensional and three-dimensional suturing: Is there a difference in a robotic surgery setting? *J Endourol* 2005;19:1212–5.

36. Byrn JC, Schluender S, Divino CM, Conrad J, Gurland B, Shlasko E, Szold A. Three-dimensional imaging improves surgical performance for both novice and experienced operators using the da Vinci Robot System. *Am J Surg* 2007;193:519–22.

37. DASH retraction sponge. Available at: http://www.ezsurgical.com/Products.asp?Page=Dash

38. Matsouka S, Kikuchi I, Kitade M, Kumakiri J, Jinushi M, Tokita S, Taked S. Utility of an organ retraction sponge (endoractor) in gynecologic laparoscopic surgery. *J Minim Invasive Gynecol* 2011;18:507–11.

39. Tortora G, Ranzani T, De Falco I, Dario P, Menciassi A. A miniature robot for retraction tasks under vision assistance in minimally invasive surgery. *Robotics* 2014;3:70–82.

40. Weber PA, Merola S, Wasielewski A, Ballantyne GH. Telerobotic-assisted laparoscopic right and sigmoid colectomies for benign disease. *Dis Colon Rectum* 2002 Dec;45(12):1689–94.

41. Barbash G, Glied SA. New technology and health care costs—The case of robot-assisted surgery. *N Engl J Med* 2010 Aug 19;363(8):701–4.

42. Memon S et al. Robotic versus laparoscopic proctectomy for rectal cancer: A meta-analysis. *Ann Surg Oncol* 2012;19(7):2095–101.

43. Lin S et al. Meta-analysis of robotic and laparoscopic surgery for treatment of rectal cancer. *World J Gastroenterol* 2011;17(47):5214–20.

44. Kim JY et al. A comparative study of voiding and sexual function after total mesorectal excision with autonomic nerve preservation for rectal cancer: Laparoscopic versus robotic surgery. *Ann Surg Oncol* 2012;19(8):2485–93.

45. Hagn U, Nickl M, Jörg S, Passig G, Bahls T, Nothhelfer A et al. The DLR MIRO: A versatile lightweight robot for surgical applications. *Ind Robot* 2008;35(4):324–36.

46. Tobergte A, Passig G, Kuebler B, Seibold U, Hagn UA, Fröhlich FA et al. MiroSurge—Advanced user interaction modalities in minimally invasive robotic surgery. *Presence: Teleop Virt* 2011 Jul 6;19(5):400–14.

47. Titan Medical. Available at: http://www.titanmedicalinc.com

48. Bogue R. Robots in healthcare. *Ind Robot* 2011 May 3;38:218–23.

49. Hwang MJ, Evans T, Lawrence G, Karandikar S. Impact of bowel cancer screening on the management of colorectal cancer. *Colorectal Dis* 2014;16(6):450–8.

50. Keshava A, Young CJ, Richardson GL, De-Loyde K. A historical comparison of single incision and conventional multiport laparoscopic right hemicolectomy. *Colorectal Dis* 2013;15(10):e618–22.

51. Vestweber B, Galetin T, Lammerting K, Paul C, Giehl J, Straub E, Kaldowski B, Alfes A, Vestweber KH. Single-incision laparoscopic surgery: Outcomes from 224 colonic resections performed at a single center using SILS. *Surg Endosc* 2013 Feb;27(2):434–42.

52. Gonzalez AM, Rabaza JR, Donkor C, Romero RJ, Kosanovic R, Verdeja JC. Single-incision cholecystectomy: A comparative study of standard laparoscopic, robotic, and SPIDER platforms. *Surg Endosc* 2013 Dec;27(12):4524–31.

53. Horise Y, Nishikawa A, Sekimoto M, Kitanaka Y, Miyoshi N, Takiguchi S, Doki Y, Mori M, Miyazaki F. Development and evaluation of a master-slave robot system for single-incision laparoscopic surgery. *Int J Comput Assist Radiol Surg* 2012 Mar;7(2):289–96.

54. Ostrowitz MB, Eschete D, Zemon H, DeNoto G. Robotic-assisted single-incision right colectomy: Early experience. *Int J Med Robot* 2009 Dec;5(4):465–70.

55. Yagci MA, Kayaalp C. Transvaginal appendectomy: A systematic review. *Minim Invasive Surg* 2014;2014:384706.

56. Morino M, Risio M, Bach S, Beets-Tan R, Bujko K, Panis Y et al. Early rectal cancer: The European Association for Endoscopic Surgery (EAES) clinical consensus conference. *Surg Endosc* 2015;29(4):755–73.

57. Tasende MM, Delgado S, Jimenez M, Del Gobbo GD, Fernández-Hevia M, DeLacy B, Balust J, Lacy AM. Minimal invasive surgery: NOSE and NOTES in ulcerative colitis. *Surg Endosc* 2015;29(11):3313–8.

58. Aigner F, Hörmann R, Fritsch H, Pratschke J, D'Hoore A, Brenner E et al. Anatomical considerations for transanal minimal-invasive surgery: The caudal to cephalic approach. *Colorectal Dis* 2015;17(2):O47–53.

59. McLemore EC, Coker AM, Devaraj B, Chakedis J, Maawy A, Inui T et al. TAMIS-assisted laparoscopic low anterior resection with total mesorectal excision in a cadaveric series. *Surg Endosc* 2013 Sep;27(9):3478–84.

60. Atallah SB, Larach S, deBeche-Adams TC, Albert MR. Transanal minimally invasive surgery (TAMIS): A technique that can be used for retrograde proctectomy. *Dis Colon Rectum* 2013 Jul;56(7):931.

61. Wood JJ, Lord AC, Wheeler JM, Borley NR. Laparo-endoscopic resection for extensive and inaccessible colorectal polyps: A feasible and safe procedure. *Ann R Coll Surg Engl* 2011;93(3):241–5.

62. Dighe S, Purkayastha S, Swift I, Tekkis PP, Darzi A, A'hearn R, Brown G. Diagnostic precision of CT in local staging of colon cancers: A meta-analysis. *Clin Radiol* 2010;65:708–19.

63. CRUK. 2007. *Bowel Cancer Statistics—Key Facts.* Available at http://info.cancerresearchuk.org/cancerstats/types/bowel/

64. Resch A, Langner C. Lymph node staging in colorectal cancer: Old controversies and recent advances. *World J Gastroenterol* 2013 Dec 14;19(46):8515–26. doi: 10.3748/wjg.v19.i46.8515.

65. van der Zaag ES, Kooij N, van de Vijver MJ, Bemelman WA, Peters HM, Buskens CJ. Diagnosing occult tumour cells and their predictive value in sentinel nodes of histologically negative patients with colorectal cancer. *Eur J Surg Oncol* 2010;36:350 7.

66. van der Zaag ES, Bouma WH, Tanis PJ, Ubbink DT, Bemelman WA, Buskens CJ. Systematic review of sentinel lymph node mapping procedure in colorectal cancer. *Ann Surg Oncol* 2012;19:3449–59.

67. Retter SM, Herrmann G, Schiedeck TH. Clinical value of sentinel node mapping in carcinoma of the colon. *Colorectal Dis* 2011;13:855–9.

68. Moesta KT, Ebert B, Handke T, Rinneberg H, Schlag PM. Fluorescence as a concept in colorectal lymph node diagnosis. *Recent Results Cancer Res* 2000;157:293–304.

69. Kusano M, Tajima Y, Yamazaki K, Kato M, Watanabe M, Miwa M. Sentinel node mapping guided by indocyanine green fluorescence imaging: A new method for sentinel node navigation surgery in gastrointestinal cancer. *Dig Surg* 2008;25(2):103 8.

70. Cahill RA, Anderson M, Wang LM, Lindsey I, Cunningham C, Mortensen NJ. Near-infrared (NIR) laparoscopy for intraoperative lymphatic road-mapping and sentinel node identification during definitive surgical resection of early-stage colorectal neoplasia. *Surg Endosc* 2012 Jan;26(1):197–204.

71. Ankersmit M, van der Pas MH, van Dam DA, Meijerink WJ. Near infrared fluorescence lymphatic laparoscopy of the colon and mesocolon. *Colorectal Dis* 2011 Nov;13(Suppl 7):70–3.

72. Stummer W et al. Counterbalancing risks and gains from extended resections in malignant glioma surgery: A supplemental analysis from the randomized 5-aminolevulinic acid glioma resection study. *J Neurosurg* 2011;114:613–23.

73. Stenzl A et al. Detection and clinical outcome of urinary bladder cancer with 5-aminolevulinic acid-induced fluorescence cystoscopy. *Cancer* 2011;117:938–47.

74. Babu R, Adamson DC. Fluorescence-guided malignant glioma resections. *Curr Drug Discov Technol* 2012 Dec;9(4):256–67.

75. Lykke MR, Nielsen TK, Ebbensgaard NA, Zieger K. Reducing recurrence in non-muscle-invasive bladder cancer using photodynamic diagnosis and immediate post-transurethral resection of the bladder chemoprophylaxis. *Scand J Urol* 2015;49(3):230–6.

76. https://www.ukctg.nihr.ac.uk/trials?query=%257B%2522query%2522%253A%2522fluorescence%2520lymph%2520node%2522%257D

77. Jafari MD, Wexner SD, Martz JE, McLemore EC, Margolin DA, Sherwinter OA, Lee SW, Senagore AJ, Phelan MJ, Stamos MJ. Perfusion assessment in laparoscopic left-sided/anterior resection (PILLAR II): A multi-institutional study. *J Am Coll Surg* 2015;220:82–92.

Index